Case Studies in Biometry

Case Studies in Biometry

Edited by

NICHOLAS LANGE
National Institutes of Health
Bethesda, Maryland

LOUISE RYAN
Harvard University and
Dana-Farber Cancer Institute
Boston, Massachusetts

LYNNE BILLARD
University of Georgia
Athens, Georgia

DAVID BRILLINGER
University of California, Berkeley
Berkeley, California

LOVEDAY CONQUEST
University of Washington, Seattle
Seattle, Washington

JOEL GREENHOUSE
Carnegie Mellon University
Pittsburgh, Pennsylvania

Sponsored by

The Eastern and Western North American Regions of the
International Biometrics Society

A Wiley-Interscience Publication
JOHN WILEY & SONS, INC.
New York • Chichester • Brisbane • Toronto • Singapore

Rn

This text is printed on acid-free paper.

Library of Congress Cataloging in Publication Data:
Case studies in biometry / edited by Nicholas Lange.
       p.   cm. — (Wiley series in probability and mathematical
  statistics. Applied probability and statistics)
   "A Wiley-Interscience publication."
   Includes bibliographical references (p.   ) and index.
   ISBN 0-471-58885-7(cloth : acid-free paper). — ISBN 0-471-58925-X
(paper : acid-free paper)
   1. Biometry — Case studies.   I. Lange, Nicholas, 1952–
II. Series.
QH323.5.C367   1994
574'.01'5195 — dc20   94-13156

Printed in the United States of America

10 9 8 7 6 5 4 3 2

FTW
AHK9452

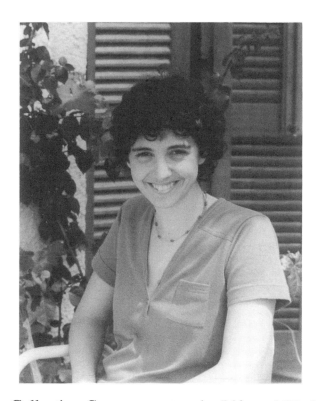

This Collection Commemorates the Life and Work of
Myrto Lefkopoulou
1957–1992

Contents

Contributors

CHERYL L. ADDY, Department of Epidemiology and Biostatistics, University of South Carolina, Columbia, SC 29208

A. JOHN BAILER, Department of Mathematics and Statistics, Miami University, Oxford, OH 45056-1641

PHILLIP L. C. BANKS, Ross Laboratories, Columbus, OH 43215

SHELLEY BULL, Samuel Lunenfeld Research Institute, and Department of Preventive Medicine and Biostatistics, University of Toronto, Toronto, Ontario M5G 1X5, Canada

JOHN P. BUONACCORSI, Department of Mathematics and Statistics, University of Massachusetts at Amherst, Amherst, MA 01003

W. HANS CARTER, JR., Department of Biostatistics, Virginia Commonwealth University, Richmond, VA 23298-0032

LARRY C. CLARK, Department of Family and Community Medicine, University of Arizona, Tucson, AZ 85716

DENNIS L. CLASON, Department of Experimental Statistics, New Mexico State University, Las Cruces, NM 88003-0003

JOE N. CORGAN, Department of Agronomy and Horticulture, New Mexico State University, Las Cruces, NM 88003-0003

JOHN A. CRAWFORD, Department of Fisheries and Wildlife, Oregon State University, Corvallis, OR 97331-3803

CATHY M. CRYDER-WILSON, Shamrock Seed Company, Las Cruces, NM 88003

MARIE DIENER-WEST, Department of Biostatistics, The Johns Hopkins University, Baltimore, MD 21205

MARTIN S. DRUT, Department of Fisheries and Wildlife, Oregon State University, Corvallis, OR 97331-3803

MARK D. ECKER, Department of Statistics, University of Connecticut, Storrs, CT 06269

SCOTT S. EMERSON, Arizona Cancer Center, University of Arizona, Tucson, AZ 85724

BETTY J. FLEHINGER, Mathematical Sciences Department, IBM T. J. Watson Research Center, Yorktown Heights, NY 10598

CAROL Z. GARRISON, Department of Epidemiology and Biostatistics, University of South Carolina, Columbia, SC 29208

CHRIS GENNINGS, Department of Biostatistics, Virginia Commonwealth University, Richmond, VA 23298-0032

BRENDA W. GILLESPIE, Department of Biostatistics, University of Michigan, Ann Arbor, MI 48109-2029

JINKO GRAHAM, Department of Biostatistics, University of Washington, Seattle, WA 98195

MICHAEL T. HALPERN, Medical Technology Assessment and Policy Research Program, Batelle Memorial Institute, Arlington, VA 22201

JAMES F. HELTSHE, Department of Computer Science and Statistics, University of Rhode Island, Kingston, RI 02881

KIRBY L. JACKSON, Department of Epidemiology and Biostatistics, University of South Carolina, Columbia, SC 29208

MAREK KIMMEL, Department of Statistics, Rice University, Houston, TX 77251

ALISON J. KIRBY, Department of Epidemiology, The Johns Hopkins University, Baltimore, MD 21205-1999

NANCY LANE, Department of Medicine, University of California—San Francisco, San Francisco, CA 94143

L.-J. SALLY LIU, Department of Environmental Health, Harvard School of Public Health, Boston, MA

BILLY R. MARTIN, Department of Pharmacology and Toxicology, Virginia Commonwealth University, Richmond, VA 23298-0032

MARTI MCCRACKEN, Department of Statistics, Oregon State University, Corvallis, OR 97331-4606

ROBERT E. MCKEOWN, Department of Epidemiology and Biostatistics, University of South Carolina, Columbia, SC 29208

B. MICHELE MELIA, The Wilmer Ophthalmological Institute, The Johns Hopkins Medical Institutions, Baltimore, MD 21205

CARL N. MORRIS, Statistics Department, Harvard University, Cambridge, MA 02138 and Department of Health Care Policy, Harvard Medical School, Boston, MA 02115

PHILIP NASCA, Bureau of Cancer Epidemiology, New York State Department of Health, Albany, NY 12237

JOHN D. NEILSON,* Pelagic and Reef Fisheries Resource, Kingston, Islands of St. Vincent and the Grenadines

EDWARD C. NORTON, Research Triangle Institute, Center for Economic Research, Research Triangle Park, NC 27709

JAMES T. ORIS, Department of Zoology, Miami University, Oxford, OH 45056

A. JOHN PETKAU, Department of Statistics, University of British Columbia, Vancouver, British Columbia V6T 1Z2, Canada

FRED L. RAMSEY, Department of Statistics, Oregon State University, Corvallis, OR 97331-4606

JOHN O. RAWLINGS, Department of Statistics, North Carolina State University, Raleigh, NC 27695-8203

PENNY S. REYNOLDS,† Department of Zoology,, University of Wisconsin—Madison, Madison, WI 53706

WILLIAM J. RIPPLE, Department of Forest Resources, Oregon State University, Corvallis, OR 97331-5703

STEPHEN J. SMITH, Department of Fisheries and Oceans, Bedford Institute of Oceanography, Dartmouth, Nova Scotia B2Y 4A2, Canada

DAVID J. SPIEGELHALTER, MRC Biostatistics Unit, Institute of Public Health, University Forvie Site, Cambridge, CB2 2SR, United Kingdom

SUSAN E. SPRUILL,‡ Department of Statistics, North Carolina State University, Raleigh, NC 27695-8203

BRUCE W. TURNBULL, School of Operations Research and Industrial Engineering, Cornell University, Ithaca, NY 14853

*Present address: Department of Fisheries and Oceans, Biological Station, St. Andrews, New Brunswick, Canada E0G 2X0
† Present address: Division of Biological Sciences, University of Montana, Missoula, MT 59812
‡ Present address: Pharmaceutical Product Development, Inc., Morrisville, NC 27560

N. SCOTT URQUHART, Department of Statistics, Oregon State University, Corvallis, OR 97331-4606

KEN G. WAIWOOD, Department of Fisheries and Oceans, Biological Station, St. Andrews, New Brunswick E0G 2X0, Canada

JENNIFER L. WALLER, Department of Epidemiology and Biostatistics, University of South Carolina, Columbia, SC 29208

LANCE A. WALLER, Division of Biostatistics, University of Minnesota, Minneapolis, MN 55455

KENNETH E. WARNER, Department of Public Health Policy and Administration, University of Michigan, Ann Arbor, MI 48109-2029

SUZANNA WONG, Syntex Laboratories, Inc., Palo Alto, CA 94304

DAVID WYPIJ, Department of Biostatistics, Harvard School of Public Health, Boston, MA 02115

XIAO H. ZHOU, Indiana University School of Medicine, Department of Medicine, Division of Biostatistics, Indianapolis, IN 46202

Foreword

Modern science has developed from the confluence of two major streams of thought: the philosophical tradition of ancient Greece and the empirical approach to problem solving that was reborn in renaissance Europe. Academic mathematics is neatly divided along these same lines. Pure mathematics departments follow the philosophical tradition of axioms, proofs, and an internally constructed universe. Statistics departments, and other practitioners of applied mathematics, naturally turn toward the real world, and in doing so tend to favor the heuristic spirit of empirical analysis.

This is a book about the problems of the real world and how to solve them. Biometry doesn't include the entire real world, of course, and these twenty-one case studies don't include all of biometry. Nevertheless, the range of interests is breathtaking. How do hummingbirds learn their geometry so well? What factors influence the lengths of time the elderly spend in nursing homes? Can halibut survive being caught and returned to the ocean? Which histological changes predict cervical cancer?

Those of us who work in statistics become inured to its amazing range of applicability. In fact, there is no a priori reason to believe that any one mathematical method could shed light on hummingbirds, old people, halibut, and cancer cells. As the editors point out, the secret is that statistics is a way of thinking, not just a collection of techniques.

Statistical thought focuses on the accumulation of information from many sources (many hummingbirds, for example), when no single source is particularly informative. How is the act of accumulation carried out? That is what *Case Studies in Biometry* concerns. A smart person stuck on a desert island with this book (and a personal computer) could learn most of modern statistics by following these twenty-one analyses.

Thirteen years ago, Rupert Miller, Byron Brown, Lincoln Moses, and I published a collection of case studies in biostatistics. These have been used gratifyingly often as examples in the statistics literature. *Case Studies in Biometry* has chosen a wider subject area and a more ambitious collection of techniques. I believe it will have a correspondingly larger influence on the literature. More importantly, it will reinforce, by good example, the proper role of statistics as the facilitator of scientific inference. There is plenty of philosophy underlying these analyses, but there is even a larger amount of effective problems solving.

BRADLEY EFRON

Stanford University

Preface

Case Studies in Biometry (CSB) aims to provide students, faculty, and practicing statisticians with detailed analyses that address important scientific questions. What you will find here are twenty-one biometric studies at the intersection of theory and application in a wide variety of fields. This collection thus lies somewhere between a textbook and a set of journal articles.

Applied statistics is only an afterthought to some subject-matter scientists who do not realize how much modern statistical thinking has to offer them. Far more than the development and application of methods, statistical science is a way of thinking. This book contains a sample of approaches taken by statistical scientists to tackle important biometric problems in six general areas: environmental hazards; fisheries, forestry, genetics; habitat and animal studies; health care and public health policy; clinical trials; and epidemiology and toxicology. These scientists' use of statistical theory, computational algorithms (both pre-coded and tailor-made), and hard-core data analysis yields practical results and useful conclusions in all six areas.

As teachers, we struggle to make our subject come alive in the classroom. Many textbook examples are too brief, too stylized: this book contains no such examples. Through its detailed case-based approach, *CSB* brings to an applied audience certain recent developments in statistical theory; it also serves to introduce substantive research areas not usually addressed in statistics courses. Some students in our introductory courses are surprised to learn that ours is a creative, *dynamic* endeavor. Some need to retool their thinking to meet the careful, quantitative analytic requirements. Others are surprised to find that there doesn't usually exist one correct answer. These discoveries do not surprise us. Yet how much do applications of our different tools (graphs, methods, and models, etc.) to a given scientific context yield different substantive conclusions? Detailed study of this book will help to address preceding issues as they arise in twenty-one real-life cases.

Most of *CSB*'s chapters are divided internally into five sections: *1. Motivation and Background, 2. Data, 3. Methods and Models, 4. Results*, and *5. Conclusions*. Each chapter also contains a *Questions and Problems* section, and a short paragraph of *Software Notes and References* when appropriate. Subsections within these main sections differ from chapter to chapter.

We have included all data sets used by the *CSB* authors on an accompanying diskette. These data sets are also available through *statlib*, a general electronic resource for statistical software and data accessible nationwide through the Internet and Bitnet. Please read the appendix and the DOS-compatible diskette itself for more detail. We have included a sample of each data set in the first tables for each chapter. We expect that your use of the original data from each of these case studies will enhance greatly this book's usefulness as a research and teaching tool.

CSB began in 1991 when, at the spring meetings of the Eastern North American Region of the International Biometric Society, Barbara Tilley (then president), Tom Louis (then president-elect), and Jim Dambrosia (then regional advisory board chair) liked our idea and encouraged a formal proposal. Our proposal soon gained financial support from the Eastern North American Region, the Western North American Region joined in the enterprise, and the editorial board was identified.

We also decided at this point that no one should receive any financial benefit from *CSB* and that any royalties would go back to the International Biometric Society to help sponsor future similar projects. Abstract solicitations were sent to all society members in North America. Our letter invited contributions from a very wide range of applications areas, even wider than the present selection. At one point, we turned down a suggestion to title the book *Case Studies in Biostatistics*, thinking that "biostatistics" has too much of a medical connotation and would thus limit our intended scope. The invitation was well received: over 100 abstracts were submitted in a relatively short period of time.

All abstracts were reviewed blindly with regard to author, gender, race, and institution. We chose to blind our review to maintain our overall fairness, and also as somewhat of an experiment. Our administrative assistant kept a master copy and provided us and the other editors with blinded abstracts identified only by a neutral code. After review by the entire board, forty authors were invited to submit a full manuscript for consideration, with the understanding that only approximately one-half of that number would be published. Most submitted abstracts and manuscripts indicated high-quality work. Some were not selected for this volume because their contexts were not biological or medical, or due to overall topics coverage considerations. The result of this two-phase selection procedure is thus a truly peer-reviewed volume with an acceptance rate of 19 percent, a rate similar to that of many high-quality journals in various fields.

The blinding experiment produced some interesting results. Twenty-nine percent of abstract first authors were female. Of these women, 45 percent were invited to submit a full-length chapter; the corresponding rate for males was 38 percent. Eighty percent of abstracts were from academic institutions. Seven students submitted abstracts as first authors: *all* students were invited to submit a manuscript, and four did! By the end of 1992, we received thirty-six complete manuscripts. After review by the editors, again blinded, nineteen were selected, eventually to become *CSB*. Two additional papers were solicited to cover important topics not represented in the original submissions.

What would we do differently? Not much! We are happy with most aspects of *CSB* and encourage others interested in similar projects to:

1. Cast a wide net: let the response dictate eventual content.
2. Blind your selection process, if possible.
3. Make your effort truly peer reviewed.
4. Be strict when it comes to development and production target dates.
5. Make it clear from the start that substantial editors' prerogative will be involved in order to arrive at a cohesive collection.

One thing we would change is to require everyone to use the same word-processing program. Electronic submissions pay off: a great deal of effort went into the editing process to produce the final version on our end, and this was much easier when we could edit on-line.

We've enjoyed producing this collection and are grateful to all who've contributed and helped out. In particular, we thank Karen Abbett for her expert administrative assistance, Sarah and Nick for some proofreading and on-line editing in a pinch, and Kate Roach, Senior Editor at John Wiley & Sons. Who knows? Some of us may actually *use CSB* to help solve real-world problems.

NICK LANGE AND LOUISE RYAN

Cambridge, Massachusettes

Case Studies in Biometry

PART I

Environmental Hazards

CHAPTER 1

Spatial Pattern Analyses to Detect Rare Disease Clusters

Lance A. Waller, Bruce W. Turnbull, Larry C. Clark, and
Philip Nasca

1 MOTIVATION AND BACKGROUND

The spatial distribution of incident cases of a disease may indicate possible
causes. For instance, one may observe an increased incidence of respiratory
problems in persons living downwind from an incinerator. Particular differences
in the risk of contracting a disease due to environmental exposures may manifest themselves in differences in the incidence rate of the disease in areas with
different exposures to these environmental factors. An early example of the
use of the spatial distribution of disease incidence to determine the etiology
of a disease involves the work of Dr. John Snow, a London physician who is
often regarded as the father of modern epidemiology. Snow was intrigued by
a neighborhood epidemic of cholera occurring in 1854 in London. He plotted
the cholera deaths for September 1854 on a map and noted that many of the
deaths occurred in the vicinity of the water pump on Broad Street (see Figure
1). Snow called for the removal of the handle to the Broad Street pump, ended
the epidemic, and proceeded to show that drinking water contaminated with
sewage was a primary cause of cholera (Gilbert, 1958).

   Similar problems exist today, where the diseases of interest often include
chronic conditions such as cancers. In the United Kingdom, questions concerning possible elevated rates of childhood leukemia near nuclear installations
have stirred considerable controversy (Openshaw et al., 1988; Cook-Mozaffari
et al., 1989; Doll, 1989; Ewings et al., 1989; Gardner, 1989; Wakeford et al.,
1989; Wheldon, 1989; Wakeford, 1990; Doll et al., 1994). Another well-publi-

Case Studies in Biometry, Edited by Nicholas Lange, Louise Ryan, Lynne Billard,
David Brillinger, Loveday Conquest, and Joel Greenhouse.
ISBN 0-471-58885-7 © 1994 John Wiley & Sons, Inc.

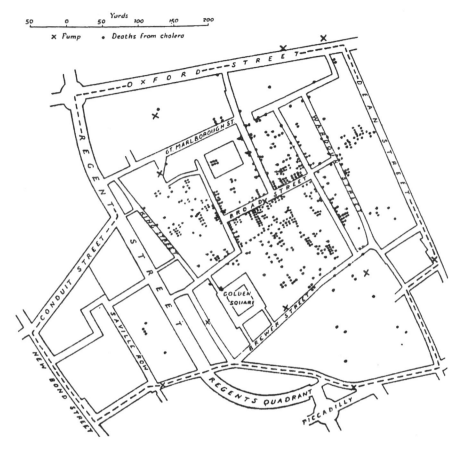

Figure 1. Dr. John Snow's map of cholera deaths for September 1894. Cholera deaths are indicated by dots; water pumps are indicated by crosses (from Tufte, 1983, p. 24).

cized and controversial case concerned hazardous waste disposal in the town of Woburn, Massachusetts. There Lagakos et al. (1986) found a statistically significant relationship between the incidence of leukemia in children aged 0 to 19 years and exposure to wells contaminated with the volatile organic compound (VOC) trichloroethylene (TCE). The latter case prompted the Department of Health in the neighboring state of New York in the summer of 1986 to initiate a series of meetings of statisticians, epidemiologists, and public health officials to discuss policy regarding the monitoring of the geographical distribution of cancer cases in their state. The Department of Health was interested in developing surveillance methodology to use in conjunction with the Cancer Registry to scan for possible clusters or aggregations of incident cases of cancer. Such a procedure is called *proactive* since any "hot spots" so found will be identified prior to or without regard to local reports of a cluster. In fact, state departments of public health expend sizable resources investigating many hundreds of reported disease clusters each year, only a few of which eventually turn out to be of justifiable concern. Such investigations are termed *reactive*. There is clearly a need to have in place a proactive system which would provide an objective way to detect, prioritize, and monitor the occurrence of possible disease clusters. Such a program would enable timely response to lay reports of perceived clusters.

Initially, in order to develop and compare various statistical clustering techniques, it was decided to examine leukemia incidence in the five-year period 1978–1982 in an eight-county region in upstate New York. The region is shown in Figure 2. According to the 1980 U.S. Census, the region contained a population of a little over 1 million people; from the state Cancer Registry there were 592 cases of leukemia reported in this period in this region. Leukemia was selected because of its remarkably uniform distribution, although apparent clusters have been known to occur, possibly as the result of point-source environmental exposures, such as might have occurred in Woburn.

The eight-county region was divided up into 790 subregions or cells, for which we have population counts and leukemia incidence counts. These cells were defined by using U.S. Census block groups for all counties except Broome, where the geocoding by the state Cancer Registry permitted only the larger cen-

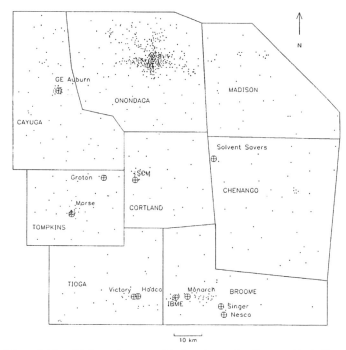

Figure 2. Map of New York study area with locations of cell centroids indicated by · and hazardous waste sites containing trichloroethylene indicated by ⊕ (from Waller et al., 1992).

sus tract unit to be used as a cell. (Typically, a census tract contains 1000 to 4000 people and comprises between two and five block groups.) The centroids of the 790 cells are also displayed in Figure 2. Since census districts were originally defined to contain roughly the same number of people, the spatial distribution of the centroids shown in Figure 2 gives an approximation of the spatial distribution of the population at risk. We see that the area is largely rural and the population is concentrated about two cities in the study area: Syracuse in Onondaga County and Binghamton in Broome County. Three smaller cities are also apparent: Auburn in Cayuga County, Cortland in Cortland County, and Ithaca in Tompkins County. From the Cancer Registry, the counts of incident cases of leukemia in each cell were collected. (Because of confidentiality concerns, the precise locations of incident cases are not generally available; for similar reasons, age, gender, and race information on the cases is also not generally available.) Hence the cases in each cell are assumed to occur at the centroid, and these are plotted in Figure 3. When Figures 2 and 3 are compared, it is clear that varying population density must be accounted for in assessing

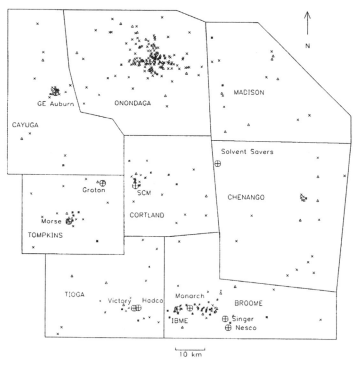

Figure 3. Map of New York study area, location of leukemia cases, 1978–1982. Cell centroids with fewer than one case are not shown, centroids of cells with one or more but fewer than two reported cases are indicated by ×, centroids of cells with two or more but fewer than three reported cases are indicated by △, and centroids of cells with three or more reported cases are indicated by * (from Turnbull et al., 1990).

visual appearance of the spatial patterns of disease incidence. For this purpose, one may consider the use of cartograms or density-equalized map projections (Schulman et al., 1988) whereby the map is distorted so that land areas are proportional to population size. Levison and Haddon (1965) display such a map for the state of New York. However, such maps are not uniquely constructed, nor do they help directly with the quantitative assessment of possible clustering effects.

The population data consist of an array with 790 rows, one for each cell, and five columns. The population data corresponding to the first five cells are displayed in Table 1. The first column is a label identifying the cell. The second and third columns are x- and y-coordinates, indicating the location of the centroid of the cell. The x- and y-coordinates are defined by the 1980 U.S. Census and represent deviations from the geographic centroid of the study area in the east-west and north-south directions. The fourth and fifth columns give the population count and disease case count of the cell, respectively. Recall that due to limitations of the data, we are making the approximating assumption that all the population and all the cases are concentrated at the cell centroid. The location data for the inactive hazardous waste sites containing TCE are displayed in Table 2.

The population data are summarized in Table 3. For a small fraction of the cases, the residence could only be located to a group of possible cells. These cases were divided fractionally among the candidate cells, with fractions being proportional to the population of these cells; hence the disease counts are not necessarily all integers. By assigning cases proportional to population, the data will appear less clustered, but different assignment schemes had little effect on the results presented here (cf. Turnbull et al., 1990). Less than 10% of the cases had to be fractionally allocated to cells. However, a very small proportion of these cases was identified only by county, which means, unfortunately, that almost every cell has a fraction added to its observed leukemia incidence count.

Table 1 First Five Data Records: x- and y-coordinates of Cell Centroids, Population Sizes, and Leukemia Incidence in Upstate New York, 1978–1982

Cell	x	y	Population Size	Incident Leukemia Cases[a]
70001000	4.07	−67.35	3540	3.08
70002000	4.64	−66.86	3560	4.08
70003000	5.71	−66.98	3739	1.09
70004000	7.61	−66.00	2784	1.07
70005000	7.32	−67.32	2571	3.06

[a]Fractional maximum for cases due to the method of handling incomplete data (see text).

Table 2   Location Data for Inactive Hazardous Waste Sites Containing Trichloroethylene (TCE)

x	y	Name
−0.14	−67.19	Monarch Chemicals
−4.47	−67.65	IBM Endicott
11.98	−71.61	Singer
13.03	−75.34	Nesco
−46.60	24.43	GE Auburn
9.30	−5.82	Solvent Savers
−19.04	−15.37	Smith Corona
−19.41	−67.39	Victory Plaza
−17.97	−67.16	Hadco
−41.99	−30.90	Morse Chain
−30.37	−14.39	Groton

We wish to test for randomness, that is, that each person in the population has an equal chance of being a case. When we have no particular alternative in mind, a statistical test of this hypothesis will be called a general test. The application of such procedures to our data is considered in the next section. Sometimes we might have a particular alternative hypothesis in mind in which disease incidence rates will be higher in the vicinity of prespecified potential sources of hazard (foci); the resulting test procedures will be called focused. [The terms *general* and *focused* were introduced by Besag and Newell (1991).] Such focused tests are discussed in Section 3, where, for the foci, we will be using 11 hazardous waste sites in the region classified by the New York State Department of Environmental Conservation (1987) as containing TCE. More details are given in Section 3.

It should be noted that there is a very large literature on the general subject of disease clustering. Marshall (1991) provides an excellent review of the disease clustering tests and methodologies that appear in the statistical literature. For a discussion of the modeling aspect, the reader is referred to Diggle (1990). Here we concentrate on empirical assessment techniques that are based on the observed spatial distribution of incidence and population cell counts such as we have described.

Table 3   Data Summary: Leukemia Incidence in 790 Census Areas in Upstate New York, 1978–1982

	Total	Minimum	Maximum	Mean
Cases	592	0	9.29[a]	0.749
Population	1,057,673	3	12,221	1339

[a]Fractional maximum for cases due to the method of handling incomplete data (see text).

2   GENERAL TESTS OF RANDOMNESS

We begin by examining the question of whether the data are consistent with a hypothesis of randomness. Formally this null hypothesis is:

> H_0: Every person is equally likely to contract the disease
> independently of other cases, and of the location
> of their residence.

First we must define some notation. Suppose that the study area is subdivided into I cells. We denote the population of cell i by $n_i, i = 1, \ldots, I$, and the total number of persons in the study area by $n_+ = \sum_{i=1}^{I} n_i$. The number of incident cases of the disease in cell i can be considered a random variable C_i with observed value denoted by c_i. The total number of cases will be denoted by $c_+ = \sum_{i=1}^{I} c_i$. For our application $I = 790$, $n_+ = 1,057,673$, and $c_+ = 592$.

For a rare disease, if we use the Poisson approximation to the multinomial distribution, the null hypothesis above is equivalent to

> H_0: the $C_i, i = 1, \ldots, I$, are independent
> Poisson random variables with $E(C_i) = \lambda n_i$,

where λ denotes the risk of any one individual contracting the disease, assumed constant under H_0. This probabilistic model assumes no genetic factors or contagion in the disease of interest; however, such features could be added to the model by incorporating covariates or more sophisticated features such as extra-Poisson variation (Breslow, 1984). We see that under H_0 the expected number of cases in each cell is simply the baseline risk of disease for an individual multiplied by the number of individuals residing in cell i. We begin testing for clustering of the cases by testing H_0 versus the general alternative hypothesis H_1: not H_0.

Shortly after the initial meetings at the New York Department of Health, Alice Whittemore at a regional meeting of the International Biometric Society discussed her recent study on clustering by census tract of residence of 63 cases of rectal cancer occurring in San Francisco between 1973 and 1981 (see Whittemore et al., 1987). Since the form of these data was similar to ours, it seemed natural to start by trying to apply this new method. The test statistic is the mean distance between all pairs of cases. This method was developed for precise location data; however, the approximation involved in placing the cases at the cell centroids does not unnecessarily complicate the analysis. The variance and expected value of the test statistic are computed using the population data (i.e., the n_i's). Whittemore et al. (1987) show that their test statistic is asymptotically normally distributed under the null hypothesis. For the New York study area under consideration, the observed mean distance between all pairs of cases is 60.24 km, compared to the expected value of 59.01 km with a standard deviation of 0.96 km. Hence, the standardized test statistic has value $Z = (60.24 - 59.01)/0.96 = 1.28$, which is not significant at the $\alpha = 0.05$ level compared to the standard normal distribution.

There are two major drawbacks to the use of the method proposed by Whittemore et al. (1987). First, the method merely gives a statistic reflecting the degree of clustering in the entire study area and does not detect any particular clusters or give the location of the areas most likely to represent clusters of excess cases. Second, although the null distribution of the test statistic takes into account the heterogeneous population density, the statistic's value depends on the position of the cases only through their pairwise distances. This may be a problem since clusters of many nearby cases may be due to high population density (i.e., many people at risk) or due to a truly elevated incidence rate (i.e., a true cluster). The statistic does not readily provide a way to differentiate between these possibilities.

Shortly after the paper by Whittemore et al. (1987), an article appeared in the British medical journal *Lancet* by Openshaw et al. (1988) on a graphical procedure they called the *geographical analysis machine* or GAM, which they applied to the spatial distribution of 853 cases of childhood leukemia in northern England diagnosed between 1968 and 1985 in a population which in 1981 comprised 1,544,963 children. Application of the GAM method to the New York data is described in Turnbull et al. (1990). The method proceeds by examining a large number of overlapping circular regions and noting those with particularly high rates. Specifically, the algorithm proceeds as follows:

1. Select a radius r (e.g., 1, 2, or 4 km).
2. Lay down a square lattice over the study region with grid points evenly spaced at intervals $r/5$ apart. Label the grid points $i = 1, 2, \ldots, K(r)$.
3. Consider each of the $K(r)$ grid points in turn. For the ith grid point, compute C_{ir}, the number of cases in a circle of radius r and centered at that grid point. Draw in the circumference of that circle if the observed value of C_{ir} is two or more and exceeds the 99.8th percentile of a Poisson distribution with mean $\mu = P_{ir}c_+/n_+$, where P_{ir} is the population contained in the circle centered at the ith grid point.
4. Return to step 1 and repeat the procedure for the next higher value of r.

Using these three values of r (1, 2, 4 km), we examined 83,587 circles in the New York data; the map in Figure 4 shows the 503 (0.6%) found significant at the $p = 0.002$ level. While it is a good descriptive tool, the GAM procedure does not offer a quantitative assessment of the significance of an observed pattern. Many circles are considered, and the circles overlap to the extent that if one circle is drawn, many neighboring circles (often containing many of the same cases) will be drawn. The use of an α level of 0.002 rather than a more conventional value of 0.01 or 0.05 is a recognition of the multiplicity problem, but this value seems to have been chosen in an *ad hoc* way. Even under the

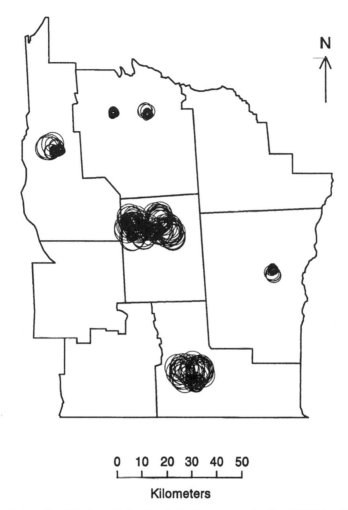

Figure 4. Circles of radii 1, 2, and 4 km found significant at nominal level 0.2% by GAM method of Openshaw et al. (1988) (from Turnbull et al., 1990).

null hypothesis of no clustering, it is to be expected that groups of overlapping circles will be drawn. Thus although the map perhaps indicates the existence of some clusters, it is not clear whether the method is just picking out clusters which must occur at some locations by chance. Also, with so many circles to consider, the procedure needs a lot of computer time.

Attention now turned to finding procedures which might be less computer intensive, would give a statistical assessment of the goodness of fit of the randomness hypothesis H_0 (i.e., a significance level or p-value), and would identify with some quantitative measure the most likely candidates for clusters, assuming that some exist. The GAM procedure examined disease rates (number of cases/population size) in circles of constant area, but these rates varied widely in terms of both their denominators (population sizes) and their numerators (numbers of cases). This implies that the estimated rates in the circles are not comparable, having different standard errors. Two ways of redefining the circles so that the rates are comparable are to ensure that the denominators are fixed (i.e., the new circles all contain the same population) or to ensure that the numerators are fixed (i.e., the new circles all contain the same number of cases). The former procedure was described by Turnbull et al. (1990) and the latter is essentially that of Besag and Newell (1991).

Turnbull et al. (1990) consider two-dimensional windows or balls centered at each cell centroid and containing a constant number of people at risk, termed the population *radius* and denoted by R. We use the term *ball* to differentiate from the circles of Openshaw et al. (1988). The ball for cell i is constructed by including the nearest neighboring cells until the total aggregated population around and including cell i is equal to R. The last cell added to the ball may contribute only a fraction of its population to the ball. The incident cases occurring in the ith ball are found by summing the cases observed in the cells forming the ith ball with the same fraction of cases as population from the farthest cell included in the ball. By considering a constant number of people at risk, the random variables representing the incident disease counts within each ball will be identically distributed, although the counts will not be independent since balls will overlap if the population radius is larger than the population of the cells.

A natural choice for a measure of clustering is the maximum number of cases observed in any ball of radius R. We denote this maximum divided by the fixed radius R by M_R. (The choice is a natural one because a large rate in an area might trigger an alarm to a state health department.) A test of the randomness hypothesis H_0 can be based on M_R, with H_0 being rejected for large values of M_R. How well the data fit the randomness hypothesis can be assessed quantitatively via the significance level or p-value. This is equal to the probability under H_0 of obtaining a value of M_R at least as large as the one observed. Thus we need to calculate this tail area of the distribution of M_R under H_0. This distribution could be obtained via the permutation procedures proposed by Fisher (1935); however, this would require calculating M_R for each of the possible ways of assigning the c_+ cases to the n_+ people. This calculation becomes intractable for the large values of c_+ and n_+ typically encountered in surveillance studies. Instead, we estimate the p-value via a Monte Carlo method. Such methods have been applied to spatial pattern analysis by several authors, including Ripley (1977), Besag and Diggle (1977), and Diggle et al. (1991). The Monte Carlo simulation involves placing c_+ cases at random in the I cells according to a multinomial distribution where the probability of a case being placed in cell i is proportional to the population of cell i (i.e., this probability equals n_i/n_+). The c_+ cases are assigned for each of 999 replicates for the simulation. We calculate the observed value of the statistic M_R for each replicate and obtain an estimate of the distribution of M_R under the null hypothesis.

Again, for our data, the number of cases is $c_+ = 592$, the population size is $n_+ = 1,057,673$ persons, and the number of cells is $I = 790$.

Figure 5 shows the observed values of M_R annualized (i.e., divided by 5) for four representative values of R (i.e., 2500, 5000, 10,000, and 20,000 persons at risk) as well as the upper 99th and 95th percentiles, and the lower 5th percentiles of the distributions obtained from the simulation. None of the observed values of M_R are significant at the 1% level. For $R = 20,000, M_R$ is just significant at the 5% level. However, we are using four values of R, so a Bonferonni adjustment (Miller, 1981, p. 8) may be used to account for the multiplicity of hypothesis tests, in which case the observed significance is reduced by a factor of 4. The M_R values occur at balls centered at two cells, designated M1 and H1. Both cells M1 and H1 are located in western Cortland County and are shown in Figure 6.

While the previous method considers the population at risk to be fixed in each ball, Besag and Newell (1991) propose treating the number of cases, or cluster size, as constant. That is, they consider the numerator of the incidence rate to be fixed. A cluster size k is chosen. For each cell i, we order the remaining cells by increasing distance of their centroids to the centroid of cell i. We determine the number of cells L that must be added to cell i to include the nearest k cases to the centroid of cell i. A small observed value l of L indicates that a cell centroid

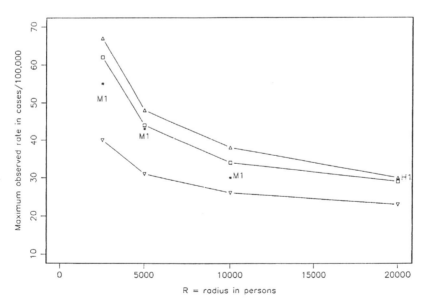

Figure 5. Empirical significance levels for method of Turnbull et al. (1990) with population radii $R = 2500$, 5000, 10,000, and 20,000 persons. $\triangle$ denotes theoretical upper 99th percentile of distribution of maximum rate, M_R; $\square$ upper 95th percentile of M_R distribution; $\triangledown$, lower fifth percentile of M_R distribution; and $*$, observed maximum rate M_R at corresponding population radius R. The symbols M1 and H1 denote cells yielding balls yielding observed maxima (from Turnbull et al., 1990).

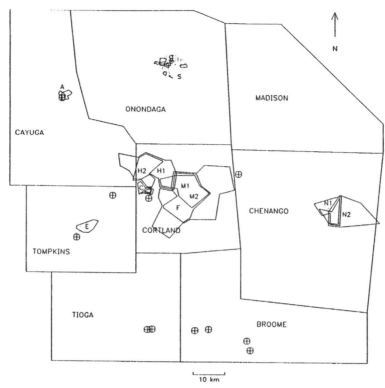

Figure 6. Clusters of $k = 8$ cases found significant at nominal level 5% using method of Besag and Newell (1991). The locations of the TCE waste sites are indicated by $\oplus$. The centroids of the cells in the center of the significant clusters are identified by the first letter of the nearest town. In the case of more than one labeled centroid near the same town, a number follows the letter.

has k cases nearby and may indicate a cluster. We may calculate the significance level of each potential cluster of the specified size by calculating the probability under H_0 that the random variable L is less than the observed value l. [This is, in fact, a slight variation of the Besag and Newell (1991) procedure, which involves looking at clusters of size k around each case considered in turn instead of around each cell centroid. The presence of fractional disease incidence cell counts motivated this adaptation of their procedure.] Let m_i represent the total of the population in cell i plus that in the cells with the l nearest centroids. The significance level associated with the observed k nearest cases to the centroid of cell i is determined by equation (1) in Besag and Newell (1991), that is,

$$\Pr(L \leq l) = 1 - \sum_{s=0}^{k-1} \frac{\exp(-m_i c_+/n_+)(m_i c_+/n_+)^s}{s!}. \tag{1}$$

Besag and Newell (1991) suggest mapping those clusters that attain some predetermined nominal significance level α (here $\alpha = 0.05$). Figure 6 shows the results with $k = 8$ when there are 31 such clusters. More precise details on how this map is drawn are given later in this section. We have chosen the largest k value used by Besag and Newell (1991) since our data contain more people at risk per cell than their data, resulting in higher expected cell counts of disease. The higher expectations (and associated variances) indicate that small clusters of two or four excess cases are not likely to be detected in our data. Comparing this with the map produced by the GAM procedure (Figure 4), we see that there is some qualitative agreement—many of the clusters with unadjusted p-values below 0.05 occur in the same areas as those where many circles were drawn by the GAM (e.g., in Cayuga and Cortland counties).

As with the GAM procedure, the presence of the subregions outlined on the maps in Figure 6 does not necessarily indicate the presence of clustering; by chance we would expect to find some cells nominally significant at a 5% level. However, we can obtain a significance level for an overall test of H_0 based on the total number T_{BN}, say, of cell centroids (out of a possible I) that are associated with clusters of size k that are significant at nominal level α. We use the adjectives *unadjusted* and *nominal* in describing the significance values since no adjustment for the multiplicity of tests is made. Again, details on various schemes for adjusting significance values to compensate for multiple tests can be found in Miller (1981). For our data, using $k = 8$ and $\alpha = 0.05$, the observed value of T_{BN} is 31. An approximation of the expectation of T_{BN} is $\alpha I = (0.05)(790) = 39.50$. This expected value is only approximate because of the discreteness of the distribution of T_{BN}. A derivation of the exact expectation of T_{BN} can be adapted from formula (2) in Besag and Newell (1991). For each cell, one successively applies equation (1) for values $l = 0, 1, \ldots$ until the significance level first exceeds α, say for $l = l^*$. The value of (1) for $l = l^* - 1$ is the true significance level α_i, say, for the cluster of k cases nearest the ith centroid. The exact expectation of T_{BN} is given by

$$E(T_{BN}) = \sum_{i=1}^{I} \alpha_i. \tag{2}$$

When this is computed with $k = 8$, the value of this exact expression (2) is 24.22, which is considerably less than $\alpha I = 39.5$. The exact expectation suggests that more clusters (31) of $k = 8$ cases were observed than would be expected under H_0, rather than the opposite conclusion, which is drawn when the approximation αI is used. Our experience suggests that the exact value (2) should be used since the accuracy of the approximation depends not only on the value of k used, but also on the population size of the cells used (i.e., the level of aggregation encountered in the data). The significance of the observed values of T_{BN} can again be determined by Monte Carlo simulation, where the cases are assigned to cells as described above for the Turnbull et al. (1990) procedure.

Using again 999 replications, we obtain a p-value for $k = 8$ of 0.18 which agrees approximately with the results of Turnbull et al. (1990) (Roughly speaking, the value of $k = 8$ here can be thought of as corresponding to a population radius of $R = kn_+/c_+ = 14,293$ persons.) As a check on the simulation program, the mean of the (999) simulated T_{BN} values should approximately equal the value given by expression (2). In our case, this was extremely close (24.21), which is well within the sampling error of the simulation.

The cell with the lowest unadjusted p-value for the application of the method of Besag and Newell (1991) (i.e., the cell most likely to be a cluster) is the cell labeled M1 mentioned earlier for $k = 8$ cases. Cell M1 is in Cortland County and its centroid is located near the symbol M1 in Figure 6. The centroids of cells whose associated unadjusted p-values are less than 0.05 are also shown in Figure 6. The labels A, N1, and C represent three, four, and five centroids, respectively, that are very near each other geographically. We use single labels to indicate their general location while maintaining the readability of Figure 6. There are also 12 clusters near the label S in Onondaga County in Figure 6. These cells are in the city of Syracuse and are smaller geographically due to the higher population density found in an urban setting. Each of the remaining labels in Figure 6 represents a single centroid. The contours of a cluster represent the border of the union of the Voronoi polygons of the centroids of those cells included in a cluster. The Voronoi polygon of a centroid is defined to be the border of the collection of points that are closer to the centroid than to any other centroid (Ripley, 1981, p. 38). These contours are adjusted slightly so that the borders do not overlap, again to improve the readability of Figure 6. A similar map could be drawn with contours representing those borders of the balls with observed cases exceeding some nominal significance value for the method of Turnbull et al. (1990).

Our overall conclusion is that the evidence of clustering of the cases is rather weak, although there is some suggestion that there may be a mild effect when one considers larger radii in the method of Turnbull et al. (1990). Of course, failing to reject H_0 does not necessarily imply that the randomness hypothesis is true. By trying to maintain a type I error rate in the face of so many multiple tests (i.e., to control the probability of wrongly declaring *any* subregion to be the site of a cluster), the power of the procedures must necessarily be very low. That is, to appear statistically significant, a clustering effect must be very strong. It may seem that low statistical power is inevitable for surveillance situations of this kind. However, a standard way in statistical theory to develop more powerful test procedures is to define a more limited set of interesting alternative hypotheses and ask for test statistics that are required to be powerful only against these alternatives. By reducing power against unlikely or uninteresting alternatives, increased power can be achieved for the specified ones. This leads us to the idea of focused tests, in which the alternative hypothesis of interest is that disease rates are elevated in the vicinity of sources of some environmental exposure. Such tests are discussed in the next section.

3 TESTING FOR CLUSTERING ABOUT PRESPECIFIED LOCATIONS

We next turned our attention to considering statistical procedures which would examine the question of whether disease cases tend to cluster around prespecified sources of environmental hazard. In order to test and compare the procedures, we took for our putative sources of hazard the 11 hazardous waste sites in the study area listed as containing the chemical TCE (New York State Department of Environmental Conservation, 1987). The locations of these 11 sites are shown in Figure 2. The TCE-contaminated sites were chosen as the model foci for the following reasons. A common groundwater contaminant, TCE has been associated with leukemia incidence, although the evidence is weak (Kimbrough et al., 1985). Contaminated drinking water often contains TCE as well as other VOCs whose human carcinogenicity is more firmly established (e.g., tetrachloroethylene) (Brown et al., 1984; Andelman, 1985; McKone, 1987; Cothern, 1988; U.S. Department of Health and Human Services, 1991; McKone and Bogen, 1991, 1992). Hence we used TCE as a surrogate for exposure to VOCs in groundwater in general. Such chemicals were also present in the contaminated wells in the Woburn study mentioned earlier (Lagakos et al., 1986). Of course, as usual, any significant results cannot be interpreted as evidence of a necessarily causal association between TCE and leukemia, due to the fact that the individuals in the study were potentially exposed to many environmental contaminants, as well as other confounding factors. The original analysis of the upstate New York leukemia data and the TCE waste sites appears in Waller et al. (1992).

An obvious first approach is to compare the locations of the waste sites (Figure 2) to the circles drawn on Figures 4 and 6. However, it is hard to assess the correspondence between them. Some of the clusters of circles in Figures 4 and 6 coincide with some of the waste site locations—others do not. We need a quantitative assessment of association between the locations of the waste sites and the spatial incidence pattern of the leukemia cases. Also, the procedures that produced Figures 4 and 6 did not use the information about these putative sources of hazard and so will not be as sensitive in detecting associations, as pointed out at the end of the preceding section.

We can apply a focused version of the method of Besag and Newell (1991) by examining the sets of k cases around each TCE waste site. Again we find the number of nearest cells l needed to find the k nearest cases to a focus and use (1) to determine the unadjusted p-value by finding the probability that L is greater than l. We list the unadjusted p-values for each focus in Table 4 for $k = 6$, 8, and 10. We use several values for k to illustrate that the significance values will change depending on how many cases are considered to define a cluster. Additional values of k may also be used with the general method of Besag and Newell, but this is left as an exercise for the reader. Note that only two foci have unadjusted p-values less than $\alpha = 0.05$, one focus for $k = 6$ and one focus for $k = 10$. The two foci are different, and considering the number

Table 4   Results of Focused Tests for Leukemia in Upstate New York, 1978–1982[a]

Focus	Besag and Newell's (1991) p-Value[b]			T_{Stone} (p-Value[c])	$U*$ (p-Value[d])
	$k = 6$	$k = 8$	$k = 10$		
Monarch Chemicals	0.069	0.072	0.013	2.50 (0.011)	4.12 (<0.001)
IBM Endicott	0.227	0.056	0.072	2.53 (0.036)	3.39 (<0.001)
Singer	0.665	0.725	0.470	1.48 (0.245)	2.47 (0.007)
Nesco	0.665	0.725	0.470	1.48 (0.245)	2.46 (0.007)
GE Auburn	0.108	0.133	0.143	2.13 (0.156)	2.06 (0.020)
Solvent Savers	0.551	0.254	0.168	1.77 (0.502)	0.29 (0.386)
Smith Corona	0.337	0.258	0.120	2.13 (0.162)	2.56 (0.005)
Victory Plaza	0.013	0.492	0.237	3.37 (0.102)	1.97 (0.024)
Hadco	0.769	0.490	0.284	1.52 (0.572)	1.87 (0.031)
Morse Chain	0.843	0.726	0.879	1.19 (0.784)	−0.78 (0.782)
Groton	0.847	0.875	0.722	1.60 (0.385)	0.81 (0.209)
Combined foci	0.315	0.602	0.334	1.88 (0.207)	3.54 (<0.001)

[a]No adjustments are made for multiple foci in any of the three methods.
[b]Unadjusted p-value obtained for each focus following (1).
[c]Analytic p-value from (3) and (4).
[d]Asymptotic p-value obtained from standard normal distribution (see text).

of foci and the number of k-values used, this method does not show strong evidence that the cases are clustered about any of the TCE waste sites.

Stone (1988) proposed a method to test for clustering about a single focus. We order the cells by increasing distance of their centroids to the focus, so that the cell whose centroid is nearest to the focus is cell 1, and the cell with its centroid farthest from the focus is denoted cell I. We test the null hypothesis H_0 as before against the alternative that the incidence rate decreases with increasing distance from the focus. The test statistic is

$$T_{Stone} = \max_{1 \leq j \leq I} \frac{\sum_{i=1}^{j} C_i}{\sum_{i=1}^{j} E_i},$$

where $E_i = n_i c_+/n_+$ is the expected number of cases in cell i under $H_0, i = 1, \ldots, I$. This statistic has the intuitive interpretation of being the maximum estimated relative risk among geographic areas about the source composed of the j closest cells over the possible values of $j = 1, \ldots, I$. Hence, the value of j where the maximum is obtained is the number of nearest cells about the source within which the estimated relative risk is maximized. This test is different from the focused version of the method of Besag and Newell (1991) in that the data define both the cells most likely to be a cluster, and the number of cases in the detected cluster.

The distribution of T_{Stone} under the null hypothesis is obtained by considering a two-dimensional random walk in the plane defined by the cumulative observed and cumulative expected numbers of cases. The significance value for the test of H_0 is the probability of a random walk beginning at the origin traversing above a line passing through the origin with slope equal to the observed value of T_{Stone}. The significance value associated with the observed value $T_{Stone} = t$ is $\Pr(T_{Stone} > t) = 1 - \Pr(T_{Stone} \leq t)$, where

$$
\Pr(T_{Stone} \leq t) = \Pr\left(\sum_{k=1}^{i} C_k \leq t \sum_{k=1}^{i} E_k; \quad i = 1, \ldots, I\right)
$$
$$
= \sum_{j=0}^{E} q(I, j) \tag{3}
$$

for

$$
q(v, j) = \Pr\left[\left(\sum_{k=1}^{v} C_k = j\right) \cap \left(\sum_{k=1}^{i} C_k \leq t \sum_{k=1}^{i} E_k\right); \quad i = 1, \ldots, v\right],
$$

and $E = \lfloor t \sum_{i=1}^{I} E_i \rfloor$ is the largest integer less than or equal to $t \sum_{i=1}^{I} E_i$. Note that the summations are in terms of the indices of the cells and values are summed *in order of decreasing exposure to the focus*. The upper limit of summation in (3) represents a minor correction to the formula given by Stone (1988, p. 654). The probabilities $q(v, j)$ may be interpreted as the probability that the v closest cells to the focus contain j cases and that the cumulative ratio is less than t. These probabilities are obtained recursively from the backward equations associated with the random walk mentioned above, and are defined under H_0 by

$$
q(v, j) = \begin{cases} \displaystyle\sum_{k=0}^{j} \dfrac{q(v-1, j-k)\, \exp(-E_v)(E_v)^k}{k!} & j = 0, \ldots, E', \\ 0 & j > E', \end{cases} \tag{4}
$$

with $q(0, 0) = 1$ and $E' = \lfloor t \sum_{i=1}^{v} E_i \rfloor$.

The results for applying the method of Stone (1988) to the leukemia data for each of the TCE sites are shown in Table 4. We see two significant values among the results, namely those given by the Monarch Chemicals and IBM Endicott sites in Broome County. The two sites are close together, but the areas around the sites containing the maximum estimated relative risks (i.e., the detected clusters) do not have any cells in common. We note that, again, we are conducting multiple tests, so that the significance values should be adjusted to compensate for multiple analyses of the data.

As well as ordering the cells by their distance to a single focus, we may also order the cells by their distance to *any* focus and obtain a test of whether the leukemia cases appear to be clustered around the TCE sites as a group. Of course, we are treating the foci as if the relationship with exposure and geographic distance were the same for all of the foci and that the foci do not interact to increase exposure. Specific exposure data would be needed to account for any heterogeneity or synergism between the foci. The results of Stone's (1988) test using the distance to any source are listed as combined foci in Table 4. The method of Besag and Newell (1991) may also be applied to the set of foci as a whole, again by ordering the cells by the distance of their centroids to the nearest focus. The results of applying the method of Besag and Newell (1991) in this manner also appear in Table 4 as combined foci.

The final focused test we consider here was developed for use when a quantitative measure of the exposure to the foci for each individual is available, denoted by g_i for an individual in cell i. Of course, for large-scale surveillance studies, precise estimates of exposure are unlikely to be available, so as a surrogate, we take g_i to be the reciprocal of the distance from the focus to the centroid of cell i. Other inversely related functions of distance for g_i were tried, but results were essentially identical to those presented below for the simple reciprocal function.

Following Breslow et al. (1983), Waller et al. (1992) and Lawson (1993) propose using the sum of the deviations of the observed disease incidence in each cell from its expectation under H_0, weighted by the exposure as a test statistic, that is,

$$U = \sum_{i=1}^{I} g_i(C_i - E_i),$$

where $E_i = n_i c_+/n_+$ is the expected number of cases in cell i under H_0. It turns out that this test is a score test which is uniformly most powerful (UMP) against the focused clustering alternative:

$$H_A: E(C_i) = n_i \lambda(1 + g_i \epsilon),$$

where ϵ is positive but unspecified. Under this alternative, the expected number of cases in cell i is increased proportional to the exposure of individuals in cell i to the foci. (Under H_A the disease counts remain independent.) Note that the null hypothesis corresponds to $\epsilon = 0$. The UMP property (see, e.g., Cox and Hinkley, 1974, pp. 101–102) implies that the probability that this test will reject the null hypothesis when the alternative H_A is true will be greater than or equal to the probability that any other test will reject H_0 when H_A is true. We will refer to this test as the UMP test. Note that the alternative H_A is more specific than the one Stone (1988) considered, since it is based on a probability model relating incidence to an exposure measure in a particular way.

Under H_0, the test statistic U has expectation zero and variance equal to the Fisher information, which is approximately

$$\text{Var}(U) = \sum_{i=1}^{I} g_i^2 E_i.$$

The standardized statistic $U^* = U/[\text{Var}(U)]^{1/2}$ has an asymptotic standard normal distribution (Cox and Hinkley, 1974, p. 113). This normal approximation is generally quite accurate. The results for the New York leukemia data with exposure to the TCE sites defined as the inverse distance of the cell centroids to the foci are presented in Table 3. As before, we may investigate the effect of the foci as a homogeneous collection by using the inverse distance to the nearest focus as the exposure surrogate. We list this result under combined foci in Table 4. Note that several of the tests yield significant results. The multiplicity of tests cannot alone account for the significant results. While the significance values for the UMP test are quite different from those obtained from the tests of Besag and Newell (1991) and Stone (1988), we see some qualitative agreement, since the Monarch Chemical site is again the focus of the most likely cluster. The reason for the quantitative discrepancy between the UMP test and the other two focused tests in Table 4, in particular the much greater significance attached to the Monarch site, can be discerned upon closer examination of the data. Whereas the method of Besag and Newell (1991) looks only at clusters of k cases and that of Stone (1988) only at the maximum incidence rate over neighborhoods of a focus, the UMP test statistic takes into account the fact that the incidence rate is high and sustained over a wide family of neighborhoods of the Monarch site (see Waller et al., 1992).

4 DISCUSSION

The results of the analyses in Section 2 of the upstate New York leukemia data indicate that there is not strong evidence of the cases clustering, although there is some suggestive clustering, most notably in Cortland County. However, it is not clear if these somewhat negative results are due to an actual absence of clustering or due to a lack of statistical power to detect deviations from the null hypothesis by the tests used. The results in Section 3 of the focused tests for the hazardous wastes sites containing TCE do give some indication of a clustering effect (e.g., near the Monarch Chemicals site). This particular cluster is not apparent simply by comparing the general clusters to the locations of the TCE waste sites. We discovered, after the analysis, that the Monarch Chemicals site is near the Town of Vestal Water Supply Well 4-2, a Federal Superfund Site, classified by the New York Department of Environmental Conservation (1987) as a "significant threat to public health" because of TCE contamination. Well 4-2 was taken out of service in 1983, and the drinking water in the area (now from different wells) was classified as presenting no significant health risk. However, the well was in service prior to and during the 1978–1982 study period so that exposure of the nearby resident population is possible. The contamination of Well 4-2 may not be due to Monarch Chemicals; we only note that the location of the well is near this particular waste site. We also note that the ordering of cells with respect to possible exposure to the well will not precisely match the ordering with respect to inverse distance to the Monarch Chemicals site used to obtain the results above. The well is located near the Susquehanna River and only those cells south of the river received water from the well, while the nearest cell centroid to the Monarch Chemicals site is north of the river. A detailed follow-up epidemiologic investigation using an ordering based on estimated exposure to drinking water from Well 4-2 could be conducted using exposure estimates similar to those used by Lagakos et al. (1986).

The tests of clustering applied to the upstate New York data were applied in a manner consistent with a large-scale or macroscopic surveillance for potential disease clusters. The results may be used to prioritize areas, in the case of general tests, or to prioritize prespecified foci, in the case of focused tests, for follow-up action on a more local, or microscopic level. Such local action should involve more precise exposure measurements, and additional data on possible confounding factors, such as the age distribution, occupational exposures, and so on, associated with both cases and noncases. The local studies will be able to provide a clearer picture of any causal pathways that may exist by controlling for confounding factors with data that are generally not available on a large-scale basis. The goal of surveillance studies should be to indicate where local studies would best be conducted, and which cells should be considered to provide the best allocation of limited resources. This project is still continuing. At the moment the emphasis is on the efficient and timely registering and geocoding of the incidence data. Demographic information will be updated using the 1990 U.S. Census.

Finally, it should be remarked that clustering problems arise in a variety of other applications, including biology and geology. The statistical theory is closely connected with the study of coincidences (Diaconis and Mosteller, 1989). Fienberg and Kaye (1991) describe many interesting legal examples of clusters and coincidences.

QUESTIONS AND PROBLEMS

1. Define an exposure function for the UMP test that considers only those cells within a specified radius of the foci to be exposed. How does such a change in the definition of exposure change the results?

2. The general test of Besag and Newell (1991) was applied only for $k = 8$. Apply the method as described in the text for other values of $k = 6$ and $k = 10$. Do the results change? Are the significant clusters in locations different from those shown in Figure 6?

3. Use equation (1) to relate the choice of the value of k to the population size of the cell whose centroid is the center of the cluster. For a given population size in a cell, are there cluster sizes (values of k) that cannot be declared significant at a given level (say, $\alpha = 0.05$)? What does this say about the possible choices of k?

4. The general tests seem to indicate that some of the most likely clustering of cases occurs in Cortland County while the focused tests indicate the most likely focused clustering occurring about foci in Broome County. Discuss possible reasons for this difference.

CHAPTER 2

Assessing Toxicity of Pollutants in Aquatic Systems

A. John Bailer and James T. Oris

1 MOTIVATION AND BACKGROUND

The study of toxicants in the aquatic environment grew out of the post-World War II industrial age and the advent in the use of synthetic pesticides and fertilizers, the use of synthetic detergents and their additives, the use of increasing amounts of fossil fuels and their derived industrial products, and the use of fissionable materials and their generated waste products. The degradation of aquatic resources became readily apparent during the 1950s and 1960s, and public recognition of a need to protect the environment from toxic insult reached a peak during the period after 1970, when the U.S. Environmental Protection Agency (EPA) was formed.

Between World War II and the present, most of the current environmental legislation was developed (see, e.g., Foster, 1985; West Publishing, 1991). A select few of these laws have had significant impacts on the field of aquatic toxicology and for background purposes are introduced below. In this introduction, several acronyms are defined even though they may not subsequently appear in the text. However, these laws and their amendments have had a profound impact on environmental safety assessments, and the acronyms are in common usage among environmental scientists and regulatory agencies.

The Federal Water Pollution Control Act (FWPCA) was enacted in its current form in 1948, and was the first act to approach the prevention of water pollution in a comprehensive manner, promoting the study of water pollution issues through joint state and federal programs and providing financial assistance for these studies. The primary focus of the FWPCA was the discharge of sewage and nutrients, until the passage of amendments in 1977 and 1978 referred to as the Clean Water Act. The Clean Water Act dealt not only with sewage and nutri-

Case Studies in Biometry, Edited by Nicholas Lange, Louise Ryan, Lynne Billard,
David Brillinger, Loveday Conquest, and Joel Greenhouse.
ISBN 0-471-58885-7 © 1994 John Wiley & Sons, Inc.

ents but also with the discharge of toxic materials. The legislation provides for the permitting and limitation of point-source effluent discharges (National Pollutant Discharge Elimination System (NPDES) permits) to inland waters and to waters within the 3-mile boundary of the territorial sea. The act also provides for the development of water quality criteria, toxic and pretreatment effluent standards, ocean discharge criteria, and permitting for dredged or fill materials. The Federal Insecticide, Fungicide and Rodenticide Act (FIFRA) was enacted in 1947. FIFRA, and its revisions of 1972 under the Federal Environmental Pesticide Control Act, requires that all pesticide products used in the United States be registered with the EPA. This legislation requires the registrant to submit information on the composition, intended use, and efficacy of the product, along with a comprehensive database establishing that the material can be used without causing unreasonable adverse effects on humans or the environment. The Marine Protection, Research and Sanctuaries Act of 1972 empowered the EPA to regulate the transport of materials for ocean disposal by requiring permits based on an evaluation of the potential ecological impact of the applicant's material on the marine environment. The Safe Drinking Water Act of 1974 directed the EPA to promulgate National Revised Primary Drinking Water Regulations for organic, inorganic, microbial, and radionuclide contaminants in drinking water. The Toxic Substances Control Act (TSCA) of 1976 provides the EPA the authority to require testing of chemicals and to regulate commercial chemicals (new or existing) other than pesticide products that present a hazard to human health or the environment. Manufacturers are required to submit information to the EPA to allow for the identification and evaluation of the potential hazards of a chemical prior to its introduction into commerce (Pre-Manufacture Notification). The act also provides for the regulation of production, use, distribution, and disposal of chemicals. The focus, approach, and development of standard methodology in aquatic toxicology have been driven to a major extent by these important pieces of legislation in part because they require the routine testing of a very large number of chemicals and effluents.

The need to develop and to refine standard toxicity test methodology was recognized during the First Annual Symposium on Aquatic Toxicology, held in 1976 in conjunction with the American Society for Testing and Materials (ASTM). In an introductory overview at that symposium (Mount, 1977), three major points were made which have since greatly influenced the field of aquatic toxicology:

1. That the chronic or life-cycle test should be used as the mainstay of the profession. At this point in time a reasonable database on whole life-cycle testing had been developed by the Duluth laboratory of the EPA, and there was a great interest and need to develop shortened, partial life-cycle tests. Currently, the EPA (cf. Weber et al., 1989) requires the use of a battery of short-term methods for estimating the chronic toxicity of effluents and receiving waters to aquatic organisms.

2. That perhaps a new professional society should be founded to address the needs of this new and growing field of endeavor. The Society of Environmental Toxicology and Chemistry was subsequently founded in 1978–1979, with the goal of maintaining balance and communication among academia, government, and industry. The primary focus of the society during its early years of development was aquatic toxicology. The current society, however, holds interests in all aspects of environmental toxicology, chemistry, and hazard assessment, and has grown into an international organization with nearly 2500 members.

3. That whereas several chronic toxicity test methods were well developed at the time, the methods were far ahead of the ability to apply the results and that a major emphasis should be directed toward analyzing the data derived from the tests. A major interest during the late 1970s, which continues to a large extent today, was merely to obtain the data from toxicity tests for the purpose of complying with federal and state environmental legislation. Indeed, one of the top five all-time Science Citation Classics is the description of an apparatus used to conduct concentration–response tests in flow-through aquariums (Mount and Brungs, 1967).

In the spirit of point 1 above and in an effort to protect freshwater resources from industrial and municipal effluents, regulatory agencies are developing programs which require dischargers to conduct an increasing number and frequency of toxicity tests (USEPA, 1990). As currently recommended, protocols for acceptable toxicity tests require time commitments ranging from 2 to 7 days. The toxicity test battery is designed to encompass a range of biological ecosystem components (i.e., plants, invertebrates, vertebrates) and a variety of endpoints, such as mortality, growth, reproductive success, and birth defects (teratogenicity). These tests include acute mortality tests, an algal (*Selenastrum capricornutum*) growth test, an invertebrate zooplankton (*Ceriodaphnia dubia*) survival and reproduction test, a vertebrate (fathead minnow) embryo–larval survival and growth test, and a vertebrate (fathead minnow) embryo–larval survival and teratogenicity test (Weber et al., 1989).

The most common endpoints in the tests mentioned above are growth and reproductive output. These endpoints generally are expressed on a relative basis, with the control group performance considered as the benchmark to which the dosage groups' performances are compared. Although the shape of the concentration–response relationship can be complex and is not usually known a priori, the concentration–response curves can be grouped into one of three classes: linear, threshold, or nutritive (Figure 1). Chemicals demonstrating a linear concentration–response are nonessential materials that interfere with biological processes at extremely low concentrations. Threshold toxicants are those which are nonessential materials which over a range of concentrations can be homeostatically regulated before detrimental effects are observed. A threshold response is one that does not occur unless the concentration of a toxicant exceeds a particular level, labeled the *threshold* of the toxicant. The nutritive chemicals are those which at low concentrations are essential for the growth, survival, and reproduction of the organism, but which are toxic at concentrations which exceed the ability of the organism to regulate the chemical homeostatically. Thus, at low concentrations the investigator often observes an enhancement of dosage group performance relative to the control group prior to the onset of toxicity. Because these responses can be characterized in a general sense, it would be useful to develop a flexible model of concentration–response relationships from aquatic toxicity tests that could be used to calculate point estimates for the potency of chemicals and effluents regardless of the shape of the concentration–response curve. Furthermore, it would be beneficial to the regulatory community to develop methods to estimate the variance of (and hence confidence limits around) these point estimates for use in the establishment of water quality criteria. The development, application, and discussion of such a potency estimator provide the focus for this case study. For the development that follows, we focus on reproductive toxicity response in studies of *Ceriodaphnia dubia.*

Ceriodaphnia dubia is a small (0.2 to 1.5 mm; juvenile to adult) freshwater invertebrate zooplankton (phylum Arthropoda, subphylum Crustacea, class Brachiopoda, order Diplostraca, suborder Cladocera, family Daphnidae), which

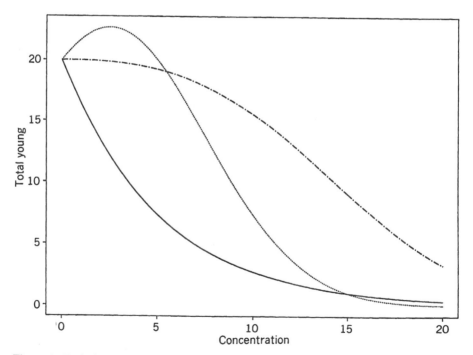

Figure 1. Typical concentration–response patterns exhibiting linear effects (solid line), nutritive effects (dotted line), and threshold effects (chain dotted line).

feeds by filtering microscopic algai and particulate organic material from the water column. This and related species of zooplankton are common and important members of freshwater ecosystems throughout the world and form the basis of food chains for the higher invertebrates and for fish and birds. Under optimal environmental conditions, only females are present in a population of *C. dubia*; adult females reproduce asexually, producing eggs that develop without fertilization and giving birth to female offspring. Individuals attain sexual maturity and give birth within 72 to 96 hours of hatching. Up to 35 eggs are carried internally within a brood pouch. Eggs develop and hatch within 48 hours and are released from the brood pouch in coordination with the molting cycle of the adult female (24- to 48-hour cycle). Thus the typical *C. dubia* hatches, matures, and produces three or four broods of offspring within the first 7 days of its lifespan (approximately 30 days).

The *C. dubia* survival and reproduction toxicity test is an accepted standard method in the assessment of the toxicity of effluents, environmental samples, and single chemicals (Weber et al., 1989). A typical test is initiated with <12-hour-old juveniles and measures the survival and reproductive output of 10 individuals in each of four concentrations of toxicant plus a control for a 7-day period (50 organisms per test). This period of time is sufficient for the growth and maturation of the animals and for the production of three broods of offspring.

2 DATA

Nitrofen (2,4-dichlorophenyl 4-nitrophenyl ether; CAS 1836-75-5) is a selective contact herbicide that was used for the control of broad-leaved and grass weeds in cereals and rice (Hartley and Kidd, 1987). Even though it is relatively nontoxic to adult mammals (Hartley and Kidd, 1987; Kimbrough et al., 1974), nitrofen is a significant teratogen (Costlow et al., 1983; Francis, 1989) and mutagen (Draper and Casida, 1983). In addition, it is both acutely toxic and reproductively toxic to cladoceran zooplankton (Oris et al., 1991). Because of the risk of human exposure (Francis, 1989) and its persistence in aquatic systems (Lee et al., 1976), nitrofen is no longer in commercial use in the United States. Nitrofen was the first pesticide to be withdrawn from commercial use because of teratogenic effects (Francis, 1989).

The reproductive toxicity test was conducted at measured nitrofen concentrations of 0, 80, 160, 235, and 310 μg/L. The observed number of offspring born in three broods to each of the 10 *C. dubia* in each of the concentration groups are reported and summarized in Table 1. Summary statistics (means and variances) along with observed percentage reproduction inhibitions in total offspring per brood relative to control reproduction are reported in Table 2. From observations of the means and variances, it appears that nitrofen has a minimal effect at low concentrations and then becomes toxic at higher doses.

Table 1 Number of Offspring Produced by *C. dubia* in a Reproductive Toxicity Test of Nitrofen

Animal No.	Concentration (µg/L)	Number of Offspring			
		Brood 1	Brood 2	Brood 3	Total
1	0	3	14	10	27
2	0	5	12	15	32
3	0	6	11	17	34
4	0	6	12	15	33
5	0	6	15	15	36
6	0	5	14	15	34
7	0	6	12	15	33
8	0	5	13	12	30
9	0	3	10	11	24
10	0	6	11	14	31
11	80	6	11	16	33
12	80	5	12	16	33
13	80	6	11	18	35
14	80	5	12	16	33
15	80	8	13	15	36
16	80	3	9	14	26
17	80	5	9	13	27
18	80	7	12	12	31
19	80	5	13	14	32
20	80	3	12	14	29
21	160	6	12	11	29
22	160	6	12	11	29
23	160	2	8	13	23
24	160	6	10	11	27
25	160	6	11	13	30
26	160	6	13	12	31
27	160	6	12	12	30
28	160	5	10	11	26
29	160	6	13	10	29
30	160	6	12	11	29
31	235	4	13	6	23
32	235	6	10	5	21
33	235	2	5	0	7
34	235	6	0	6	12
35	235	6	13	8	27
36	235	6	0	10	16
37	235	7	0	6	13
38	235	4	2	9	15
39	235	6	8	7	21
40	235	7	0	10	17
41	310	6	0	0	6

Table 1 (*Continued*)

Animal No.	Concentration (μg/L)	Number of Offspring			
		Brood 1	Brood 2	Brood 3	Total
42	310	6	0	0	6
43	310	7	0	0	7
44	310	0	0	0	0
45	310	5	10	0	15
46	310	5	0	0	5
47	310	6	0	0	6
48	310	4	0	0	4
49	310	6	0	0	6
50	310	5	0	0	5

Table 2 Summary Statistics for a *C. dubia* Reproductive Toxicity Test of Nitrofen

Concentration (μg/L)	Mean (Variance)[a]	Percent Inhibition Relative to Control Reproduction[b]
0	31.4 (12.9)	0.0
80	31.5 (10.7)	−0.3
160	28.3 (5.6)	9.9
235	17.2 (34.8)	45.2
310	6.0 (13.8)	80.9

[a]Table values represent the mean total number of offspring produced in three broods by each female (variance is defined analogously).
[b]Percent inhibition relative to the control group is determined by $100(1-(\hat{\mu}_C/\hat{\mu}_0))\%$, where $\hat{\mu}_C$ is the mean total number of offspring produced in three broods by each female in concentration group C.

3 METHODS AND MODELS

3.1 Notation

For the derivations that follow, the following notation is employed. The total number of offspring produced in brood k to the jth animal in the ith concentration level (C_i) is denoted Y_{ijk}, where $k = 1, 2, 3, j = 1, \ldots, n_i$, and $i = 0, \ldots, L$ (concentration levels with $i = 0$ corresponding to control). For most aquatic toxicity studies of reproductive inhibition, $n_i = 10$ and the number of nonzero concentration groups (L) is five or less. The total number of animals on test is $n = n_0 + n_1 + \cdots + n_L$. For the analysis presented herein, the response of interest is the total number of offspring produced in three broods ($Y_{ij1} + Y_{ij2} + Y_{ij3}$), hereafter denoted Y_{ij}. Finally, the expected total number of offspring for an animal exposed to concentration level C_i, $E(Y_{ij})$, is denoted μ_i and the variance of this total, Var (Y_{ij}), is denoted σ_i^2.

3.2 Current Potency Estimators

Currently, there are two proposed methods for analyzing and estimating inhibitory concentrations from these toxicity tests. The first method is based on successively applying statistical tests to detect treatment concentrations that differ from the control group. First, the highest concentration level where mean total number of offspring does not differ statistically from the mean total number of offspring in the control group (zero concentration group) is determined. This quantity is the no-observed effect concentration, or NOEC. Second, the lowest concentration level where the mean total number of offspring is observed to be statistically different from the mean total number of offspring in the control group is determined. This is the lowest-observed effect concentration, or LOEC. A point estimate of an estimated safe concentration, the chronic value (ChV), is then calculated as the geometric mean between the NOEC and LOEC. Depending on distributional assumptions considered for the response variable, parametric or nonparametric hypothesis tests are recommended (Weber et al., 1989). It is observed that the NOEC is generally less than 50% inhibition relative to control reproduction and the LOEC is generally greater than 50% inhibition. This behavior has been demonstrated to be a logical consequence of the experimental protocols that are currently employed in *C. dubia* tests (Oris and Bailer, 1993); that is, the behavior of this method is clearly influenced by the experimental design that has been employed.

The second method of analysis of reproduction data from these tests involves the point estimation of an inhibition concentration (IC) endpoint that causes a specified percent reduction in reproductive output (Weber et al., 1989; Oris et al., 1991; Norberg-King, 1988). This form of IC analysis assumes a monotonically decreasing reproductive output with increasing concentration of toxicant. Linear interpolation between the two nearest concentration values which produce inhibition levels above and below the specified percentage is used to calculate the point estimate endpoint. It has been observed that the 50% inhibition point (IC50) roughly corresponds to calculated ChV values and that the 25% inhibition point (IC25) corresponds roughly to NOECs from hypothesis-testing analyses (Oris et al., 1991; Norberg-King, 1988). Currently, the EPA recommends the IC25 as the preferred endpoint for compliance monitoring (USEPA, 1990).

Neither of these procedures is completely satisfactory for estimating inhibition concentrations. The ChV is an experimental design-dependent estimate of the potency of a chemical. Given its construction as a mean of two concentration levels, any experiment where L concentrations (plus a control) are tested can yield only one of L possible ChV estimates. ChV calculation is also highly dependent on the sample sizes in each concentration level, which relates to the statistical power to detect differences in mean response (Oris and Bailer, 1993). Indeed, no simple method for summarizing the variation in estimated ChV or for constructing confidence intervals for the ChV is available. Even though there exist computationally intensive statistical resampling procedures that could be used to construct a confidence interval, this interval's endpoints would be at most two of the L possible ChV estimates.

Alternatively, the IC50 is constructed by examining mean responses in concentrations that lie immediately above and immediately below 50% of the mean number of offspring observed in the control group. Confidence intervals for the IC50 can be constructed using computationally intensive statistical methods such as the bootstrap. This procedure suffers the shortcoming experienced by all tests and calculations involving means: the sensitivity of sample means to outlying observations.

3.3   Concentration–Response-Based Potency Estimation

As an alternative to the ChV and the IC procedures, a flexible model for the relationship between exposure concentration and total number of offspring is proposed. This model is then used to estimate concentrations that lead to some specified level of inhibition relative to the control group. A detailed discussion of this method of potency estimation may be found in Bailer and Oris (1993).

Concentration–Response Model and Error Distribution
The model that is proposed for relating the expected total offspring to concentration C_i is

$$\mu_i = \exp\left(\sum_{m=0}^{K} \beta_m C_i^m\right),$$

where the β's are unknown population coefficients with $\exp(\beta_0)$ corresponding to the estimate of the mean total number of offspring in the zero-concentration group and K is some positive integer (possibly equal to 0 if there is no relationship between concentration levels and reproductive outcome). This model is intrinsically linear in the model parameters in that the natural logarithm of μ_i is a linear function of the β's (i.e., a log-linear form):

$$\ln(\mu_i) = \sum_{m=0}^{K} \beta_m C_i^m = \beta_0 + \beta_1 C_i + \beta_2 C_i^2 + \cdots + \beta_K C_i^K.$$

In order to make statistical inferences about the β's after fitting this model, an assumption about the distribution of total offspring at each concentration must be made. It is commonly assumed when modeling count data in biology that observations possess a Poisson distribution (Stein, 1988). These models can readily be fit using techniques from generalized linear models, or GLIMs (McCullagh and Nelder, 1989). The Poisson distribution implies that $\mu_i = \sigma_i^2$, which is an assumption that should be evaluated when fitting such models.

To fit the log-linear model we propose, the degree of the polynomial (K) must be selected. In general, a plot of the data may suggest reasonable values of K; however, the inherent behavior of the toxicant may also suggest reasonable values of K. If there is no concentration–response (i.e., a plot of Y_{ij} versus C_i is flat), $K = 0$ is suggested. If exponential decay is exhibited (the "linear effect" of Figure 1), $K = 1$ is suggested. If the data exhibits an initial increase followed by a steady decrease (e.g., a "nutritive effect" or even a "threshold effect," as illustrated in Figure 1), $K = 2$ (or perhaps larger) is suggested.

As when fitting multiple regression models, GLIMs must be assessed for model adequacy. Residual plots (plots of $Y_{ij} - \hat{\mu}_i$ versus C_i) should be made and evaluated. Estimates of the β_m values are used to determine the $\hat{\mu}_i$, that is,

$$\hat{\mu}_i = \exp\left(\sum_{m=0}^{K} \hat{\beta}_m C_i^m\right).$$

These plots can help determine an appropriate value of K, identifying outlying observations, and indicate the absence of important predictor variables (cf. Draper and Smith, 1981). Goodness-of-fit assessments also should be conducted to evaluate model adequacy. The simplest goodness-of-fit indicator for this model is a χ^2 statistic:

$$X^2 = \sum_{i=0}^{L} \sum_{j=1}^{n_i} \frac{(Y_{ij} - \hat{\mu}_i)^2}{\hat{\mu}_i},$$

where $\hat{\mu}_i$ is the model-based estimate of μ_i and the sum ranges over all animals and all concentration levels. This statistic is approximately distributed as a χ^2 distribution with $n - K - 1$ degrees of freedom. Other statistical methods have been developed to assess the Poisson dispersion assumption (Dean and Lawless, 1989). Dean and Lawless (1989) suggested a variety of statistics for testing for overdispersion in a Poisson regression context, including

$$T_a = \frac{\sum_{i=0}^{L} \sum_{j=1}^{n_i} [(Y_{ij} - \hat{\mu}_i)^2 - Y_{ij} + \hat{h}_{ii}\hat{\mu}_i]}{\left(2 \sum_{i=0}^{L} \sum_{j=1}^{n_i} \hat{\mu}_i\right)^{1/2}},$$

where $\mathbf{H} = \mathbf{W}^{1/2}\mathbf{X}(\mathbf{X}^T\mathbf{W}\mathbf{X})^{-1}\mathbf{X}^T\mathbf{W}^{1/2}$, $\hat{h}_{ii}$ is the ith diagonal element of $\mathbf{H}$ with

$\hat{\mu}_i$ substituted for μ_i in $\mathbf{W}, \mathbf{W} = \text{diag}(\mu_0, \mu_1, \ldots, \mu_L)$ and $\mathbf{X}$ is an $(L + 1) \times (K + 1)$ matrix with i,jth element $X_{ij} = \mu_i^{-1}(\partial \mu_i / \partial \beta_j)$. A critical value from a standard normal distribution is used for a hypothesis test of overdispersion. This statistic provides a test of extra-Poisson variability. In particular, this test is sensitive to the model $\text{Var}(Y_{ij}) = \mu_i + \tau \mu_i^2$. Both T_a and X^2 were found to be generally good over situations examined by Dean and Lawless (1989).

Potency Estimation

Given an adequately characterized concentration–response relationship, it is possible to determine a reasonable estimate of the concentration required to induce a $100p\%$ level of reproductive inhibition where $0 < p < 1$. The concentration of interest is where the mean total number of offspring is a proportion $1 - p$ of the mean total number of offspring in the control group, which can be represented symbolically as the concentration C such that

$$\mu_C = (1 - p)\mu_0.$$

This implies that

$$
\begin{aligned}
1 - p &= \frac{\mu_C}{\mu_0} \\
&= \frac{\exp(\beta_0 + \beta_1 C + \beta_2 C^2 + \cdots + \beta_K C^K)}{\exp(\beta_0)} \\
&= \exp(\beta_1 C + \beta_2 C^2 + \cdots + \beta_K C^K),
\end{aligned}
$$

so

$$\ln(1 - p) = \beta_1 C + \beta_2 C^2 + \cdots + \beta_K C^K.$$

Thus, to find concentration C that induces an inhibition of $100p\%$, one determines the value of C that satisfies the following equation:

$$\beta_1 C + \beta_2 C^2 + \cdots + \beta_K C^K - \ln(1 - p) = 0. \tag{1}$$

The value of C that induces this specified level of inhibition is the *reproductive inhibition index p* (RIp).

Consider the estimation of the RI50. In other words, what is the estimate of the concentration C such that $\mu_C = 0.5\mu_0$ ($p = 0.5$, so $\ln(1 - p) = \ln(0.5) = -0.693$)? If $K = 0$, then $\hat{\mu}_i = \exp(\hat{\beta}_0)$ and RI50 cannot be determined. If $K = 1$, then $\hat{\mu}_i = \exp(\hat{\beta}_0 + \hat{\beta}_1 C_i)$ is the best-fitting model, and the estimate of the RI50 would be the value of C satisfying

$$\hat{\beta}_1 C + 0.693 = 0$$

or

$$\hat{RI50} = C = \frac{-0.693}{\hat{\beta}_1}.$$

Clearly, the RI50 is not estimated if $\hat{\beta}_1 > 0$, since this would imply that the mean total number of offspring produced is steadily increasing with higher concentrations of the toxin. If $K = 2$, then $\hat{\mu}_i = \exp(\hat{\beta}_0 + \hat{\beta}_1 C_i + \hat{\beta}_2 C_i^2)$ is the best-fitting model and the estimate of the RI50 would be the value of C satisfying

$$\hat{\beta}_2 C^2 + \hat{\beta}_1 C + 0.693 = 0.$$

The estimate of the RI50 is determined using the following roots of this quadratic equation in C:

$$\frac{-\hat{\beta}_1 - [\hat{\beta}_1^2 - 4\hat{\beta}_2(0.693)]^{1/2}}{2\hat{\beta}_2}, \quad \frac{-\hat{\beta}_1 + [\hat{\beta}_1^2 - 4\hat{\beta}_2(0.693)]^{1/2}}{2\hat{\beta}_2}.$$

The estimate of the RI50 is the maximum of the solution to the quadratic equation if the estimate of β_2 is negative. If $\hat{\beta}_2 > 0$ and $\hat{\beta}_1 < 0$, the $\hat{RI50}$ would be the minimum of the two roots of the quadratic equation. The RI50 is not estimated if $\hat{\beta}_2$ and $\hat{\beta}_1$ are both positive, since this would imply that the total number of offspring was increasing with increasing concentrations of the toxicant. If $K > 2$, an estimate of the RI50 can be calculated using Newton's method (see, e.g., Burden et al., 1978) to find the roots of equation (1).

A confidence interval for the RIp potency estimate can readily be obtained using bootstrap resampling techniques (Efron, 1982). These techniques involve repeatedly "sampling" from a discrete distribution defined by the data (Y_{ij}'s). The data from a particular concentration level are viewed as a discrete uniform distribution [i.e., $p_i(Y_{ij}) = \Pr(Y = Y_{ij}) = 1/n_i$ for $j = 1, \ldots, n_i$]. The bootstrap sample for the ith concentration is constructed by sampling with replacement n_i observations from $p_i(\bullet)$. The bootstrap samples for each of the concentration levels represent a "bootstrapping," a regeneration, of the entire experiment. Any arbitrary number of bootstrap experiments can be constructed. A RIp estimate is determined for each of the bootstrapped experiments. Thus an experiment has been "conducted" a number of times (the bootstrap experiments) and a statistic, the RIp estimate, has been calculated for each experiment. This essentially yields an estimate of the sampling distribution of the RIp estimator. Attributes of this sampling distribution, such as an interval of RIp values that occur with a certain probability, could now be considered. After sorting the RIp estimates from the bootstrapped experiments, a $100(1 - \alpha)\%$ nonparametric confidence interval can be constructed by selecting the $100(\alpha/2)$th smallest and largest RIp estimates. As an example, if 100 bootstrap experiments are selected and the associated 100 RIp estimates are calculated, a 90% confidence interval for RIp would be the fifth smallest and fifth largest RIp estimates.

A comparison of bootstrap confidence intervals with likelihood-based intervals is essentially a comparison of a nonparametric technique with a parametric method. Likelihood-based intervals are reliant on correct specification of the probability distribution of responses. Maximum likelihood estimates can be determined using weighted least-squares methods where the weights depend on the specified probability distribution (McCullagh and Nelder, 1989). If the weights are incorrectly specified (e.g., ordinary least-squares estimation used when weighted least squares should be used), the parameter estimators will no longer have minimum variance; however, they are still unbiased and consistent (see, e.g., Neter et al., 1990). Therefore, a confidence interval based on the bootstrap takes advantage of the location properties (unbiasedness) of the estimator without using an estimate of the standard error which could be incorrect.

4 RESULTS

An application of estimating thc RI50 for data from a reproductive toxicity test of nitrofen is presented in this section. Additionally, the variances are clearly not equal to the means (as the Poisson assumption suggests); however, no apparent pattern of overdispersion or underdispersion appears. From previous analyses (Oris et al., 1991), potency estimates of ChV = 194 μg/L and IC50 of 245 μg/L [95% confidence interval of (224, 258) μg/L] were determined.

The Poisson assumption was tested and the data were found to be consistent with this assumption using the test procedures described in Dean and Lawless (1989). The GLIMs with $K = 1$ and $K = 2$ were both fit to these data. A display of the results of these fits is presented in Figure 2. (A GLIM with $K = 3$ was also fit to these data; however, it did not represent a significant improvement over the $K = 2$ fit and is not shown.) The first row of Figure 2 gives the $K = 1$ model fit with the first column presenting a scatterplot of the data with a predicted curve based on the fitted GLIM and the second column presenting a standardized residual plot for this model. (A standardized residual is a residual divided by a standard error; McCullagh and Nelder, 1989.) The second row of this figure gives analogous information for the generalized linear model with $K = 2$.

As Figure 2 suggests, the $K = 1$ model is not adequate for describing these data. The fitted curve clearly does not adequately describe the pattern in the data; indeed, the standardized residual plot exhibits a revealing pattern: a "quadratic" response that suggests use of $K = 2$. Additionally, the X^2 statistic with 48 d.f. was 111.9 (p-value < 0.001), which also indicates model inadequacy.

The $K = 2$ model is a good descriptor for these data. The fitted curve does

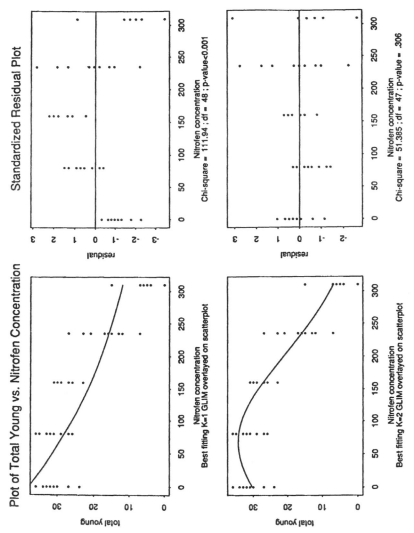

Figure 2. Plots of generalized linear model (GLIM) fits to a *C. dubia* reproductive toxicity test of nitrofen and associated residual plots. Subplots in the first column contain plots of total offspring per female plotted versus measured concentrations of nitrofen (μg/L) overlaid with the best-fitting $K = 1$ GLIM (first row). Subplots in the second column display the standardized residuals for the best-fitting GLIMs ($K = 2$ in the second row) plotted versus measured nitrofen concentration.

describe the observed data, and the standardized residual plot is unpatterned and symmetric about zero. The X^2 statistic with 47 df was 51.4 (p-value = 0.306), which indicates model adequacy. The T_a statistic did not suggest overdispersion (T_a = 1.01, p-value < 0.311 for the two-tailed alternative to τ = 0). The best-fitting K = 2 GLIM was

$$\ln(\hat{Y}_{ij}) = 3.41 + 0.00372C_i - 0.0000275C_i^2,$$

which yields an RI50 of 240 μg/L with an associated 95% confidence interval based on 100 bootstrap samples of (226, 256) μg/L. (A 95% confidence interval based on 1000 bootstrap samples was not different from the interval based on 100 bootstrap samples.) Note that the mean total number of offspring at C = 0 μg/L was 31.4 and at C = 235 μg/L was 17.2. This represents a 45.2% inhibition in reproduction relative to controls, which would suggest that any potency estimate of 50% inhibition should be somewhat larger than 235 μg/L. One would expect the RI50 to be closer to 235 μg/L than 310 μg/L since an average of six total offspring was observed at C = 310 μg/L for reproductive inhibition of over 80%.

5   CONCLUSIONS

This study has considered potency estimation for reproductive aquatic toxicology studies. By using parameter estimates from a Poisson regression model, we obtain a potency estimator of reproductive inhibition that possesses many advantages over current techniques. An attractive feature of this method is that it takes advantage of all the available data and the nature of the concentration–response relationship in its derivation. Additionally, this method allows for the estimation of the concentration associated with any selected level of reproductive inhibition. To use this method, it is assumed that an adequate model fit can be obtained. If the data are highly variable (i.e., depart significantly from a Poisson distribution), it may not be possible to obtain an adequate model. If this were to occur, more complicated statistical models may be needed which explicitly address this overdispersion (Breslow, 1984; Wedderburn, 1974).

SOFTWARE NOTES AND REFERENCES

Computer software to fit the GLIM models described in this chapter is readily available (e.g., the GLIM macro in the NLIN procedure of SAS).

QUESTIONS AND PROBLEMS

1. Under what circumstances would using the bootstrap-based confidence intervals be ill advised?

2. Derive an expression for a large-sample likelihood-based confidence interval for the RIp when $K = 1$. (*Hint:* Use the delta method to obtain an estimate of the variance in terms of the variances and the covariances of the estimators of the β values.)

3. Repeat Question 2 for $K = 2$.

4. If Y_{ijk} is distributed as a Poisson random variable with mean λ_{ik} and $Y_{ij} = Y_{ij1} + Y_{ij2} + Y_{ij3}$, will $E(Y_{ij}) = \text{Var}(V_{ij})$? If not, this suggests that the Y_{ij} can not be Poisson. How does this affect the bootstrap confidence intervals for the RIp?

CHAPTER 3

Prediction Models for Personal Ozone Exposure Assessment

David Wypij and L.-J. Sally Liu

1 MOTIVATION AND BACKGROUND

Millions of Americans are routinely exposed to ozone in the ambient air at levels which are known to cause adverse health effects, including increased incidence of cough, chest pain, or other respiratory symptoms and decrements in lung function (McDonnell et al., 1983; Kulle et al., 1985; Koenig et al., 1987; Lippmann, 1989). While there is a great deal of knowledge about outdoor ozone concentrations, little is known about indoor concentrations and even less about personal exposures. Measurements of personal exposures are important in that estimates based on ambient concentrations alone may result in substantial misclassification of the exposure status of study subjects (Dockery and Spengler, 1981). A small passive ozone sampler recently developed by Koutrakis et al. (1993) has made possible assessment of personal ozone exposures in large field studies. However, this passive sampler has only been tested in controlled chamber conditions, and validation of the sampler in the ambient environment is important.

In this chapter we present results from a pilot study conducted during the summer of 1991 in State College, Pennsylvania, a college town located approximately 240 km east of Pittsburgh. Extensive indoor, outdoor, and personal ozone measurements were collected for 23 children using passive ozone samplers. Detailed time–activity information was also collected for these children. These data were used to validate the new passive ozone sampler and to identify factors that affect personal ozone exposures. The primary goal was to develop multi-

Case Studies in Biometry, Edited by Nicholas Lange, Louise Ryan, Lynne Billard, David Brillinger, Loveday Conquest, and Joel Greenhouse.
ISBN 0-471-58885-7 © 1994 John Wiley & Sons, Inc.

ple regression and time-weighted personal exposure models to predict personal ozone exposures in the children.

The passive ozone sampler, developed by Koutrakis et al. (1993), consists of a badge clip supporting a barrel-shaped device (weight = 7 g, size = 2 cm diameter × 3 cm). The sampler contains two glass-fiber filters coated with potassium carbonate (K_2CO_3) and sodium nitrite ($NaNO_2$). The sampling technique is based on the oxidation reaction of nitrite (NO_2^-) by ozone (O_3) to form nitrate (NO_3^-) and oxygen (O_2). The limit of detection for the passive sampler was 17.5 ppb for 12-hour measurements. The passive ozone sampler was used at indoor and outdoor home sites, at a stationary site, and to measure personal exposures of individual children.

For validation purposes, outdoor ozone concentrations at a stationary site were measured continuously by the U.S. Environmental Protection Agency designated ozone analyzer (weight = 7.26 kg, size = 58 cm × 23 cm × 13 cm). The limit of detection of this method is 2 ppb with a precision of 2 ppb (Thermo-Environmental Instruments Inc., Franklin, Massachusetts).

2 DATA

Ozone concentrations were measured in State College, Pennsylvania, from July 8 through August 27, 1991. Ozone samples were collected on days exhibiting a wide range of ozone concentrations. Indoor, outdoor, and personal samples were collected for 23 children (ages 10 to 11), all living in nonsmoking households in one of six residential regions (Figure 1). Monitoring was conducted at each child's home for up to a six-day period. Up to three children were monitored each period. Regions 1 (downtown), 2, 4, and 5 are densely populated, while regions 3 and 6 are less populated communities, having been only recently developed.

Outdoor ozone concentrations were measured at the State College National Dry Deposition Network site approximately 6 km west of downtown State College. At this stationary site, 12-hour average samples were collected twice daily (8 A.M. to 8 P.M. and 8 P.M. to 8 A.M.) using both passive ozone samplers and continuously using a photometric ambient ozone analyzer. Continuous monitoring also allows collection of 1-hour average measurements. At each home, indoor samples were collected over 12 hours for both daytime (8 A.M. to 8 P.M.) and nighttime (8 P.M. to 8 A.M.) periods using passive samplers. These samplers were placed in the main activity room of the child's home, at least 1 meter away from walls, windows, and air conditioners or other ventilation devices, and 1.2 meters above the floor. Outdoor ozone concentrations were measured using passive samplers placed outside homes, at least 1 meter from walls, trees, or other large objects. Outdoor samples were collected for 24-hour periods beginning at 8 A.M.

Personal exposures were measured during the day (8 A.M. to 8 P.M.) using passive samplers. Samplers were pinned to the strap of a backpack worn by each

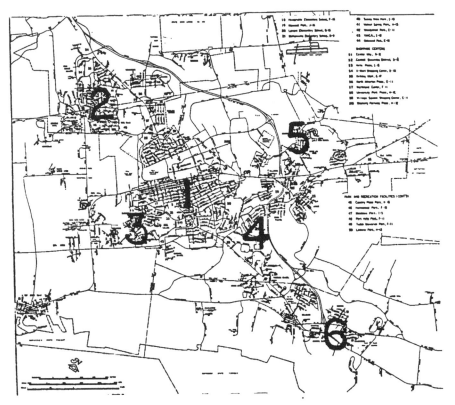

Figure 1. Six geographic regions in State College, PA. Regions 1, 2, 4, and 5 are densely populated, while regions 3 and 6 are less populated.

participant throughout the monitoring period. Each participant also recorded his/her activities in a notebook during daytime monitoring periods. These entries were later aggregated into half-hour periods and were transferred onto formatted time–activity sheets by field technicians.

Before proceeding further, we first establish notation. The response variable is the 12-hour average daytime personal ozone concentration (Y) for participants on different days. The covariate values (X) have the subscript "1" for measured ozone concentrations, "2" for microenvironmental prediction values, or "3" for data extracted from the time–activity diaries. The superscripts are mnemonic, with "D" for daytime, "N" for nighttime, "C" for continuous sampling, "P" for passive sampling, "O" for outdoor, "I" for home indoor, "H" when based on hourly values, and "S" for staying near the home.

A total of 101 passive samples (both day and night) and 301 indoor, outdoor, and personal samples were collected at the stationary and home sites, respectively. Table 1 displays the validation data collected at the stationary ambient monitoring site during the first five days of the study. At this site, 12-hour

Table 1   Validation Data from First Five Days of Observation

Date	X_1^{DC}	X_1^{DP}	X_1^{NC}	X_1^{NP}
7/8/91	47.33	52.82	19.58	17.78
7/9/91	42.58	53.25	9.42	6.06
7/10/91	59.55	56.32	19.83	14.81
7/11/91	52.92	50.06	15.08	9.75
7/12/91	55.25	59.50	28.75	27.21

average daytime and nighttime continuous (X_1^{DC} and X_1^{NC}) and daytime and nighttime passive (X_1^{DP} and X_1^{NP}) samples were collected.

Table 2 displays the personal ozone exposure data from the first two participants in the study, including subject numbers (ranging from 1 to 23), date, and home region (regions 1 to 6). In addition to using the continuous ozone concentrations at the stationary site (X_1^{DC} and X_1^{NC}), exposure data from the home sites consisted of 24-hour average outdoor (X_1^O) and 12-hour average daytime and nighttime indoor (X_1^{DI} and X_1^{NI}) ozone concentrations. Prediction values from a microenvironmental model based on hourly ozone concentrations (X_2^H) are discussed below. Information on fraction of time spent anywhere outdoors (X_3^O), at home indoors (X_3^I), and whether or not the child stayed near the home for the entire day ($X_3^S = 1$ when yes, and 0 when no) was extracted from the time–activity diaries. It is possible to have $X_3^O + X_3^I < 1$ when a child spends a portion of a day in an indoor environment other than their home (e.g., shopping mall, friend's home).

3   METHODS AND MODELS

There were two primary questions of interest in this study. First, did the passive samplers at the stationary site measure the same levels of ozone as the EPA-designated ozone analyzer? The EPA-designated continuous ozone analyzer has high reliability, is calibrated weekly, and serves as the standard with which to compare. To answer this question, Pearson's correlation coefficients and paired t-tests were used to compare the measurements obtained using the passive and continuous ozone monitors. The relative error of the passive sampler measurements was studied using the relative root-mean-square statistic.

The second major goal was to identify factors that affect personal ozone exposures. Could we utilize the different ozone measurements as well as the time–activity information to better predict personal ozone exposures? Personal exposure models were developed using multiple linear regression analyses and time-weighted exposure models. Regression diagnostics were used to examine the aptness of the modeling assumptions.

Table 2 Personal Ozone Monitoring Data from First Two Subjects

Subject No.	Date	Region	Response Variable, Y	X_1^{DC}	X_1^{NC}	X_1^{O}	X_1^{DI}	X_1^{NI}	X_2^{H}	X_3^{O}	X_3^{I}	X_3^{S}
1	7/8/91	2	26.29	47.33	19.58	25.36	22.29	13.51	29.01	0.57	0.43	1
	7/9/91	2	14.63	42.58	9.42	26.74	13.97	10.11	39.33	0.90	0.06	0
	7/10/91	2	21.45	59.55	19.83	33.20	18.96	6.55	32.78	0.55	0.23	0
	7/11/91	2	43.07	52.92	15.08	27.62	—	2.37	32.12	0.46	0.16	0
2	7/9/91	1	11.18	42.58	9.42	—	10.17	0.87	18.75	0.62	0.34	1
	7/10/91	1	3.30	59.55	19.83	22.91	22.27	9.77	25.13	0.17	0.49	0
	7/11/91	1	12.52	52.92	15.08	—	22.20	3.19	23.31	0.10	0.56	0

Demographic Information — Subject No., Date, Region
Measured Ozone Variables — X_1^{DC}, X_1^{NC}, X_1^{O}, X_1^{DI}, X_1^{NI}
Hourly Microenvironmental Model Variable — X_2^{H}
Time-Activity Diary Information — X_3^{O}, X_3^{I}, X_3^{S}

We assume that all observations are independent, even observations from adjacent days or from the same home or individual. Although this may not be completely realistic, the number of observations per subject is relatively small and the within-person correlations are not too large. In other settings adjustment for correlated responses may be required for correct inference.

4 RESULTS

4.1 Validation of the Passive Sampler

Ozone concentrations measured by the continuous and passive monitors at the stationary site are displayed in Figure 2 (overlaid with a 45° line). High correlations between continuous and passive sampling measurements were evident for daytime (Pearson's correlation coefficient $r = 0.73$), nighttime ($r = 0.82$), and combined samples ($r = 0.90$), with $p < 0.001$ for each. Passive monitoring yielded slightly smaller measurements on average (for continuous daytime monitoring, 54.8 ± 15.1 ppb (mean ± standard deviation); passive daytime, 54.1 ± 18.3 ppb; continuous nighttime, 20.0 ± 10.1 ppb; and passive nighttime, 19.1 ± 8.9 ppb). Paired t-tests showed that these differences were not significantly different from zero for daytime ($p = 0.69$), nighttime ($p = 0.21$), or combined samples ($p = 0.37$). The relative error can be studied using the relative root-mean-square statistic, obtained by taking the square root of the mean of the squared differences between the passive and continuous samples (to get a measure of absolute error), then dividing by the mean of the continuous samples (to get a measure of relative error). For daytime comparisons we calculate

$$\frac{[\sum_{j=1}^{n} (X_{1,j}^{DP} - X_{1,j}^{DC})^2 / n]^{1/2}}{\overline{X}_1^{DC}},$$

where $X_{1,j}^{DP}$ is the passive sample for day j, $X_{1,j}^{DC}$ is the continuous sample for day j, $\overline{X}_1^{DC}$ denotes the average of the $X_{1,j}^{DC}$ measurements, and n is the number of measurements, with similar calculations for night or combined samples. The relative errors observed were fairly low (0.23 for daytime, 0.30 for nighttime, and 0.26 for combined samples). The higher relative error for nighttime samples may be due to the low nighttime ozone concentrations.

Overall, the passive sampler appears to perform well compared to the continuous sampler at the stationary site. A few observations far from the 45° line in Figure 2 indicate excessive variability or possibly laboratory errors in the passive sampler measurements. Assessment of possible outliers and how they affect inferences is left as an exercise.

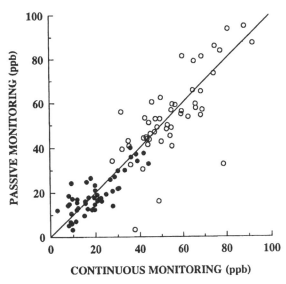

Figure 2. Passive vs. continuous ozone measurements at the stationary site, overlaid with a 45° line. Open circles denote 12-hour daytime values, filled circles denote 12-hour nighttime values.

4.2   Prediction Models for Personal Exposure

Comparisons were made between indoor and outdoor daytime concentrations and the personal ozone monitoring. Since 12-hour average passive outdoor home measurements were not made, average daytime outdoor home concentrations (denoted by X_1^{DO}) were estimated for each home and day by

$$X_1^{DO} = X_1^O \cdot \frac{X_1^{DC}}{(X_1^{DC} + X_1^{NC})/2},$$

multiplying the 24-hour average outdoor home concentration by a proportion equal to the average 12-hour daytime concentration of ozone exposure at the stationary site divided by the average 24-hour concentration of ozone exposure at the stationary site. Personal ozone exposures, Y, were highly correlated with both indoor exposures, X_1^{DI}, ($r = 0.55, p < 0.001$), and outdoor exposures, X_1^{DO} ($r = 0.37, p = 0.002$). Personal exposures were significantly lower than the corresponding outdoor concentrations (mean difference = -20.9 ± 21.4 ppb, $p < 0.001$ using a paired t-test), but higher than indoor concentrations (mean difference = 4.1 ± 14.0 ppb, $p = 0.011$).

Model-Building Results
To set notation, consider the general multiple linear regression model, which permits the mean of the response variable to depend on one or more covari-

ate values. Suppose that the data collected are $(X_1, Y_1), (X_2, Y_2), \ldots, (X_n, Y_n)$ where Y_i is the scalar response from the ith observation and $X_i = (X_{i1}, \ldots, X_{i,p-1})$ is the collection of variables that are thought to affect the ith response. Thus, there are n observations and p parameters (including an intercept) in the regression model. In particular, we assume that

$$Y_i = \beta_0 + \beta_1 X_{i1} + \cdots + \beta_{p-1} X_{i,p-1} + e_i; \qquad i = 1, \ldots, n,$$

where the error terms e_i are assumed to be independent and identically distributed from a normal distribution with mean 0 and common (unknown) variance σ^2. Using maximum likelihood or least squares to estimate $\beta = (\beta_0, \beta_1, \ldots, \beta_{p-1})^T$ gives

$$\hat{\beta} = (\mathbf{X}^T \mathbf{X})^{-1} (\mathbf{X}^T Y),$$

where Y is the $n \times 1$ vector of responses and $\mathbf{X}$ is the $n \times p$ matrix of covariates (including a column of ones for the intercept term). An unbiased estimate of σ^2 is

$$\hat{\sigma}^2 = \frac{1}{n-p} \sum_{i=1}^{n} \hat{e}_i^2$$

(sometimes denoted by MSE for mean squared error), where

$$\hat{e}_i = Y_i - \hat{Y}_i$$

is the residual for the ith observation and

$$\hat{Y}_i = \hat{\beta}_0 + \hat{\beta}_1 X_{i1} + \cdots + \hat{\beta}_{p-1} X_{i,p-1}$$

is the fitted value for the ith observation. The covariance matrix for the $\hat{\beta}$ vector, estimated by

$$\hat{\text{Var}}(\hat{\beta}) = \hat{\sigma}^2 (\mathbf{X}^T \mathbf{X})^{-1},$$

is used to construct confidence intervals and hypothesis tests about the β coefficients.

Two types of models to predict personal exposure were developed. First, stepwise regression techniques and model building were used to determine the relative influences of home indoor and outdoor concentrations and time–activity patterns on personal exposures. For these models, the measured indoor concentrations (X_1^{DI}), estimated outdoor concentrations (X_1^{DO}), the fraction of time spent outdoors (X_3^O), and the interaction terms, $X_1^{DO} \cdot X_3^O$ and $X_1^{DI} \cdot (1 - X_3^O)$, were used to predict personal ozone exposures (Y).

Stepwise variable selection techniques suggest that indoor ozone concentrations (X_1^{DI}) are the most significant predictor of personal exposures (model 1, Table 3). This is not surprising given the strong association between these variables ($r = 0.55, p < 0.001$). The interaction term $X_1^{DO} \cdot X_3^O$ was the only other important predictor variable (model 2, Table 3), suggesting that outdoor ozone concentrations are predictive only when weighted by the fraction of time spent outdoors. Model 2 explained 32.2% of the variability in personal exposures and had a slightly smaller root MSE than model 1.

Several different variable selection techniques were tried for this analysis, including forward stepwise and backward elimination procedures based on F statistics for a variable's contribution to the model if it is included and procedures based on maximizing the adjusted R^2 statistic (or equivalently, minimizing the MSE). It is interesting that for this problem, each of these procedures leads to the same final model 2. In practice, using different variable selection criteria can often lead to different final models. Draper and Smith (1981) and Neter et al. (1990) describe methods for model building and variable selection in greater detail.

Table 3   Regression Models for Predicting Personal Ozone Exposures

Model	Sample Size	Covariates	$\hat{\beta}$	se	p-Value	Root MSE	Adjusted R^2
		Stepwise Regression Models					
1	64	Intercept	9.93	3.23	0.003	13.3	0.269
		X_1^{DI}	0.69	0.14	<0.001		
2	64	Intercept	6.94	3.35	0.042	12.8	0.322
		X_1^{DI}	0.61	0.14	<0.001		
		$X_1^{DO} * X_3^O$	0.34	0.14	0.019		
3	63	Intercept	7.00	3.26	0.036	12.4	0.329
		X_1^{DI}	0.67	0.14	<0.001		
		$X_1^{DO} * X_3^O$	0.22	0.15	0.145		
		Microenvironmental Models					
4	64	Intercept	7.18	3.53	0.046	13.0	0.295
		X_2^D	0.60	0.11	<0.001		
5	80	Intercept	4.85	3.03	0.114	12.7	0.379
		X_2^H	0.70	0.10	<0.001		
6	14	Intercept	−4.22	4.27	0.342	6.4	0.744
		X_2^H	1.05	0.17	<0.001		

Regression Diagnostics

A variety of refined diagnostics for checking the adequacy of a regression model have been formulated. These diagnostics can be used to detect outliers in the covariate or response variables, observations that are overly influential on the estimated regression coefficients, and departures from the normality assumption on the errors. Studentized deleted residuals, leverages, Cook's distances, and a normal probability plot for model 2 are displayed in Figure 3.

Studentized deleted residuals (sometimes called externally studentized residuals) are used to diagnose outlying or extreme response values. If the assump-

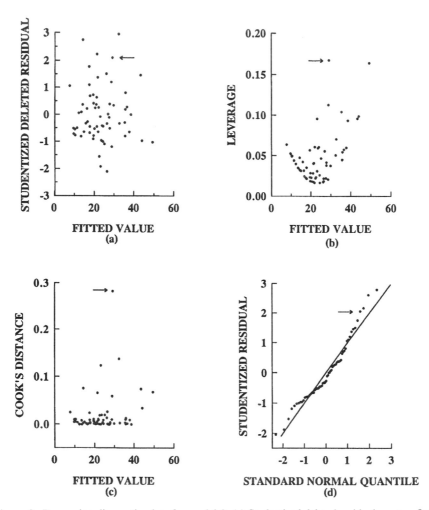

Figure 3. Regression diagnostic plots for model 2. (a) Studentized deleted residuals versus fitted values, (b) leverages versus fitted values, (c) Cook's distances versus fitted values, and (d) studentized residuals versus standard normal quantiles. The observation marked in each plot is from subject 7 on 7/22/91.

tions for the multiple linear regression model hold true, the studentized residuals, given by

$$\hat{e}_i^* = \frac{\hat{e}_i}{[\hat{\sigma}^2(1 - h_{ii})]^{1/2}},$$

should have common variance. Here h_{ii} refers to the ith diagonal element of the hat matrix,

$$\mathbf{H} = \mathbf{X}(\mathbf{X}^T\mathbf{X})^{-1}\mathbf{X}^T.$$

Deleted residuals refers to measuring the ith residual when the fitted regression is based on the cases excluding the ith one, which may be advantageous when assessing the influence of the ith case. The studentized deleted residuals are given by

$$\hat{d}_i^* = \frac{\hat{e}_i}{[\hat{\sigma}_{(i)}^2(1 - h_{ii})]^{1/2}},$$

where $\hat{\sigma}_{(i)}^2$ is the MSE when the ith case is deleted in fitting the regression function. Although they are not independent, studentized deleted residuals follow a t distribution with $n - p - 1$ degrees of freedom. Thus, observations with studentized deleted residuals of large absolute value are outliers in the response space. From Figure 3a, we see that a few observations have large studentized deleted residuals, with observed values much higher than predicted. Residual plots can also be used to assess graphically the nonlinearity of the regression function (by plotting residuals versus covariates included in the model), to help decide whether to add a variable to the model (by plotting residuals versus possible covariates to include in the model), to assess constancy of variance, and to look for nonindependence of error terms (by plotting residuals versus a time sequence).

Hat matrix leverages h_{ii} provide a useful indicator in the multivariate regression setting of whether or not an individual observation is outlying with respect to its covariate values. Observations with large leverages exercise substantial influence in determining the fitted value for that particular observation. It can be shown that the leverages always fall between 0 and 1 and sum to p, so it follows that the average leverage value is p/n. Often, leverages greater than $2p/n$ are considered to be outlying cases in terms of their covariates. For model 2, $n = 64$ and $p = 3$, so $2p/n = 0.094$. Several observations have leverage values near this cutoff in Figure 3b, and two observations have particularly high leverage.

Cook's distance provides an overall measure of the combined impact of an observation on all of the estimated regression coefficients. Cook's distance is calculated by

$$\hat{D}_i = \frac{1}{p\hat{\sigma}^2} [\hat{\boldsymbol{\beta}} - \hat{\boldsymbol{\beta}}_{(i)}]^T X^T X [\hat{\boldsymbol{\beta}} - \hat{\boldsymbol{\beta}}_{(i)}],$$

where $\hat{\boldsymbol{\beta}}_{(i)}$ is the estimated regression coefficient vector obtained when the ith case is deleted. One observation (from subject 7 on 7/22//91) appeared particularly influential on the regression coefficients in Figure 3c. This observation, which also had a relatively large studentized deleted residual and large leverage, is marked in each of the diagnostic plots.

Studentized residuals can also be used to assess the normality assumption of the error terms. Here each residual is plotted against its expected value when the distribution is normal (the normal quantiles). A good approximation to the expected value of the ith smallest observation in a random sample of size n of a standard normal random variable is

$$\Phi^{-1} \left[\frac{i - 0.375}{n + 0.25} \right].$$

A normal probability plot that is nearly linear suggests agreement with normality. A few observations lie away from the line in Figure 3d, suggesting that some observations have larger than expected studentized deleted residuals. A χ^2 goodness-of-fit test or the Kolmogorov–Smirnov test could be used to test the normality assumption formally.

Deleting the single observation with overly large influence on the regression coefficients yields a better-fitting model (model 3, Table 3), but with reduced significance of the $X_1^{DO} * X_3^{O}$ coefficient. Thus, our inferences depend on whether or not this observation is included. Looking back through the records, there was no reason to suspect that this observation was anamolous in any way. Careful attention must be paid to this and other potentially influential observations, as it is difficult to justify deleting observations that do not fit well unless they can be shown to be the result of a gross measurement error.

Other regression diagnostics can be used to assess influence on individual regression coefficients, the covariance matrix of the estimated coefficients, and the fitted values. Belsley et al. (1980), Cook and Weisberg (1982), and Neter et al. (1990) discuss regression and influence diagnostics, multicollinearity, and heteroscedasticity in greater detail. Remedial measures include the deletion of particular observations, data transformations, the use of weighted least squares, and ridge regression.

Microenvironmental Exposure Models
The models resulting above do not have an intuitive interpretation, so a second type of model was constructed utilizing the simple microenvironmental

exposure concept (Duan, 1982). A reasonable prediction of daytime personal exposure would be

$$X_2^D = X_1^{DO} \cdot X_3^O + X_1^{DI} \cdot (1 - X_3^O),$$

the time-weighted average of the outdoor and indoor exposures. The linear regression model incorporating an intercept term together with the calculated X_2^D predictor variable is summarized as model 4, Table 3. This model has a similar fit to that of the single-variable model 1. A simplified model using the X_2^D variable as our prediction of personal exposure would require the intercept to be zero and the slope to be 1. The F-test of the composite null hypothesis that the X_2^D slope is 1 and the intercept is zero has a p-value <0.001, enough evidence to reject this hypothesis. This simplified microenvironmental model has root MSE = 14.5 and does not fit as well.

Since ozone concentrations exhibit a distinct diurnal pattern (i.e., concentrations vary systematically over the day), when an individual spends time outdoors may be an important predictor of personal exposures. To incorporate hourly variation into the time-weighted model, concentration and activity data were divided into 1-hour intervals. Hourly average outdoor concentrations were estimated for each home using

$$X_1^O(k) = \frac{X_1^O \cdot X_1^{DC}(k)}{(X_1^{DC} + X_1^{NC})/2},$$

where $X_1^{DC}(k)$ denotes the 1-hour average continuous outdoor ozone concentration measured at the stationary site during hour k. Similarly, hourly average indoor concentrations were estimated by

$$X_1^{DI}(k) = \frac{X_1^O(k) \cdot (X_1^{DI})}{X_1^{DO}},$$

multiplying the 1-hour average outdoor ozone concentration by the ratio of indoor to outdoor ozone concentrations at the home site. The microenvironmental prediction for personal exposure based on hourly information is then

$$X_2^H = \frac{1}{12} \sum_{k=1}^{12} [X_1^{DI}(k) \cdot X_3^I(k) + X_1^O(k) \cdot X_3^O(k)],$$

where $X_3^I(k)$ and $X_3^O(k)$ are the fraction of time spent indoors and outdoors in the kth hour, respectively. This variable is included in the data set.

The model incorporating an intercept and the X_2^H predictor variable is summarized as model 5, Table 3. This hourly microenvironmental model explained a higher percentage of the variability in personal exposures and had a smaller root MSE than the simpler microenvironmental model using X_2^D. An F-test rejects the composite null hypothesis that the X_2^H slope is 1 and the intercept is zero with $p = 0.001$.

Further improvements to the accuracy of the hourly microenvironmental model could be achieved by accounting for the contribution of diverse outdoor and indoor environments to personal ozone exposures. Support for this is given by noting that model 5 predicted values were more accurate for participants who stayed at or near their home at least 95% of the day (so having $X_3^S = 1$) than for those who did not (Figure 4). Fitting the analogue of model 5 only to the 14 observations from participants who stayed at or near their home at least 95% of the day resulted in explaining 74.4% of the variability in personal ozone exposures (model 6, Table 3), a substantial improvement. A more complete analysis of these data would incorporate additional regression diagnostics and assessment of outlying or inaccurate covariate values.

5   CONCLUSIONS

Our results showed that the new passive sampler measurements gave quite consistent readings as compared to the continuous monitor. A few passive sampler measurements were relatively far from the corresponding continuous monitor

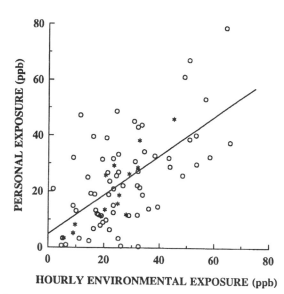

Figure 4. Personal ozone exposures versus hourly microenvironmental model predictions, overlaid with the fitted regression line (model 5). Observations from subjects who stayed at or near their home at least 95% of the time are plotted with asterisks.

measurement, suggesting some excessive variability in the passive sampling measurements. With more experience with the passive sampler, the laboratory may analyze the passive monitoring more accurately.

Personal exposures were correlated with both home outdoor and indoor measurements. The ability to predict personal exposures from outdoor and indoor measurements was relatively poor, however, even when daytime time-weighted concentrations were used. The accuracy of the predictions was improved somewhat when considering hourly time-weighted concentrations. The inability of the microenvironmental models to estimate personal exposures may result from the consideration of only two environments, indoor home and outdoor home. Ozone concentrations from these microenvironments may not accurately represent the ozone concentrations of other indoor and outdoor microenvironments. When analyses were restricted to observations from children who stayed near their home, the accuracy of the hourly microenvironmental model improved substantially. Contributions from diverse microenvironments must be considered in order to estimate personal ozone exposures accurately, as using passive samplers for each child can be prohibitively expensive in a large epidemiologic study. Needless to say, to be effective, good model building is a team effort that requires both statistical sophistication and scientific insight into the plausible effects of the variables under study.

Liu et al. (1993) give more details and present further analyses of a modified version of these data, including study of diurnal (day versus night) and temporal variations in the data. They study spatial variations in ozone concentrations among the six residential regions and the stationary monitoring site. Compared to rural or wooded areas, nitric oxide (NO) concentrations have been shown to be higher near residential areas, due to increased auto exhausts and other NO sources. Thus, more NO may be available to react with and remove ozone in residential environments, resulting in lower ozone concentrations near homes. Yet many health studies use stationary ozone monitoring sites, and assume that all subjects are effectively exposed to the same level of ozone exposure. Liu et al. (1993) also characterize the distribution of the effective ozone penetration rates, expressed as the mean ratio of indoor to outdoor ozone concentrations.

ACKNOWLEDGMENTS

This work was supported by U.S. EPA Cooperative Agreement CR816 740-02 and by Electric Power Research Institute Contract RP 1630-59. The authors acknowledge the helpful assistance received from Petros Koutrakis, Helen H. Suh, and J. Michael Wolfson of the Harvard School of Public Health.

QUESTIONS AND PROBLEMS

1. Continuous ozone monitoring is very reliable, but it is possible that there are laboratory errors in the new passive sampling measurements. Describe meth-

ods for detecting outliers in the validation study, and recalculate the validation measures after any outlying measurements have been deleted. Discuss your inferences.

2. Compare ozone measurements from the stationary site to those from the six residential regions, and the outdoor home sites or residential regions among each other. How can you quantify the spatial variation? Should differences or ratios in the measurements be used to quantify the variation?

3. Since indoor ozone originates mainly from outdoor sources, the indoor/outdoor ozone ratio can be viewed as the effective penetration rate of ozone from outdoor to indoor environments. Compare the effective penetration rates among the 23 homes.

4. Carry out a detailed regression analysis of the personal exposure measurements using all available covariate information. Discuss your inferences.

5. Study the effect of measurement errors in the covariates on the resulting regression inferences.

PART II

Forestry, Fisheries, Genetics

CHAPTER 4

Measurement Error Models for Gypsy Moth Studies

John P. Buonaccorsi

1   MOTIVATION AND BACKGROUND

In many regression problems, particularly those arising in ecological studies, one must deal with the presence of large measurement errors in some of the variables. Such errors often arise in ecological settings because the problem of interest involves variables which are impossible to measure exactly due to time and cost constraints. Often there are spatial units, and estimates of the variables of interest are obtained via some sampling scheme on the units. As in the examples treated here, this often involves some method of sampling subunits within the main unit. In addition, the variance in the measurement error changes with the quantity being estimated in many of these problems.

Despite their increasing use, measurement error/errors-in-variables techniques in regression problems are still greatly underutilized in many disciplines. There are a number of reasons for this. One is the lack of exposure in the applied books used by many researchers and statisticians. The coverage is often brief, if treated at all, and the models treated too simple to apply in many contexts. The exception to this is the seminal work of Fuller (1987). This book is wide ranging in its coverage and has many interesting examples but is a bit theoretical for many applied statisticians and practitioners. An additional hindrance is the lack of computing routines in any of the major statistical packages.

In this chapter we illustrate some of the available methods when accounting for measurement error in simple linear regression where replicate subsamples are available on each unit and the measurement error variability is allowed to change across units. The data come from two studies involving gypsy moth egg

Case Studies in Biometry, Edited by Nicholas Lange, Louise Ryan, Lynne Billard, David Brillinger, Loveday Conquest, and Joel Greenhouse.
ISBN 0-471-58885-7 © 1994 John Wiley & Sons, Inc.

mass densities and their relationship to other variables. Although the illustrations are through ecological problems, the methodology is readily applicable to many disciplines where similar data occur.

2 DATA

Two different data sets will be analyzed which are related by the fact that both contain the density of gypsy moth egg masses as one of the variables. Together they illustrate a variety of different issues which can arise when applying measurement error methodology. Knowledge of gypsy moth egg mass densities is important because it determines subsequent damage as the insects emerge to destructive stages. However, the estimation of egg mass densities via traditional sampling methods (selecting certain areas and counting all egg masses on those areas) is very time consuming and often prohibitive. The first data set involves assessment of an easier method to estimate egg mass densities while the second is concerned with the relationship between egg mass densities and defoliation.

2.1 Burlap Data

This data set comes from a study which investigates various issues concerning gypsy moths, directed by J. Elkinton at the University of Massachusetts at Amherst. For this part of the data, the objective was to see how well counts of gypsy moth egg masses found under burlap bands on trees can be used to predict the egg mass density for a larger area. The data involve 11 different wooded stands, each 9 ha in size, located in Massachusetts and Maryland. Data were collected over a six-year period, but each stand does not have data for all years. On each stand there is a 7 by 7 grid of 49 circular subplots each 0.0177 ha in size. Egg mass densities were estimated on 21 of these subplots. A complete count of egg masses was not obtained for each of the 21 subplots but rather, involved a combination of ground counts and further subsampling of trees within the subplot using a prism point method (Wilson and Fontaine, 1978). The result is an estimated egg mass density on each subplot. On 12 other subplots the 25 trees nearest the center of the plot were banded and counts of egg masses recorded under the bands.

The data are presented in Table 1, with each record corresponding to a stand in a particular year. Given is the mean burlap count (averaged over 12 subplots), the mean egg mass density per acre (averaged over 21 subplots) and the standard error for the mean egg mass density computed by treating the 21 subplot values as a random sample. As discussed in Section 3, the standard error squared is used as an estimate of the measurement error variance for true egg mass density.

Table 1   Burlap Data

Mean Burlap	Mean Egg	$\hat{s}e(eg)^a$	Mean Burlap	Mean Egg	$\hat{s}e(egg)^a$
7.0833	13.0000	7.6000	0.3333	9.5000	9.5200
22.2500	3545.7000	455.2500	2.3333	0.0000	0.0000
0.4167	8.5000	5.8300	2.0000	1.4000	1.4200
9.0000	0.0000	0.0000	24.9167	60.8000	25.4700
11.6667	1290.3000	584.4400	22.0833	820.0000	268.6400
0.5833	14.8000	10.3400	46.9167	197.5000	46.9800
0.0000	3.0000	2.1300	9.4167	182.1000	44.8000
0.0000	0.0000	0.0000	0.0000	0.0000	0.0000
0.0000	0.3000	0.2900	8.1667	302.6000	97.5200
6.5833	986.9000	210.0400	13.3333	1472.4000	216.0900
12.6667	313.2000	72.6000	0.0000	0.0000	0.0000
0.0833	0.0000	0.0000	0.0000	0.2000	0.1800
0.2222	0.0000	0.0000	4.8333	93.8000	52.4000
3.9167	0.0000	0.0000	0.0833	0.0000	0.0000
0.3333	0.0000	0.0000	0.8333	0.0000	0.0000
1.0000	0.0000	0.0000	2.0000	9.5000	9.5200
0.4167	3.4000	2.6500	6.7500	17.4000	12.9800
11.1667	127.6000	68.1600	1.9167	4.3000	2.8300
0.3846	42.5000	25.8900	3.9167	25.0000	11.5100
0.0000	4.0000	3.9500	0.0000	0.4000	0.4200
84.0000	2095.6001	281.9500	38.5833	4430.5000	1318.7800
19.6667	202.4000	99.3800	0.0000	0.4000	0.4200
144.5000	5908.7998	694.1500	38.8462	2196.8000	706.7000
1.5833	20.0000	5.6600	0.0000	0.0000	0.0000
34.1667	690.5000	163.6700	118.1538	3561.8000	1042.9500
0.5000	3.2000	1.5800			

$^a\hat{s}e(egg)$ is the estimated standard error of mean egg mass density.

The standard error clearly increases with the egg mass density and can be quite large at high densities. A plot of the mean values appears in Figure 1 with further details and analysis following in Section 4.

2.2   Defoliation Data

The second data set is one piece of a U.S. Department of Agriculture (USDA) Forest Service study investigating the relationship between gypsy moth egg mass densities and subsequent defoliation. Table 2 shows values arising from sampling six stands/units in the George Washington National Forest in 1988, each stand being 60 ha in size. Twenty circular subunits, 0.1 ha in size were sampled systematically within each stand. On each of these subunits an estimate of the egg mass densities was obtained in a manner similar to that used in the burlap data. Subsequently, on the same 20 subunits, a measure of defoliation,

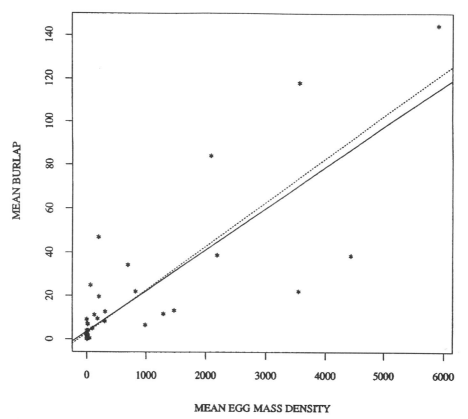

Figure 1. Plot of mean burlap versus mean egg mass density for the burlap data with fitted lines from least squares (——) and unweighted measurement error analysis (- - - -).

expressed as a percentage, was obtained. For each unit, Table 2 gives the means and standard errors for each variable and the estimated covariance between the two means, obtained by treating the 20 replicate values within the unit as a random sample. A scatterplot of the means appears in Figure 2.

There are some difficult applied issues surrounding the defoliation measure which are not completely addressed here. Defoliation is difficult to measure. The values used are subjective measures of percent defoliation formed visually on each subunit. Using the mean over the subunits to estimate the mean defoliation for the unit is only suitable when the potential area to be defoliated is relatively constant across subunits. If not, some sort of weighted average is needed. The methods applied here use the mean; however, the methods can easily be adapted to handle weighted averages. This would require different expressions than those given in Section 3.2.

Table 2   Defoliation Data[a]

Mean Def.	ŝe(def)	Mean Egg	ŝe(egg)	Ĉov(def, egg)
45.5	6.13	69.5	12.47	13.20
100	0	116.3	28.28	0
25	2.67	13.85	3.64	1.64
97.5	1.23	104.95	19.54	0.7566
48	2.77	39.45	7.95	−2.74
83.5	4.66	29.6	6.47	12.23

[a]Mean Def., mean defoliation; ŝe(def), estimated standard error of mean defoliation; Mean Egg, mean egg mass density; ŝe(egg), estimated standard error of mean egg mass density; Ĉov(def, egg), estimated covariance among mean defoliation and egg values.

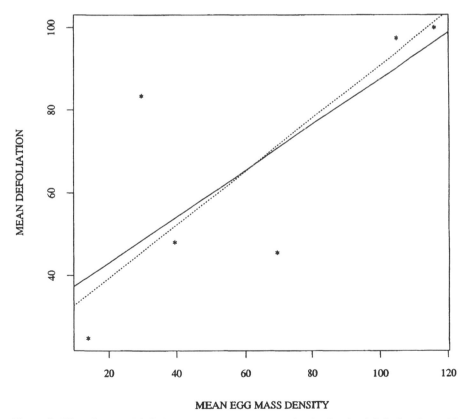

Figure 2. Plot of mean defoliation versus mean egg mass density for the defoliation data with fitted lines from least squares (——) and unweighted measurement error analysis (- - - -).

3   METHODS AND MODELS

3.1   Regression Model for True Values

Let y_i and x_i denote the true values of the variables of interest for the ith unit in the sample. The main concern is with the standard simple linear regression model in terms of the true values

$$y_i = \beta_0 + \beta_1 x_i + \epsilon_i, \qquad i = 1, \ldots, n, \tag{1}$$

where the ϵ_i are assumed independent and identically distributed with mean 0 and constant variance σ^2. The term ϵ_i is referred to as the *error in the equation.*

It is often important to distinguish between cases where the x_i's are fixed values, the *functional* case, or the x_i's are random, the *structural* case. This distinction is often downplayed in regression problems without measurement error since the resulting analysis for the regression coefficients is the same under appropriate assumptions, although the meaning of the model changes. In measurement error problems the difference can be more important. Except where mentioned otherwise in part of the defoliation analysis, the x's are treated as fixed.

3.2   Measurement Error Models

The observed values on the ith unit are denoted by Y_i and X_i, for which it is assumed that

$$Y_i = y_i + w_i \qquad \text{and} \qquad X_i = x_i + u_i. \tag{2}$$

Thus, w_i is the measurement error in Y_i as an estimate of y_i and similarly, u_i is the measurement error in X_i as an estimate of x_i. The measurement errors are assumed to have the following properties:

$$E(u_i) = 0, \qquad \text{Var}(u_i) = \sigma_{ui}^2, \qquad E(w_i) = 0,$$
$$\text{Var}(w_i) = \sigma_{wi}^2, \qquad \text{and} \qquad \text{Cov}(u_i, w_i) = \sigma_{uwi}, \tag{3}$$

where E denotes expected value, Var denotes variance, and Cov denotes covariance. It is also assumed that the measurement errors are independent across units and that all measurement errors are uncorrelated with errors in (1). These are reasonable assumptions with preset subsampling schemes carried out independently within each unit.

Either of the variables may be observed exactly, in which case the appropriate measurement error is set to 0, as are the corresponding variance and the covariance. In the burlap example the dependent variable will be the observed mean burlap count, which does not involve measurement error. In this case, $Y_i = y_i$ so $w_i = 0$, $\sigma_{wi}^2 = 0$ and $\sigma_{uwi} = 0$, $i = 1, \ldots, n$.

Equation (3) says that the observed values are unbiased estimates for the true values and that the variances and covariance can change over i. The latter fact is a key feature of the model. In correcting for measurement error, estimates of the measurement error variances and covariances are needed. These will be denoted by $\hat{\sigma}_{ui}^2$, $\hat{\sigma}_{wi}^2$ and $\hat{\sigma}_{uwi}$, respectively.

In problems with subsampling, the X_i and Y_i values are unbiased estimates for the true values on the ith unit, and the subsampling scheme will determine the measurement error variances and how they are estimated. This allows for a wide variety of subsampling techniques. For the examples here a unit is a stand and there are n_i subsamples within unit i with values $X_{i1}, \ldots, X_{in_i}$ and/or $Y_{i1}, \ldots, Y_{in_i}$, depending on which variables are measured with error. When there is measurement error in both variables, the X's and Y's will be paired. On the ith unit, the estimates of the true values are the means

$$X_i = \sum_{j=1}^{n_i} \frac{X_{ij}}{n_i} \quad \text{and} \quad Y_i = \sum_{j=1}^{n_i} \frac{Y_{ij}}{n_i}.$$

With simple random sampling or systematic sampling within the unit, this produces unbiased estimates of the true values. However, with systematic sampling within the unit, as is done in both examples, one cannot effectively estimate the variance of X_i or Y_i. As an approximation, assume that the replicates arise from a simple random sample of size n_i from a collection of N_i subunits. Cochran (1977, p. 212) has some discussion which indicates that this approach would be reasonable if the area within a stand is relatively homogeneous. Assuming simple random sampling, we have

$$\sigma_{ui}^2 = \frac{f_i \tau_{ui}^2}{n_i}, \qquad \sigma_{wi}^2 = \frac{f_i \tau_{wi}^2}{n_i}, \qquad \text{and} \qquad \sigma_{uwi} = \frac{f_i \tau_{uwi}}{n_i},$$

where τ_{ui}^2, τ_{wi}^2 and τ_{uui} represent, respectively, the among subunit variation in X values, the among-subunit variation in Y values, and the among-subunit covariance among X and Y values on unit i. The quantity $f_i = 1 - (n_i/N_i)$ is the finite population correction factor (Cochran, 1977). In the burlap example f is approximately 0.96, and in the defoliation example approximately 0.99. The correction factor is ignored in the computations.

The estimated measurement error variances and covariance are

$$\hat{\sigma}_{ui}^2 = \frac{f_i s_{ui}^2}{n_i}, \qquad \hat{\sigma}_{wi}^2 = \frac{f_i s_{wi}^2}{n_i}, \qquad \text{and} \qquad \hat{\sigma}_{uwi} = \frac{f_i s_{uwi}}{n_i},$$

where

$$s_{ui}^2 = \sum_{j=1}^{n_i} \frac{(X_{ij} - X_i)^2}{n_i - 1},$$

$$s_{wi}^2 = \sum_{j=1}^{n_i} \frac{(Y_{ij} - Y_i)^2}{n_i - 1},$$

and

$$s_{uwi} = \sum_{j=1}^{n_i} \frac{(X_{ij} - X_i)(Y_{ij} - Y_i)}{n_i - 1}$$

are the among-unit sample variances and sample covariance on unit i. The square roots of the estimated variances are the standard errors which appear in Tables 1 and 2.

The formulas above ignore any further subsampling within a subplot as arises in both data sets when measuring egg mass density (through the selection of trees with the prism point method). This works here since the number of sub-units is a small fraction of the possible subunits (see Cochran, 1977, p. 279). If this were not the case, additional terms in the variance expressions are needed to account for the lower level of subsampling.

3.3   Estimation

Approximate inferences are obtained by applying the methods of Fuller (1987, Section 3.1). The results there are given in matrix forms designed to handle general multiple regression. While the general expressions will not be reproduced here, some simplified expressions are given for the simple linear regression setting. Define the sample covariance of X and Y and the sample variance of X as

$$S_{XY} = \frac{\sum_{i=1}^{n} (X_i - \overline{X})(Y_i - \overline{Y})}{n - 1} \quad \text{and} \quad S_{XX} = \frac{\sum_{i=1}^{n} (X_i - \overline{X})^2}{n - 1},$$

where $\overline{X} = \sum_{i=1}^{n} X_i/n$ and $\overline{Y}$ is similarly defined. With no measurement error, the usual least-squares estimate of the slope is S_{XY}/S_{XX}.

There are two methods of obtaining estimated coefficients which correct for measurement error, an unweighted and a weighted version, both of which are special cases of equation (3.1.6) of Fuller. Fuller also gives an α-modification, which will not be discussed here. The unweighted estimator for the slope result-ing from equation (3.1.19) in Fuller can be rewritten as

$$\frac{S_{XY} - [\sum_{i=1}^{n} \hat{\sigma}_{uwi}/(n-1)]}{S_{XX} - \sum_{i=1}^{n} \hat{\sigma}_{ui}^2/(n-1)}.$$

A slightly modified version is used here with

$$\hat{\beta}_1 = \frac{S_{XY} - \sum_{i=1}^{n} \hat{\sigma}_{uwi}/n}{S_{XX} - \sum_{i=1}^{n} \hat{\sigma}_{ui}^2/n}. \tag{4}$$

One reason for the modification is that in the case of constant measurement error variances and covariance, it yields the "usual" measurement error estimators [e.g., equations (2.2.12) and (1.2.3) in Fuller]. Also, the modified version is such that the expected value of the numerator of (4) is $\beta_1 S_{xx}$ and of the denominator is S_{xx} where S_{xx} is the among-x variability defined appropriately for x's fixed or random. Note though that this does not mean that $\hat{\beta}_1$ is unbiased for β_1. (For those interested, in general the modifications used here can be described in terms of equation (3.1.6) of Fuller by replacing $\hat{\Sigma}_{aatt}$ by $[(n-1)/n]\hat{\Sigma}_{aatt}$.) This modification does not affect the asymptotic properties. For reasonably large n and/or where the measurement error variances are small relative to S_{xx}, it will not matter much which form is used. This raises the unanswered question as to what is the best thing to do with small sample sizes. The results are based on asymptotic properties which are not altered by interchanging n and $n-1$, or even $n-2$, which enters in some places.

The unweighted estimator of the intercept is $\hat{\beta}_0 = \overline{Y} - \hat{\beta}_1 \overline{X}$ and an estimate of σ^2 from equation (3.1.22) in Fuller is

$$\hat{\sigma}^2 = \sum_{i=1}^{n} \frac{r_i^2}{n-2} - \sum_{i=1}^{n} \frac{\hat{\sigma}_{wi}^2 + \hat{\beta}_1^2 \hat{\sigma}_{ui}^2 - 2\hat{\beta}_1 \hat{\sigma}_{uwi}}{n},$$

where $r_i = Y_i - (\hat{\beta}_0 + \hat{\beta}_1 X_i)$.

Weighted estimators are obtained from equation (3.1.26) of Fuller (with the same kind of modification used for the unweighted estimator). They are based on the fact that $v_i = Y_i - (\beta_0 + \beta_1 X_i) = \epsilon_i + w_i - \beta_1 u_i$ has variance

$$\sigma_{vi}^2 = \text{Var}(\epsilon_i) + \sigma_{wi}^2 + \beta_1^2 \sigma_{ui}^2 - 2\beta_1 \sigma_{uwi}. \tag{5}$$

The weight used for the ith observation is $1/\hat{\sigma}_{vi}^2$, where

$$\hat{\sigma}_{vi}^2 = \hat{\sigma}^2 + \hat{\sigma}_{wi}^2 + \hat{\beta}_1^2 \hat{\sigma}_{ui}^2 - 2\hat{\beta}_1 \hat{\sigma}_{uwi}. \tag{6}$$

The weighted estimates are not simply weighted least-squares estimates but rather, use the weights in combination with a correction for measurement error. Asymptotically, the weighted estimator should be better, but in practice this may not be the case, due to the extra uncertainty in estimating σ_{vi}^2.

It is worth commenting that even with the corrections for measurement error the estimators of the coefficients are not unbiased. The argument for their use is that under certain conditions they are consistent. The simple least-squares estimators are not only biased for finite sample size but are typically inconsistent.

3.4   Approximate Inferences

Inferences are based on the approximate normality of $\hat{\beta}_0$ and $\hat{\beta}_1$ as given by Fuller (1987, Theorem 3.1.1). For this, an estimated covariance matrix of $(\hat{\beta}_0, \hat{\beta}_1)$ is needed. This is arranged as

$$
\mathbf{C} = \begin{bmatrix} \hat{\mathrm{V}}\mathrm{ar}(\hat{\beta}_0) & \hat{\mathrm{C}}\mathrm{ov}(\hat{\beta}_0, \hat{\beta}_1) \\ \hat{\mathrm{C}}\mathrm{ov}(\hat{\beta}_0, \hat{\beta}_1) & \hat{\mathrm{V}}\mathrm{ar}(\hat{\beta}_1) \end{bmatrix}.
\tag{7}
$$

In the usual jargon, $\hat{s}e(\hat{\beta}_1) = \hat{\mathrm{V}}\mathrm{ar}(\hat{\beta}_1)^{1/2}$ is the estimated standard error of the estimated slope $\hat{\beta}_1$ with $\hat{s}e(\hat{\beta}_0)$ similarly defined as the estimated standard error for $\hat{\beta}_0$. The term $\hat{\mathrm{C}}\mathrm{ov}(\hat{\beta}_0, \hat{\beta}_1)$ is important in forming prediction (or inverse-prediction) intervals or confidence bands for the regression line.

There are two ways for obtaining $\mathbf{C}$, both applicable for either unweighted or weighted estimators. The expression in equation (3.1.12) of Fuller does not use normality assumptions, while the expression in (3.1.23) of Fuller does. These are referred to as the nonnormal and normal estimates of the covariance matrix, respectively.

If one considers a problem with *no measurement error*, it is the normal estimate which produces the results obtained from a standard least-squares analysis. This estimate is known, though, to be correct even without normality assumptions. The nonnormal-based $\mathbf{C}$ yields essentially a robust estimate of the covariance matrix which does not assume equal variances for the ϵ_i. This estimator, denoted $\mathbf{AC}$, is due to White (1980) and is such that the nonnormal estimate of $\mathbf{C}$ is $n/(n-2)\mathbf{AC}$. Remember that this is the case for which there is no measurement error in x. This suggests that there may be more than just the dropping of the normality assumption involved and that the nonnormal estimate of $\mathbf{C}$ may be robust to unequal variances in the ϵ's.

3.5   Residual Analysis

In any regression problem, a typical approach is to begin with a relatively simple model, such as (1) with $\mathrm{Var}(\epsilon_i)$ constant, and then to check the assumptions via residual analysis. The ith residual is defined in terms of the observed values as

$$r_i = Y_i - (\hat{\beta}_0 + \hat{\beta}_1 X_i). \tag{8}$$

Without measurement error, an evaluation of the assumptions is made by plotting the residual or some function of it versus X_i or the fitted Y value. The use of these plots is based in spirit on the behavior of ϵ_i (which of course is not observed) under model violations. See Draper and Smith (1981), Carroll and Ruppert (1988), or other regression texts for a more complete discussion.

With measurement error present there are additional complications. Carroll and Spiegelman (1992) provide a discussion and references regarding residual analysis in measurement error problems closely related to the ones under discussion here. Examples and further discussion are also found in Fuller. The main problem is that even with known regression coefficients the quantity $v_i = Y_i - (\beta_0 + \beta_1 X_i) = \epsilon_i + w_i - \beta_1 u_i$ is correlated with X_i due to the common measurement error u_i entering in both quantities. Hence, a plot of the residual r_i (which estimates v_i) versus X_i can be misleading. However, v_i is uncorrelated with the quantity $x_i^* = X_i + [(\beta_1 \sigma_{ui}^2 - \sigma_{uwi}) v_i]/\sigma_{vi}^2$. As developed by Fuller (p. 21) this particular quantity arises by considering the β's as known and obtaining a generalized least-squares estimator of x_i. The x's here are treated as fixed, while Carroll and Spiegelman (1992) have random x values. Under normality, v_i and x_i^* are independent and the expected value of v_i given x_i^* is $E(\epsilon_i)$. A plot of v_i versus x_i^* will aid in assessing the linearity assumption. Obviously, neither of these quantities can be observed, so r_i is used in place of v_i and

$$\hat{x}_i = X_i + \frac{(\hat{\beta}_1 \hat{\sigma}_{ui}^2 - \hat{\sigma}_{uwi}) r_i}{\hat{\sigma}_{vi}^2}$$

is used instead of x_i^*, where $\hat{\sigma}_{vi}^2$ is given in equation (6). This is a modified estimator of x_i using information from the fitted regression.

An examination of (5) shows that changes in the variance of v_i (this variance being estimated by r_i^2) do not necessarily reflect changes in the variance of ϵ_i because of the changing measurement error variances/covariance. A plot of r_i, or functions of it, versus $\hat{x}_i$ will not then be useful in detecting changes in the variance of ϵ_i. A simplistic approach to correcting the problem is to use a *modified squared residual*

$$\text{msr}_i = r_i^2 - \hat{\sigma}_{wi}^2 - \hat{\beta}_1^2 \hat{\sigma}_{ui}^2 + 2\hat{\beta}_1 \hat{\sigma}_{uwi}. \tag{9}$$

This modification is new here. If, in fact, the β's and all the σ's were known, the expected value of the modified squared residual is simply $\text{Var}(\epsilon_i)$. A trend in the plot of msr_i versus $\hat{x}_i$ suggests a changing variance for the error in the equation. While the modified squared residual suffers from the problem of possibly being negative, it is preferable to using simply the squared residual. When the measurement error variances/covariance are relatively small, there will not be much difference between the two.

As noted by Carroll and Spiegelman (1992), when the errors in the equation have an asymmetric distribution, there can be problems in assessing heteroscedasticity using the plots just described. They discuss this further and also provide some alternative residual plots that can be useful.

4 RESULTS

4.1 Burlap Data

For the burlap data, the prime objective is the development of a point and interval estimate for the egg mass density on a future unit based on observed burlap counts. It is important to note that the results are limited to cases where future burlap counts are obtained from 12 subplots with trees banded in the same way as in the original data set. There are some approaches that can be implemented when the future unit has a different kind of subsampling, but they will not be discussed here.

The first issue is deciding whether to regress the mean burlap count on true egg mass density, or vice versa. It seems more natural to think of the conditional distribution of the mean burlap count given the true egg mass density, and this is the approach taken here. This also allows illustration of the methods when there is measurement error in x. (If one chooses to regress in the other direction, account still needs to be made for the measurement error in egg mass density. The analysis is exactly like that in the next section for predicting defoliation.) The true egg mass densities are treated as fixed and (1) is used to model $y_i = Y_i$, the mean burlap count from the 12 subplots, given x_i, the true egg mass density. There is no measurement error in the y variable since it is just the mean on the 12 subplots upon which the estimation of egg mass density will be based. The functional model with the egg mass densities treated as fixed is used because the stands were not randomly chosen and the behavior of random egg mass densities over stands and years is complicated due to spatial and temporal effects.

Table 3 shows both the least-squares and measurement error analyses using all the data. The fitted lines from the least-squares fit and the unweighted measurement error fit are displayed in Figure 1. Approximate confidence intervals and tests for the coefficients proceed in a standard way based on approximate normality. For example, an approximate $100(1 - \alpha)\%$ confidence interval for β_1 uses $\hat{\beta}_1 \pm z_{1-\alpha/2}\hat{se}(\hat{\beta}_1)$, where $z_{1-\alpha/2}$ is the appropriate percentile from the standard normal distribution; (e.g., $z_{1-\alpha/2} = 1.96$ for $\alpha = 0.05$). An approximate size α test of the hypothesis $H_0: \beta_1 = 0$ rejects H_0 if 0 is not in the confidence interval or, equivalently, if $|Z| > z_{1-\alpha/2}$ where $Z = \hat{\beta}_1/se(\hat{\beta}_1)$; a p-value can also be computed.

Table 3   Analysis of Burlap Data Using All Values

Method[a]	$\hat{\beta}_0$	$\hat{\beta}_1$	$\hat{se}(\hat{\beta}_0)$	$\hat{se}(\hat{\beta}_1)$	$\hat{Cov}(\hat{\beta}_0, \hat{\beta}_1)$	$\hat{\sigma}^2$
LS	3.4943	0.01882	2.5165	0.00184	−0.0019	268.403
ME-UW, NN	2.8462	0.01997	1.5098	0.00428	−0.00245	234.0632
ME-UW, N			2.4429	0.00274	−0.00269	
ME-W, NN	3.203	0.02013	1.3700	0.00420	−0.00163	
ME-W, N			2.394	0.00246	−0.00222	

[a]LS, least squares; ME, measurement error analysis; UW, unweighted; W, weighted; N, normal-based estimate of standard errors and covariance; NN, nonnormal-based estimate of standard errors and covariance.

There are some differences between the least-squares and measurement error results and within the measurement error analyses, differences between the weighted and unweighted approaches. As expected from the theory, the measurement error analysis increases the estimated slope and decreases the estimate of the variance around the regression. The weighted analysis produces somewhat smaller standard errors than the unweighted analysis and there are rather large differences between the nonnormal estimate of the covariance matrix and the normal-based one. As discussed earlier, this could be due to changing variance in the error in the equation as well as a violation of the normality assumptions. For both the weighted and unweighted measurement error estimators, use of the nonnormal approach results in a smaller standard error for the intercept but a larger standard error for the slope.

In problems like this with measurement error in x only, the key factor as to how important it is to correct for measurement error is not the absolute magnitude of the measurement error variances but how large they are relative to the variability in the x values. While some of the measurement error variances are very large, the huge spread in egg mass densities makes accounting for the measurement errors less important. This is illustrated by running the analysis on just those observations for which X_i is less than 500 as given in Table 4.

Table 4   Analysis of Burlap Data Using Cases with $X_i < 500$

Method[a]	$\hat{\beta}_0$	$\hat{\beta}_1$	$\hat{se}(\hat{\beta}_0)$	$\hat{se}(\hat{\beta}_1)$	$\hat{Cov}(\hat{\beta}_0, \hat{\beta}_1)$	$\hat{\sigma}^2$
LS	1.8466	0.06598	1.255	0.0137	−0.0078	50.042
ME-UW, NN	1.340	0.07674	0.7111	0.03121	−0.011	45.21
ME-UW, N			1.2795	0.02046	−0.01309	
ME-W, NN	1.2764	0.08742	0.6290	0.03331	−0.00957	
ME-W, N			1.242	0.0195	−0.01109	

[a]LS, least squares; ME, measurement error analysis; UW, unweighted; W, weighted; N, normal-based estimate of standard errors and covariance, NN, nonnormal-based estimate of standard errors and covariance.

The changes from the least-squares to the measurement error analyses are now more substantial, the result of the measurement error variances being larger relative to the spread in egg mass densities. The apparent differences between the coefficients here and those resulting from the full analysis also suggest that the relationship is different at small versus larger values of the egg mass density. This is also suggested by the subsequent residual analysis.

The issue of how important the differences among the various methods are depends on the objective of the analysis. Here the main goal is to estimate egg mass density on a future unit. With the x's as fixed, this is just the so-called calibration or inverse prediction problem but with measurement error in the x's. See Osborne (1992) for a review of calibration. Assuming that the model is correct, suppose that there is a new unit with unknown egg mass density x_o on which a mean burlap value Y_{obs} is obtained. By inverting (1), the estimated egg mass density is $\hat{x}_o = (Y_{\text{obs}} - \hat{\beta}_0)/\hat{\beta}_1$. With no measurement error, a confidence region for x_o can be obtained as described by Graybill (1976, p. 280); it follows from applying Fieller's theorem for a ratio of means. By approximating the variance of $\hat{x}_o$, an approximate $100(1 - \alpha)\%$ confidence region for x_o is given by the collection of x's such that

$$\frac{(\hat{x}_0 - x)^2}{A(x)} \leq z^2_{1-\alpha/2},$$

where $A(x) = \hat{\beta}_1^{-2}[\hat{\sigma}^2 + \hat{\text{V}}\text{ar}(\hat{\beta}_0) + x^2\,\hat{\text{V}}\text{ar}(\hat{\beta}_1) + 2x\,\hat{\text{C}}\text{ov}(\hat{\beta}_0, \hat{\beta}_1)]$. The result will be an interval, expressible in terms of the roots of a particular quadratic equation, as long as $[\hat{\beta}_1^2/\hat{\text{V}}\text{ar}(\hat{\beta}_1)] \geq z^2_{\alpha/2}$. Figure 3 shows 95% confidence intervals for x_o resulting from using standard least squares and the unweighted measurement error estimates with the normal **C** based on all the data. The intervals are one at a time in that the 95% applies to a single future unit and not to many units simultaneously. As the burlap count increases, the two methods begin to differ markedly. With either analysis, however, the result indicates that burlap counts do not produce precise estimates of egg mass density. Two items are mainly responsible for the width of the interval; one involves the variance $\hat{\sigma}^2$ while the other is due to uncertainty in the regression coefficients which enters through **C**. It is the former that is the dominant term leading to the wide intervals.

Residual Analysis
A plot of the residual r_i versus $\hat{x}_i$, which is used to assess linearity, is given in Figure 4. Especially if better resolution near small values of $\hat{x}_i$ is used, there is indication of some difficulty with the model at small values of the egg mass density. This was also suggested by the analysis in Table 4 using only units with smaller egg mass values. Figure 5 depicts the modified squared residual versus $\hat{x}_i$. There is some trend upward as $\hat{x}_i$ increases, indicating changing variance for the errors in the equation, but this is tempered by the value farthest to the

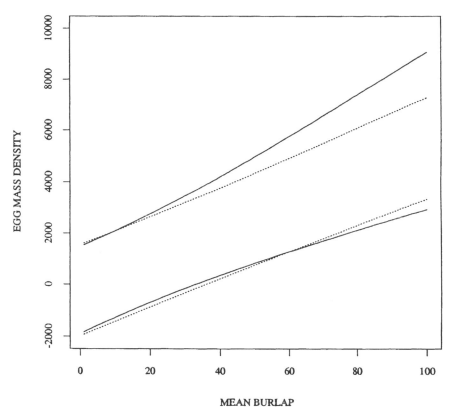

Figure 3. Confidence interval for egg mass density based on observed burlap mean using all data; least squares (——) and unweighted measurement error analysis with normal **C** (- - - -).

right. One of the difficulties here is the amount of variability in the modified squared residuals due to the various estimated quantities in (9).

The model assumes that state and year do not influence the conditional distribution of burlap counts given egg mass density. Although not given here, the residuals were examined as a function of year and state, resulting in some suggestion that the model differed between the two states.

Model Violations

The residual analysis leads to the problem of what to do if the model assumptions are violated. The various options cannot be explored in detail here, but some general comments can be made. Many of these areas need further investigation.

To account for the lack of fit, one could try piecewise linear regression or a nonlinear model. Most of the literature allowing errors in variables in nonlinear models treats only the case of constant measurement error variances (see Fuller, 1987, Chapter 3).

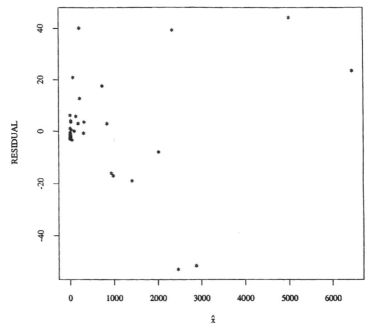

Figure 4. Plot of r_i versus $\hat{x}_i$ for all burlap data.

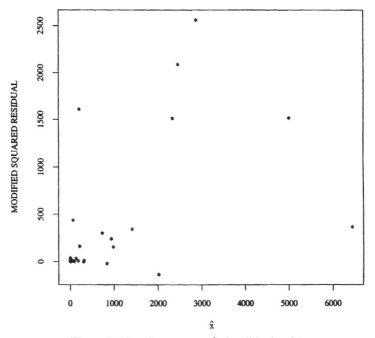

Figure 5. Plot of msr$_i$ versus $\hat{x}_i$ for all burlap data.

Alternatively, one might consider a linear regression after transforming both variables, say using logarithms or square roots. There is a long tradition in entomology and other disciplines of routinely using logarithms of both variables before using simple linear regression. The log-log transformation is known both to linearize the regression if the original relationship is of the form $\gamma_0 x^{\gamma_1}$ with multiplicative errors and to homogenize variance if the standard deviation equals the mean. With measurement error present, using transformations poses further difficulties. For example, when using logarithms, although X_i is unbiased for x_i as a result of the sampling scheme, $\log(X_i)$ is not unbiased for $\log(x_i)$ and the bias may not be negligible, as it depends on the measurement error variance. Additionally, the variance of $\log(X_i)$ and an estimate of it are required. This could be handled by approximating $\text{Var}[\log(X_i)]$ in standard ways. Additional complications arise with the presence of zeros.

For the heteroscedasticity problem, where $\text{Var}(\epsilon_i)$ changes over i, the nonnormal $\mathbf{C}$ should be investigated further for robustness properties suggested in Section 3.4. Hasabelnaby and Fuller (1991) investigate an iterative weighting method, but it requires a functional form for $\text{Var}(\epsilon_i)$ as a function of x_i and other parameters. Without a functional form, perhaps other types of weighting could be developed.

4.2 Analysis of Defoliation Data

Predicting Defoliation
There are a couple of different objectives which can be pursued with the defoliation data. One is to predict true defoliation based on an estimated egg mass density from 20 subunits. Whether the true egg mass densities are treated as fixed or random is important here. The problem is first addressed assuming that the six units are a random sample of units from some population and prediction is to be made on a future unit sampled from the same population. In this case the regression of y (true defoliation) on $x = X$ (observed mean egg mass density on 20 subunits) can be used. Hence, there is no measurement error in x while y_i equals the true defoliation on unit i and Y_i is the measured defoliation on the 20 subunits. It might appear, then, that this is a standard regression problem with no need for dealing with the measurement error in the dependent variable. However,

$$Y_i = \beta_0 + \beta_1 X_i + v_i,$$

where $v_i = w_i + \epsilon_i$ has a variance $\sigma_{wi}^2 + \sigma^2$ which leads to a heteroscedastic regression model. Even if σ_{wi}^2 were constant in i, inferences about the regression coefficients from the usual least-squares analysis will be correct, but one must account for the measurement error in y in order either to estimate σ^2 or to obtain a prediction interval for defoliation on a future unit. A standard least-squares regression of Y on X will, on average, overestimate σ^2 and lead to prediction intervals that are too big, since the measurement error in y has not been removed.

With σ_{wi}^2 changing in i, the measurement error in y must also be accounted for in estimating the coefficients, since Var (v_i) is changing in i. This is a well-treated problem in regression with the two main options being to continue to use least squares but correct the covariance matrix or to use weighted least squares. The first two lines of Table 5 depict a standard least-squares analysis on the observed mean values, while the next four lines result from running the measurement error analysis with no measurement error in x but measurement error in y. For the coefficients, the key issue is the change in the standard errors to account for the heteroscedasticity. The unweighted measurement error analysis produces least-squares estimates of coefficients, but the estimated covariance matrix differs. The nonnormal $\mathbf{C}$ matrix is $(\frac{6}{4})$ times the robust $\mathbf{AC}$ from least squares, while the normal-based $\mathbf{C}$ uses explicitly the fact that Var $(v_i) = \sigma^2 + \sigma_{wi}^2$. The weighted measurement error analysis is equivalent to running weighted least squares using weight $1/(\hat{\sigma}^2 + \hat{\sigma}_{wi}^2)$ for the ith observation. Notice also that the estimate of σ^2 has decreased from 543.41 to 530.8 by accounting for measurement error in y.

With the estimated covariance matrix of the coefficients expressed as in (7), an approximate $100(1 - \alpha)\%$ prediction interval for the defoliation based on a new unit with mean egg density X_{obs} is

$$\hat{\beta}_0 + \hat{\beta}_1 X_{obs} \pm z_{1-\alpha/2}[\hat{\sigma}^2 + \hat{V}ar(\hat{\beta}_0)$$
$$+ X_{obs}^2 \hat{V}ar(\hat{\beta}_1) + 2X_{obs}\hat{C}ov(\hat{\beta}_0, \hat{\beta}_1)]^{1/2}.$$

Table 5   Analysis of Defoliation Data

Method[a]	$\hat{\beta}_0$	$\hat{\beta}_1$	$\hat{se}(\hat{\beta}_0)$	$\hat{se}(\hat{\beta}_1)$	$\hat{C}ov(\hat{\beta}_0, \hat{\beta}_1)$	$\hat{\sigma}^2$
LS	31.916	0.5567	18.223	0.2496	−3.8783	543.406
LS with **AC**			16.334	0.1618	−2.4730	
ME in y only						
UW, NN	31.916	0.5567	20.005	0.1982	−3.7096	530.799
UW, N			18.196	0.2479	−3.8451	
W, N	31.683	0.5619	19.759	0.1944	−3.6081	
W, N			18.194	0.2479	−3.8449	
ME in both						
UW, NN	26.49	0.6438	22.736	0.2384	−5.1702	452.219
UW, N			20.365	0.3153	−5.6753	
W, NN	28.605	0.6148	22.054	0.2438	−5.0016	
W, N			19.18	0.2968	−4.9455	

[a]LS, least squares; LS with AC uses robust estimate of standard errors; ME, measurement error analysis; UW, unweighted; W, weighted; N, normal-based estimate of standard errors and covariance, NN, nonnormal-based estimate of standard errors and covariance.

If there is no measurement error in y and $z_{1-\alpha/2}$ is replaced by $t_{1-\alpha/2}(n - 2)$, the corresponding table value from a t-distribution with $n - 2$ degrees of freedom, the prediction interval above agrees with standard regression results under normality (Draper and Smith, 1981, p. 31).

In summary, this first objective leads to a regression problem with measurement error only in the y variable, which must be taken into account in conducting certain analyses. Although the residual analysis is not provided here, notice that for assessing homogeneity of variance for the error in the equation the modified squared residual removes the changing measurement error variance in y.

The analysis above assumed a random sample of units. With the units and associated true egg mass densities fixed, the conditional distribution of y given X is just the distribution of y given the true egg mass density, and predictions must be based on an estimate of the latter conditional distribution; see Fuller (1987, Section 1.6.3) for a discussion. This conditional distribution is estimated next, but the details of prediction in this context are not given.

Estimating the Relationship between True Values

As a second objective, consider assessing the relationship between true egg mass density (x) and true defoliation (y). This relationship may be of interest in its own right or, as just mentioned, it is needed for predicting defoliation when the true egg mass densities are fixed. Note that x has a different meaning than it did in the first objective, as do β_0 and β_1. For this model, there is measurement error in both variables. Furthermore, the measurement errors on a single unit are correlated because of the use of the same 20 subplots to measure defoliation and egg mass densities. The estimated measurement error variances and covariances can be obtained from the entries in Table 2.

As in the burlap example, the systematic subsample of 20 subunits is treated as a simple random sample. The last four lines of Table 5 provide the measurement error analysis with both variables measured with error. There are rather large changes in the estimates of both the coefficients and σ^2 when corrections for measurement error are used rather than least squares. Other comparisons among the methods are similar to those arising in the burlap example.

The residual analysis to assess the model assumptions proves difficult because of the small number of observations and other reasons. Figure 6 shows a plot of the residual versus the modified egg mass density, $\hat{x}_i$. There is no apparent trend, but as in standard regression problems, the assessment is difficult with so few data points. The plot of the modified squared residual versus the modified egg mass density in Figure 7 is used to assess the assumption of constant $\mathrm{Var}(\epsilon_i)$. Here a problem arises. The argument for using the modified square residual is based on the fact that if the coefficients and measurement error variances and covariance were known, it would have an expected value equal to the variance of ϵ_i. However, all of these quantities must be estimated and they are themselves subject to variability. The result is increased variability and some bias in msr_i as an estimate of $V(\epsilon_i)$ and also the potential for negative

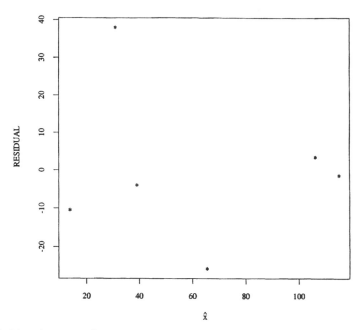

Figure 6. Plot of r_i versus $\hat{x}_i$ from analysis of defoliation data with measurement error in both variables.

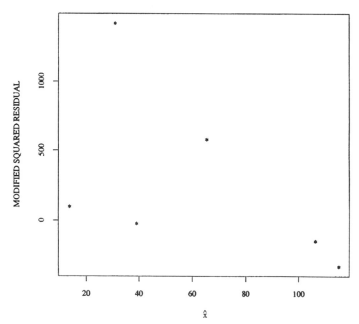

Figure 7. Plot of msr$_i$ versus $\hat{x}_i$ from analysis of defoliation data with measurement error in both variables.

values of msr$_i$. The latter potential problem is realized here, with two of the observations producing negative values for the modified squared residual. The only option is to set these values to zero, but their occurrence casts doubt on the value of the plot.

As with the first example, the question remains as to what is to be done if the model assumptions are violated. It is clear that with the dependent variable being the percent defoliated, the linear regression model with constant variance is only an approximation and it will break down at extreme defoliation values. To account for asymptotes, one could either use a nonlinear model with heteroscedasticity or try to work on a transformed scale. The reader is referred to the general discussion at the end of the analysis of the burlap data regarding these and other problems.

5 CONCLUSIONS

Two examples were used to illustrate the available methodology for handling simple linear regression problems with measurement error in one or both of the variables and subsampling. Techniques are available to handle more general multiple regression problems as described in Fuller (1987, Chapter 3). Recent work by Carroll et al. (1993) suggests some robust estimation methods. One shortcoming in the handling of the data here was the need to treat the subsamples as a simple random sample, while, in fact, systematic sampling was used. While from the statistical point of view an alternative subsampling scheme which allows estimation of the measurement error variances is desired, the systematic sampling has great logistical advantages for the scientists.

In the analyses, careful attention was given to modeling issues. In particular, it was seen that the issue of which variable(s) should be treated as having been measured with error depends on the objective of the experiment. The first objective in the defoliation analysis illustrated that sometimes one must separate out the measurement error in the dependent variable from the error in the equation. Whether the true x values are assumed fixed or random also needs careful attention.

Even though there is a need for further study of the methods, especially small-sample properties, these techniques still provide useful ways for researchers to account for measurement error. Ignoring measurement errors can lead to incorrect analyses, including biases in estimated coefficients, incorrect confidence and prediction intervals, and so on. In some cases, a failure to account for measurement error can lead to substantial changes in the qualitative conclusions.

As with any problem, carrying out an analysis in the presence of small sample sizes can be challenging. This is especially true here, as the methodology is dependent on large-sample results. While providing a nice illustration of the methods, the analysis of the defoliation example must be viewed with caution because of the small number of units involved. In many ecological studies, the large costs of sampling result in small numbers of main units in the study. The consequence of small numbers of units, along with the potential impact of measurement errors, raises the interesting design question of how to allocate limited resources among main units and subsampling within units.

ACKNOWLEDGMENTS

The author is grateful to Joe Elkinton (burlap data) and Sandy Liebhold (defoliation data) for permission to use the data, extensive and fruitful discussions on the examples, and their general encouragement and support in pursuing work on these problems. Support for this work was provided in part by cooperative agreements 23-594 and 23-735 between the USDA Forest Service and the University of Massachusetts. Chengda Yang provided some programming assistance.

SOFTWARE NOTES AND REFERENCES

There is no readily available software which easily handles problems with changing measurement error variances of the type encountered here. The EVCARP software, available from the statistical laboratory at Iowa State University, handles a variety of measurement error problems. As illustrated with examples in Fuller (1987) and in the EVCARP manual, one can make use of the functionally related covariance option in EVCARP to accommodate changing measurement error variances, but this can be cumbersome. The computations were performed in Fortran utilizing IMSL subroutines.

QUESTIONS AND PROBLEMS

1. In the analyses here, how important was it to correct for measurement error?

2. When x is measured with error, why is a plot of the residual versus the observed X possibly misleading?

3. What are the potential problems in transforming the observed X and/or Y values in trying to obtain a linear relationship?

4. If within each unit, subsampling was done using a stratified sample, how would the variances of the measurement errors and the estimates of these variances change?

CHAPTER 5

Estimating Pine Seedling Response to Ozone and Acidic Rain

John O. Rawlings and Susan E. Spruill

1 MOTIVATION AND BACKGROUND

Problems often arise when attempting to combine and analyze data from multiple experiments even when the experiments have a common objective. Although similar, the experiments may differ in many respects that affect the combined analysis. Experimental design, treatment factors, numbers of replicates, species choice, environmental factors (rainfall, temperature, etc.), and even treatment levels may vary across experiments. Failures in the basic assumptions of normality and homogeneous variances are expected. In the more extreme cases where the experiments are very dissimilar, combining information from multiple experiments may be limited to combining *p*-values associated with independent tests of particular hypotheses as suggested by Fisher (Fisher, 1958; Steel and Torrie, 1980), or to a subjective "averaging" over the individual experiments to obtain an overall response. When all experiments include a common quantitative treatment factor, and if all used a reasonably consistent experimental protocol, the information from dissimilar experiments can be combined to provide quantitative estimates of the dose–response relationship.

This case study is concerned with the combined analysis of 2-year response data generated by the Southern Commercial Forest Research Cooperative. The Southern Commercial Forest Research Cooperative originated in 1986 as part of the Forest Response Program (Bartuska and Joyner, 1987). Scientists at six sites conducted similarly designed experiments on seedlings of various genotypes of southern pines, duplicating experimental technologies across the sites with some minor variations. One objective of the Southern Commercial Forest Research Cooperative was to establish a relationship between the pollutants ozone and

Case Studies in Biometry, Edited by Nicholas Lange, Louise Ryan, Lynne Billard, David Brillinger, Loveday Conquest, and Joel Greenhouse.
ISBN 0-471-58885-7 © 1994 John Wiley & Sons, Inc.

acidic rain and the growth of commercially important pine species in the southeastern United States. Since all studies were conducted with seedlings, inferences from these studies must be restricted to the response of seedlings. The objective, however, implies that inferences made from the experiments should apply to the population of environments likely to be encountered in pine production in the southeast and to the population of commercially important pine species. For a statistically valid inference, the environments in which the studies are conducted and the genetic materials used ("sites" and "families" in this study) should be representative samples of their respective populations. A key objective is to take into account the added uncertainty that arises as a result of broadening the inference to the populations of environments and genetic material rather than the specific conditions of the present studies.

There are two approaches to combining the information on the dose–response relationships between growth and ozone and acidic rain that take into account the broader intended inference. One approach is to estimate the dose–response relationships for each site–family combination and then view the collection of fitted equations as representative of the types, and *variability*, of responses that one would obtain across the inference populations. That is, the fitted responses are considered a sample of the population of responses one might obtain. One could then use the fitted equations to estimate the population mean responses, and their standard errors, for given scenarios of ozone and acidic rain.

An alternative approach, which we use in this case study, is to combine the information from all studies to estimate a population mean response surface for each growth variable. In this approach, the "site" and "family" effects and interactions involving these effects are treated as random effects in a mixed model. The random effects induce a variance–covariance structure among the observations which is taken into account in the estimation of the fixed-effects parameters. If the variance–covariance structure has been defined correctly and if the variance components have been estimated with sufficient precision, an immediate result of the mixed model approach is that the fixed-effects parameters are estimated with greater precision *than if the covariance structure had been ignored*, as is the case when a response surface is estimated with the classical fixed-model approach. The primary motivation for using mixed models, however, is that the inference from the experiment is broadened to cover the populations of random effects that have been sampled in the studies, and the measures of precision obtained for the fitted model are more realistic for that broader inference.

While the primary purpose of this case study is to show the use of mixed models for combining information from multiple experiments, all stages of the analysis are shown. Both polynomial and nonlinear functions are used in mixed-effects models to model the mean response to ozone and acidic rain. For illustration, the results obtained from the mixed models are compared to those obtained from fixed-effects models for the polynomial mean response.

2 DATA

Six research sites—Auburn, Alabama (site 1); Clemson, South Carolina (site 2); two sites near Durham, North Carolina (sites 3 and 4); Gainesville, Florida (site 5); and Nacogdoches, Texas (site 6)—participated in the Southern Commercial Forest Research Cooperative to conduct controlled field studies on the effects of the pollutants ozone and acidic rain on pine seedling growth in southeastern United States. Ozone level in the atmosphere surrounding the growing plants was controlled by altering the ozone in the airstream being forced into the base and out the top of clear, open-topped chambers surrounding the plants. Acidic rain levels were imposed by dispensing at specified times fixed volumes of premixed solutions simulating acidic rain on all plants within each chamber. Natural rain was excluded from the chamber with movable chamber tops. Since each chamber can receive only one ozone–acidic rain treatment combination, the chamber becomes the natural whole-plot experimental unit for a split-plot experiment. All experimental designs were split-plot designs with the combinations of levels of ozone exposure and acidic rain being the whole-plot treatments. Different genetic families of particular pine species were the subplot treatments.

The studies differed from site to site in several ways (Table 1). The whole plots were arranged in randomized complete block designs at sites 1, 2, 3, and 4 and in completely random designs at sites 5 and 6. There were three replications at site 4 and two replications at all other sites. Sites 1, 2, 5, and 6 had 12 whole-plot treatments (four ozone by three acidic rain levels), whereas site 3 had 10 (5×2 factorial) and site 4 had 18 (6×3 factorial) whole-plot treatments.

The target levels of ozone are designated 1.0 for nonfiltered air, which means that the plants are being exposed to ambient levels of ozone, CF for charcoal filtered air, which removes approximately half the ambient ozone, and "$x.x$" for multiples of current ambient levels. Even though sites may have the same nominal ozone treatment (1.0, 1.7, 2.0, etc.), variations in ambient ozone levels cause the exposure levels of ozone for the same nominal treatment to be quite different between sites and to a much lesser extent between replicates within sites. The acidic rain treatments are designated by the pH of the rain solution. Because of variation in volume of rain applied, different levels of exposure are realized for the same nominal acidic rain treatments. The actual levels of exposure were provided through continual monitoring of ozone levels and rain volumes.

Loblolly pine was used at sites 1, 3, and 4; slash pine at site 5; and shortleaf pine at sites 2 and 6. The subplot treatments at each site consisted of different genetic families of these pine species. The number of families varied from two to four. Further details on the individual studies and their results are given by the investigators for the individual sites (Boutton and Flagler, 1990; Chappelka et al., 1990; Dean and Johnson, 1990; Kress et al., 1988; Paynter et al., 1991; Kress and Allen, 1991).

Table 1   Description of Experimental Design for Each Site

Site Location:	Auburn	Clemson	Duke I	Duke II	Florida	Texas
Site No.:	1	2	3	4	5	6
Species	Loblolly	Loblolly	Loblolly	Slash	Shortleaf	Shortleaf
Design[a]	RCBD[b]	RCBD	RCBD	RCBD	CRD	CRD
Replicates	2	2	2	3	2	2
Observations	48	96	60	216	96	96
Whole plot						
Ozone level[c]	0.0	0.0	0.0	0.0	0.0	0.0
	1.0	1.0	1.0	1.0	1.0	1.0
	1.7	1.7	1.5	1.3	2.0	1.7
	2.5	2.5	2.3	1.6	3.0	2.5
			3.0	2.0		
				3.0		
Rain pH	5.3	5.3	5.2	5.3	5.3	5.3
	4.3	4.3	3.5	4.3	4.3	4.3
	3.3	3.3		3.3	3.3	3.3
Subplot						
Families	2	4	3	4	4	4

[a] All studies were split-plot experimental designs in which the whole-plot designs were arranged in either randomized complete block designs (RCBDs) or completely random designs (CRDs).
[b] pH treatments were stripped across blocks at this site.
[c] 0.0, charcoal filtered air; 1.0, nonfiltered air; 1.3, 1.3 times ambient air; 1.5, 1.5 times ambient air; 1.6, 1.6 times ambient air; 1.7, 1.7 times ambient air; 2.0, 2.0 times ambient air; 2.3, 2.3 times ambient air; 2.5, 2.5 times ambient air; 3.0, 3.0 times ambient air.

A sampling of the data set is shown in Table 2. The data set contains the identification codes for site, block, replicate, ozone and acidic rain treatments, and genetic family; measurements of cumulative exposures to ozone (ppm hours) and acidic rain (vwpH) over the 2-year growth period; and measurements on the final aboveground biomass and the increment of stem diameter growth, as well as the size of the seedlings when exposures were started, initial height, and basal stem diameter. There are 612 total observations for all measurements except total biomass, for which there are only 450 observations (since only one family was measured for biomass at site 4). The response of total biomass and increment of diameter growth to ozone and acidic rain are modeled in this case study.

3   METHODS AND MODELS

The analysis of the data involved two distinct steps. First, several preliminary analyses were run for the purposes of (1) estimating residuals to check for outliers and the basic assumptions of normality and homogeneous variances, and

Table 2   A Partial Listing of the Data for This Case Study[a]

site	block	rep	ozone	rain	fam	ppmhr	vwpH	biomass	diam.	DMA	DMB	D2HA	D2HB	DMOT
1	1	.	0.0	3.3	1	50.00	-0.867	1499.72	51.25	-0.01	-0.09	0.32	-0.45	.
1	1	.	0.0	3.3	2	50.00	-0.867	1286.44	40.84	-0.01	0.09	0.32	0.45	.
1	1	.	0.0	4.3	1	51.00	0.160	1408.61	51.80	0.67	0.32	2.33	2.02	.
1	1	.	0.0	4.3	2	51.00	0.160	1911.80	49.53	0.67	-0.32	2.33	-2.02	.
1	1	.	0.0	5.3	1	49.00	1.203	1145.99	44.56	-0.12	0.52	-0.70	2.84	.
:	:	:	:	:	:	:	:	:	:	:	:	:	:	:
4	4	.	1.7	5.3	3	333.00	1.079	.	44.65	-1.31	0.44	-20.12	5.74	54.50
4	4	.	1.7	5.3	4	333.00	1.079	754.80	36.30	-1.31	-0.41	-20.12	-9.67	54.50
4	4	.	2.0	3.3	1	402.00	-0.938	.	37.95	0.29	-0.06	3.48	1.90	17.25
4	4	.	2.0	3.3	2	402.00	-0.938	.	35.05	0.29	0.04	3.48	-2.83	17.25
4	4	.	2.0	3.3	3	402.00	-0.938	1029.82	26.20	0.29	0.04	3.48	0.77	17.25
4	4	.	2.0	3.3	4	402.00	-0.938	.	41.70	0.29	-0.01	3.48	0.16	17.25
4	4	.	2.0	4.3	1	410.00	0.072	.	32.30	-0.90	0.72	-12.67	4.35	16.25
:	:	:	:	:	:	:	:	:	:	:	:	:	:	:
6	1	2	2.5	2.0	4	581.11	0.043	580.39	27.45	1.35	0.36	9.74	4.99	.
6	1	2	2.5	3.0	1	579.04	-0.961	172.88	18.85	-0.01	1.12	1.00	9.79	.
6	1	2	2.5	3.0	2	579.04	-0.961	402.64	26.15	-0.01	-0.68	1.00	-4.62	.
6	1	2	2.5	3.0	3	579.04	-0.961	397.54	29.75	-0.01	-0.47	1.00	-4.48	.
6	1	2	2.5	3.0	4	579.04	-0.961	415.67	28.15	-0.01	0.03	1.00	-0.69	.

[a] The variables *ozone*, *rain*, and *fam* are class variables denoting the levels of the three treatment factors within each site. (The coded levels are not comparable across sites.) The quantitative levels of ozone and acidic rain exposures are denoted by *ppmhr* and *vwpH*, respectively. The two response variables are *biomass* and *diam*. The covariates are denoted by *DMA* and *DMB* for the whole-plot and subplot components, respectively, for initial diameter, and similarly *D2HA* and *D2HB* for initial volume; *DMOT* is the depth-to-mottling covariate at site 4.

85

to investigate the value of alternative transformations of the response variables; (2) testing the importance of initial seedling size measurements as covariates in the control of experimental error; (3) testing for the presence of interactions between ozone, acidic rain, and genetic families; and (4) estimating experimental error variance for each site. The second step of the analysis combined the data from all sites to model the dose–response relationships, and then the results from mixed and fixed models were compared.

3.1 Definition of Covariates

Variability in seedling size at the start of the exposure treatments suggested that initial plant size measurements might be useful as covariates to control experimental error. Initial diameter (measured just before treatment exposures started) is used as the covariate for increment of diameter growth. A surrogate estimate of initial volume computed as (initial diameter^2 × initial height) was used as the covariate for biomass. The covariates were expressed as deviations from their respective site means so that all covariate adjustments would be within-site adjustments. Also, since the experimental design was a split-plot design, each covariate was partitioned into two orthogonal components; a subplot component consisting of the deviation of the covariate from the whole-plot mean and a whole-plot component consisting of the deviation of the whole-plot mean from the site mean.

Covariates were defined in the following manner. Let X_{ijklm} be the value of the particular covariate for the ith site, jth replicate, kth level of ozone, lth level of acidic rain, and mth family. Then the whole-plot and subplot components of the covariate are defined, respectively, as

$$X_{aijkl} = \overline{X}_{ijkl.} - \overline{X}_{i....} \quad \text{and} \quad X_{bijklm} = X_{ijklm} - \overline{X}_{ijkl.}, \tag{1}$$

where the bar indicates averaging over the subscripts that have been replaced with a dot. In subsequent analyses, the whole-plot and subplot covariates are labeled simply as X_a and X_b, respectively, with the understanding that the covariate is initial basal stem diameter (DMA and DMB) if increment of diameter growth is being analyzed, and initial volume ($D2HA$ and $D2HB$) if biomass is being analyzed.

After the experiment was in progress, it became apparent to the scientists at site 4 that restricted soil drainage in some areas of the field was affecting seedling growth. This led to the definition of another covariate, depth to mottling of the clay soil ($DMOT$), that quantified the soil drainage for each whole-plot at site 4. Plots of the response variables, particularly diameter, against depth to mottling suggested curvilinear relationships that appeared to be linearized with a logarithmic transformation of depth to mottling. Figure 1 shows this effect for the variable diameter. Consequently, the depth-to-mottling covariate was defined as $X_{dijkl} = \ln(DMOT_{ijkl}) - \ln(DMOT_{i...})$ for $i = 4$, and zero

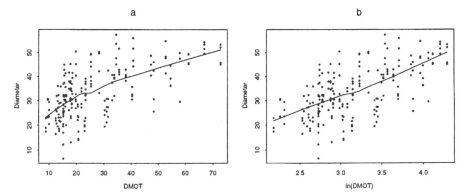

Figure 1. Increment of diameter growth versus depth to mottling (*DMOT*) at site 4 showing a curvilinear relationship (*a*), and versus ln (*DMOT*) showing a more nearly linear relationship (*b*). Each line is obtained by nonparametric smoothing.

otherwise, where the "dot" notation corresponds to means. Note that depth to mottling was measured only once for each whole plot, so there is no subplot component for this covariate. This covariate is labeled X_d in subsequent analyses.

3.2 Residuals Analysis

The residuals were estimated by fitting, for each site, the complete effects model for a split-plot design with all treatment main and interaction effects and the relevant covariates in the model. Thus, the model for the ith site is

$$
\begin{aligned}
Y_{ijklm} = \{\mu\ &+\ [rep]_j\ +\ [ozone]_k\ +\ [rain]_l\ +\ [ozone \times rain]_{kl} \\
&+\ \beta_a X_{ajkl}\ +\ \beta_d X_{djkl}\ +\ \delta_{jkl}\ +\ [family]_m\ +\ [family \times ozone]_{lm} \\
&+\ [family \times ozone \times rain]_{klm}\ +\ \beta_b X_{bjklm}\ +\ \epsilon_{jklm}\}_i,
\end{aligned}
\tag{2}
$$

where δ_{jkl} and ϵ_{jklm} are the whole-plot and subplot errors, respectively, and the other terms are self-explanatory. The bracketed model with the ith subscript outside the braces is to remind the reader that the terms in the model are site specific. The analyses of variance for biomass and incremental diameter growth are given in Tables 3 and 4. The residuals from these analyses, pooled across all sites, were plotted against the fitted values (see Figures 2a and 3a for biomass and diameter growth, respectively) and against the quantiles of the standard normal distribution to give the normal plots (Figures 2b and 3b). These plots were inspected for patterns in the residuals (nonrandomness or deviations from a straight line in the case of the normal plot) that might suggest the presence of outliers or inadequacies in the assumptions (Rawlings, 1988). In addition, the estimated observational error variances (error b) were tested for homogeneity

Table 3 Sums of Squares ($\times 10^{-2}$) from the Analyses of Variance by Site for Total Aboveground Biomass

Source[a]	Site 1[b] d.f.	Site 1[b] Sum of Squares	Site 2 d.f.	Site 2 Sum of Squares	Site 3 d.f.	Site 3 Sum of Squares	Site 4 d.f.	Site 4 Sum of Squares	Site 5 d.f.	Site 5 Sum of Squares	Site 6 d.f.	Site 6 Sum of Squares
Block	1	751	1	14	1	1,960	2	1,222	2	6,964	2	436
R	2	7,477[c]	2	186	1	893	2	4,358	3	22,233	3	4,755
O	3	6,980	3	358	4	21,611[c]	5	13,934	6	10,816	6	5,912
O × R	6	5,197	6	694	4	1,579	10	15,249	6	3,701	1	1,265
X_a	1	2,363	1	1,216[d]	1	417	1	3,958				
X_d							1	41,987[d]				
Error a	10	5,667	10	630	8	6,639	32	53,631	11	24,849	11	14,904
F	1	13	3	124	2	1,631			3	1,249	3	4,469[d]
F × O	3	1,617	9	197	8	2,202			9	4,089	9	1,661
F × R	2	2,177	6	364	2	301			6	1,954	6	2,310
O × R × F	6	4,492	18	471	8	3,203			18	9,296	18	5,969
X_b	1	4,176[c]	1	34	1	6,918[d]			1	5,022[d]	1	2,013[c]
Error b	11	6,048	35	1,154	19	13,066			35	14,762	35	11,854

[a]O, ozone treatment; R, acidic rain treatment; F, family effects; X_a, whole-plot partition of the covariate; X_b, subplot partition of the covariate. This analysis used the $\ln(D^2H)$ as the covariate, where D is the initial diameter and H is the initial height.
[b]Site 1 used a stripped plot arrangement for the rain treatments, but the stripped plot analysis showed no effect of the stripping, so the conventional split-plot analysis is shown here.
[c]Significant at $\alpha = 0.05$.
[d]Significant at $\alpha = 0.01$.

Table 4 Sums of Squares from the Analyses of Variance by Site for Increment of Diameter Growth

Source[a]	Site 1[b]		Site 2		Site 3		Site 4		Site 5		Site 6	
	d.f.	Sum of Squares	d.f.	Sum of Squares	d.f.	Sum of Squares	d.f.	Sum of Squares	d.f.	Sum of Squares	d.f.	Sum of Squares
Block	1	33	1	0	1	105	2	486	2		2	71
R	2	221	2	111	1	124[c]	2	75	2	661[c]	3	227
O	3	129	3	66	4	1,120[d]	5	4,061[d]	3	285	6	244
O × R	6	101	6	72	4	152	10	395	6	300	1	1
X_a	1	29	1	34	1	6	1	5	1	60	1	1
X_d							1	2,555[d]				
Error a	10	263	10	153	8	131	32	2,025	11	809	11	549
F	1	32	3	42[d]	2	67	3	212[c]	3	55	3	290[d]
F × O	3	65	9	9	8	191	15	211	9	178	9	117
F × R	2	41	6	43[d]	2	18	6	79	6	81	6	56
O × R × F	6	62	18	29	8	200	30	353	18	349	18	322
X_b	1	49	1	4	1	162	1	387[d]	1	144[d]	1	71[c]
Error b	11	359	35	58	19	1,140	106	2,549	35	548	35	605

[a]O, ozone treatment; R, acidic rain treatment; F, family effects; X_a, whole-plot partition of the covariate; X_b, subplot partition of the covariate. This analysis used initial diameter as the covariate.

[b]Site 1 used a stripped plot arrangement for the rain treatments, but the stripped plot analysis showed no effect of the stripping, so that the conventional split-plot analysis is shown here.

[c]Significant at $\alpha = 0.05$.

[d]Significant at $\alpha = 0.01$.

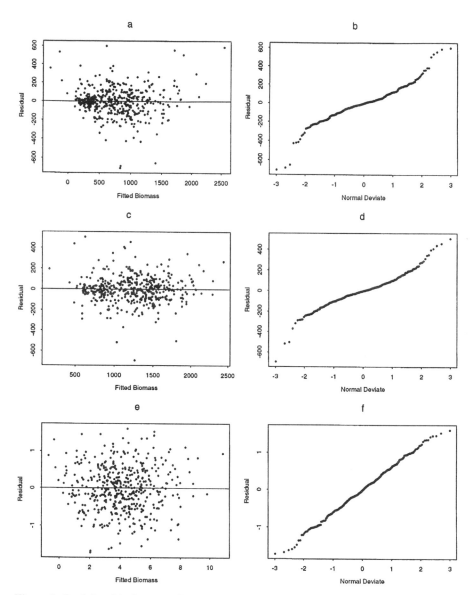

Figure 2. Pooled residuals versus fitted values (a, c, e) and normal plots of the residuals (b, d, f) for total aboveground biomass for the original data (a and b), for square-root transformed data (c and d), and for weighted analysis of the original data (e and f).

across sites using Bartlett's chi-square test of homogeneity (Steel and Torrie, 1980).

When the residuals analysis suggests failures in the underlying assumptions of normality and homogeneous variances, a power transformation of the dependent variable is sometimes useful. The Box–Cox family of power transforma-

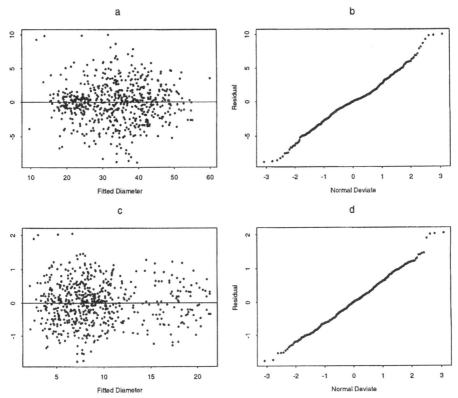

Figure 3. Pooled residuals versus fitted values (a, c) and normal plots of the residuals (b, d) for increment of diameter growth for the original data (a and b), and for weighted analysis of the original data (c and d).

tions (Box and Cox, 1964)

$$
Y_i^{(\lambda)} = \begin{cases} \dfrac{Y_i^{\lambda} - 1}{\lambda(\dot{Y})^{\lambda-1}}, & \lambda \neq 0, \\[2ex] \dot{Y}\ln(\dot{Y}), & \lambda = 0, \end{cases} \tag{3}
$$

where $\dot{Y}$ is the geometric mean of all observations, was investigated for a transformation λ for each variable that might make the error variances more nearly homogeneous and more nearly satisfy the normality assumption. The Box–Cox transformation attempts to satisfy simultaneously the expectation function of the model, and the normality and constant variance assumptions. These multiple objectives are not always compatible. For the Box–Cox analysis, the full effects model (2) was fitted to the data for each site, with the response variable being the transformed variable $Y_i^{(\lambda)}$ for $\lambda = 1, \frac{1}{2}, 0, -\frac{1}{2}$, and -1, in turn. For each

λ, the residual sums of squares SS[Res(λ)] are pooled over all sites and then plotted against λ. The transformation suggested by the analysis is the value of λ that gives the minimum pooled residual sum of squares. Most commonly, the standard power transformation, $\lambda = 1, \frac{1}{2}, 0, -\frac{1}{2}$, or -1, close to the minimum is chosen rather than the specific value of λ that yielded the absolute minimum. The analyses of variance for the individual sites were repeated using the suggested transformations and the pooled residuals reinspected and error variances retested for homogeneity across sites.

A weighted anaysis is necessary in the event that no transformation is found that makes the error variances homogeneous across sites. The appropriate weights for each variable to make the error variances constant across sites are the reciprocals of the square roots of the error mean squares for each site. Thus, the analyses are run on $Y^* = WY$, where W is a diagonal matrix with elements $w_{ii} = s_i^{-1}$, where s_i^2 is the error mean square for the ith site, and $X^* = WX$, where X is the design matrix. (One needs to be aware that some computer programs define the weight variable as w_{ii}^2. Also, the default residuals from the weighted analysis in some programs may be $e = Y - \hat{Y}$, not $e^* = Y^* - \hat{Y}^*$, so that the residuals must be reweighted, $e^* = We$, for appropriate residuals plots.)

3.3 Definition of Dose Metrics

Fitting dose–response models requires that the ozone and acidic rain treatment exposures be quantified by appropriate dose metrics (or, more correctly, exposure metrics). The problem of defining the dose metric has received considerable attention in the literature, with no clear consensus being developed. To the biologist, the primary concern is to define a metric that reflects the "effective" dose being received by the plant, but this requires a clear understanding of how the pollutant affects the physiology of the plant and how this might be related to environmental conditions such as temperature and moisture availability. To others, the dose metric should more nearly reflect definitions used in setting environmental standards, such as the number of days in which the pollutant level exceeds a given standard.

For this case study, the ozone dose metric was defined as the cumulative exposure (ppm hours) realized over 12 hours per day for the periods during which ozone was dispensed over the two seasons. All sites recorded the cumulative 12-hour daily (daytime) ozone exposure (ppm hours) for each chamber. These values were summed for each chamber over the time periods when ozone was dispensed to give the ozone dose metric. (Sites 1, 3, and 4 dispensed ozone for nine months per year, omitting the winter months, while the other sites dispensed 12 months per year. As part of the original analysis, a second ozone dose metric was also investigated, which cumulated the exposure over all 12 months at each site. Results from the two dose metrics were only trivially different.)

Computation of the acidic rain dose metric was more difficult but, again, a cumulative exposure was used. Sites varied with respect to the detail to which pH and volume of rain were recorded. Sites 1, 2, and 5 recorded pH and volume of each rain exposure for each chamber. Sites 3, 4, and 6 recorded volume and pH for every rain exposure but not by individual chambers; average pH by treatment and average volume for the entire site were recorded. The recorded values were assumed to apply equally to all chambers. A volume-weighted dose metric (vwpH) for acidic deposition was computed as

$$\text{vwpH} = -\ln\left[\sum_{j}(10^{-pH_j})(volume_j)\right], \qquad (4)$$

where summation is over all rain episodes for the chamber for the two year period of the studies. The resulting dose metric ranged from -1.119 for the lowest acidic rain treatments to 1.475 for the highest acidic rain treatments. Table 5 gives the average dose metrics by treatment and site for both ozone and acidic rain.

3.4 Dose–Response Models

The purpose is to estimate the dose–response models in a manner that will reflect the added uncertainty that accompanies the broad inference of how pine seedling growth in the southeastern United States is affected by the pollutants

Table 5 Average Cumulative Ozone and Acidic Rain Exposures by Treatment for Each Site

Treatment Code	Site					
	1	2	3	4	5	6
Cumulative Ozone Exposure (ppm hours)						
0.0	50.83	30.88	117.00	36.22	64.88	45.56
1.0	214.66	166.85	261.50	194.33	212.19	224.83
1.3–1.5			388.25	271.44		
1.7	373.66	281.71		330.22		399.08
2.0–2.6	536.83	368.20	569.75	400.66	395.70	578.55
3.0			756.00	583.78	567.96	
Cumulative Acidic Rain Exposures (vwpH)						
3.3	−0.855	−1.105	−0.385	−0.938	−1.171	−0.961
4.3	0.148	−0.116		0.072	−0.168	0.043
5.3	1.195	0.864	1.475	1.079	0.832	1.076

ozone and acidic rain. The dose–response surface obtained from a classical fixed model analysis assumes all effects other than the random error to be fixed, and as a result only the random error component of variance contributes to the measures of precision. Mixed models, on the other hand, recognize the broader inference by regarding appropriate effects as random. In this case study, effects due to sites, families in sites, blocks in sites, and interactions of sites and blocks within sites with ozone and/or acidic rain are assumed to be random effects in the mixed models. (The individual site analyses have already indicated that family within sites by ozone and/or acidic rain interactions are unimportant.) The components of variance due to these additional random effects are estimated and taken into account in the estimation of the fixed parameters and, more important, in the measures of precision of the estimates.

Two mixed models are used, a bivariate polynomial response model that is linear in all parameters and a nonlinear model that uses the Weibull function to characterize the response to ozone. (The Weibull function has been used successfully to model the response of crop plants to ozone, Lesser et al., 1990.) For comparison, the fixed-model polynomial response surface is also fitted. We describe the fixed model first.

The fixed-effects model using polynomial response functions for ozone and acidic rain had the form

$$Y_{ijklm} = \beta_{im} + \beta_1(ozone)_k + \beta_{11}(ozone)_k^2 + \beta_2(rain)_l$$
$$+ \beta_a(X_a)_{ijkl} + \beta_b(X_b)_{ijklm} + \beta_d(X_d)_{ijkl} + \epsilon_{ijklm}, \qquad (5)$$

where β_{im} is the intercept for the mth family at the ith site. The subscripts j, k, and l identify the replication, ozone treatment, and acidic rain treatment, respectively. The covariates X_a, X_b, and X_d are as defined previously. All effects are assumed to be fixed; randomness arises only from the ϵ_{ijklm} values. The model as written assumes that the response is quadratic to ozone and linear to acidic rain. The degree of polynomial needed for each variable was tested and the model modified accordingly, including the extension in the obvious way to incorporate ozone × rain interactions if needed. A weighted analysis was used as discussed previously.

The mean function for the mixed polynomial response model is

$$\mu_{ijklm} = \mu + g(ozone_k) + \beta_1(rain)_l + \beta_a(X_a)_{ijkl}$$
$$+ \beta_b(X_b)_{ijklm} + \beta_d(X_d)_{ijkl}, \qquad (6)$$

where $g(ozone_k)$ is a linear or quadratic polynomial, as determined by the data, in the ozone dose metric. A linear response to acidic rain is used in all cases; there was not sufficient response to acidic rain to detect a quadratic response or to fit a nonlinear model. The random portion of the mixed polynomial model included, in addition to the random error ϵ_{ijklm}, random effects due to sites, families within sites, blocks within sites, and all interactions of these effects with rain and ozone. The random residuals ϵ_{ijklm} are assumed to have common variances σ_i^2 within sites but possibly different among sites. The random effects are assumed to be additive to the mean function.

The mixed-effects nonlinear response model used the Weibull function to characterize the ozone response. In this model, the mean function is given by

$$\mu_{ijklm} = \{\mu + \beta_1(rain)_l + \beta_a(X_a)_{ijkl}$$

$$+ \beta_b(X_b)_{ijklm} + \beta_4(X_d)_{ijkl}\}H(x_k; \omega, \lambda) \tag{7}$$

$$= T_{ijklm}H(x_k; \omega, \lambda), \tag{8}$$

where $H(x_k; \omega, \lambda) = \exp[-(x_k/\omega)^\lambda]$, the Weibull response function with ozone dose x_k. The quantity T_{ijklm} is, conceptually, the mean response when the ozone dose is zero; the effect of increasing ozone is to decrease response by the multiplicative factor $H(\cdot)$. The behavior of the Weibull response function is described by Rawlings and Cure (1985). The model allowed for the same random effects as in the mixed polynomial model, and the random effects are assumed to be additive to the mean response model.

The mixed-effects regressions implicitly allowed for differential weighting by site by allowing each site to have its own error variance, σ_i^2. Estimates of variance components may be negative. Random effects that yielded negative estimates of variance components were dropped from the model and the reduced model was refitted. The procedures use the estimated variance components to construct an estimated variance–covariance matrix for $\mathbf{Y}$, the inverse of which is used as the weighting matrix in estimated generalized least-squares estimation (EGLS) of the fixed parameters. The standard errors of estimates of the fixed effects or functions of the fixed effects are obtained from the algebra of the EGLS estimation and using the estimated Var($\mathbf{Y}$) as the truth.

4   RESULTS

4.1   Residual Analysis

The analyses by site showed that the error variances were very heterogeneous for both variables (see Tables 3 and 4). Bartlett's chi-square test of homogeneity (Steel and Torrie, 1980) gave highly significant values of the 98.2 and 74.6 with 5 degrees of freedom for biomass and diameter, respectively. Plots of the residuals against fitted values from the fixed-model analyses of the original variables did not show any obvious problems (Figures 2a and 3a) but the normal plots tended to show some distinct curvature, particularly for biomass (Figures 2b and 3b).

The search for a power transformation on each response variable that would cause the variable more nearly to satisfy the model assumptions gave the resid-

Table 6   Residual Sums of Squares ($\times 10^{-2}$) by Site and the Pooled Across-Sites Residual Mean Square for Chosen Box–Cox Transformations (λ) of Total Aboveground Biomass[a]

Transf. λ	Site						Pooled MS
	1 (11)[b]	2 (35)	3 (19)	4 (32)	5 (35)	6 (35)	(167)
−1.0	1,136[c]	45,692	28,585	519,284	1,645	19,453	3,687
−0.5	1,586	15,033	18,742	126,310	2,422	13,747	1,065
0.0	2,329	5,657	14,146	48,529	3,983	11,398	515
0.5	3,629	2,420	12,531	36,386	7,290	10,925	438
1.0	6,048	1,154	13,066	53,631	14,762	11,854	602

[a]Error b sums of squares for all sites except site 4, for which error a is used. Site 4 had data on only one family for biomass.
[b]Degrees of freedom for each sum of squares shown in parentheses.
[c]Boxed numbers identify the Box–Cox transformation giving the minimum residual sum of squares for each site and the overall "best" transformation based on the minimum pooled residual mean square.

ual sums of squares shown in Table 6 for biomass and Table 7 for diameter. The residual sums of squares are given by site and pooled across sites for $\lambda = (1, 0.5, 0, -0.5, -1)$, where λ is the power parameter in the Box–Cox family of transformations. Since a combined analysis is intended, the same transformation must be used over all sites for a given variable, so the residual sum of squares pooled over sites was used as the criterion for choice of transformation. The transformation suggested by the pooled mean square error was never the best transformation for every site, but overall, the Box–Cox analysis suggested the square-root transformation for biomass but no transformation for diameter.

Table 7   Residual Sums of Squares by Site and the Pooled Across-Sites Residual Mean Square for Chosen Box–Cox Transformations (λ) of Increment of Diameter Growth

Transf. λ	Site						Pooled MS
	1 (11)[a]	2 (35)	3 (19)	4 (107)	5 (35)	6 (35)	(242)
−1.0	130[b]	316	1,318	9,645	282	687	51
−0.5	166	202	1,211	5,147	320	640	32
0.0	213	131	1,151	3,447	372	613	24
0.5	275	87	1,129	2,772	444	603	22
1.0	359	58	1,139	2,549	548	605	22

[a]Degrees of freedom for each sum of squares shown in parentheses.
[b]Boxed numbers identify the Box–Cox transformation giving the minimum residual sum of squares for each site and the overall "best" transformation based on the minimum pooled residual mean square.

The analyses of variance for the individual sites were repeated using the suggested transformation for biomass. The transformation may have produced slight improvements in the residuals plots (see Figures 2c,d for biomass), but the error variances remained very heterogeneous. Bartlett's chi-square test of homogeneity gave a highly significant value of 68.6 for biomass, only slightly smaller than 98.2 obtained with the original data. Since a transformation would not stabilize the variances, weighted analyses (Rawlings, 1988) of the original variables seemed to be the appropriate approach. As a final check, the residuals from the weighted analyses of the original variables were plotted and appeared to give more satisfactory normal plots for both variables than were obtained from either the original unweighted data or the transformed data (see Figures 2e,f and 3c,d for biomass and diameter, respectively). Thus, the dose–response models will be fitted to the original data using weighted analyses where the weights are determined from the individual site error variances.

The analyses by site (Tables 3 and 4) also showed that there was no convincing evidence for interactions between the pollutants and genetic families. When both variables are considered, only one out of 33 pollutant by family interactions (acidic rain $\times$ family for the variable diameter) is significant ($p \leq 0.05$); this is about the number of significant results one would expect if the null hypotheses were true. The main effects of genetic families were significant ($p \leq 0.05$) at three sites for diameter and at one site for biomass. These results provide justification for using dose–response models that allow for different levels of growth (different intercepts) for the genetic families but require a common response over families to ozone and acidic rain pollution. Neither variable showed any significant interaction ($p \leq 0.05$) between the two pollutants at any site. Finally, every covariate was significant ($p \leq 0.05$) at one or more sites and, for consistency, all covariates were retained in all subsequent analyses.

4.2 Dose–Response Models

The estimates of the parameters and their standard errors for the fixed-effects model are given in Table 8 for biomass and diameter growth. The response is quadratic for ozone and linear for acidic rain for both variables. For diameter growth, there is a significant ozone linear $\times$ rain linear interaction.

The estimates of the fixed parameters, the variance components, and the standard errors for the mixed-effects polynomial response model are shown in Table 9. As with the fixed model, the response is quadratic to ozone and linear to acidic rain. However, the mixed model did not detect a significant ozone $\times$ rain interaction. The mixed-effects nonlinear response model estimates are shown in Table 10.

The primary reason for emphasizing the mixed-model approach for combining a series of experiments is to recognize the increased uncertainty that accompanies the broader inference. Thus, while the response curves are of interest,

Table 8 Parameter Estimates (and Standard Errors[a]) for the Fixed-Effects Polynomial Regression Model for Total Aboveground Biomass and Incremental Diameter Growth Obtained from Estimated Weighted Least Squares with Separate Site–Family Intercepts and Common Response to Ozone, Acidic Rain, and Covariates

Parameter	Biomass		Diameter	
Intercepts (site/family)				
1/15-23	1200	(63)	47.01	(1.52)
1/15-91	1062	(63)	43.67	(1.52)
2/2-4	307	(21)	22.63	(0.47)
2/4-13	293	(21)	22.44	(0.47)
2/2-2	305	(21)	23.16	(0.47)
2/4-11	275	(21)	21.10	(0.47)
3/8-103	796	(77)	36.69	(2.25)
3/8-130	806	(77)	38.21	(2.25)
3/8-80	864	(77)	39.86	(2.25)
4/1-529[b]			36.28	(0.92)
4/7-107[b]			33.18	(0.92)
4/7-33[b]			34.94	(0.92)
4/8-103	846	(73)	34.76	(0.92)
5/243-56	1088	(58)	43.03	(1.10)
5/106-56	1115	(55)	43.47	(1.08)
5/6-56	1194	(55)	45.19	(1.08)
5/M-114	1128	(57)	44.12	(1.11)
6/AR-218	717	(50)	33.33	(1.13)
6/AR-146	889	(50)	38.23	(1.13)
6/TX-S2PE3	741	(50)	36.63	(1.13)
6/TX-S3PE9	791	(50)	35.32	(1.13)
Ozone linear	0.317	(0.131)	0.0120	(0.0028)
Ozone quadratic	−0.0012	(0.0002)	−0.000039	(0.000005)
Acidic rain	−38.61	(8.22)	−2.085	(0.323)
Ozone linear × rain			0.0028	(0.0011)
X_a	3.68	(0.54)	1.53	(0.18)
X_b	3.07	(0.52)	1.45	(0.21)
X_d	1069	(136)	14.00	(0.82)

[a]Standard errors are computed from the residual mean square, which assumes that all effects are fixed effects; that is, the split-plot error structure is not taken into account.
[b]These families at site 4 were not measured for TAGB.

comparisons of measures of precision between the fixed model and the two mixed models are of primary importance.

Comparison of the variance components for both mixed models (Tables 9 and 10) shows that the error variances and the site component of variance dominate in both cases. For biomass, the site component of variance is slightly larger

Table 9 Parameter Estimates (and Standard Errors) for the Mixed-Effects Polynomial Regression Model for Total Aboveground Biomass and Incremental Diameter Growth Obtained from Modified Maximum Likelihood Estimation of variance Components and Estimated Generalized Least-Squares Estimation of Fixed Parameters[a]

Parameter	Biomass		Diameter	
Fixed parameters				
Intercept	862	(133)	36.7	(3.6)
Ozone linear	0.104	(0.297)	0.0084	(0.0069)
Ozone quadratic	−0.00089	(0.00044)	−0.00003	(0.00001)
Acidic rain	−60.22	(16.64)	−1.393	(0.375)
X_a	3.23	(0.63)	1.15	(0.27)
X_b	3.02	(0.49)	1.49	(0.18)
X_d	1075	(103)	11.34	(1.01)
Variance components				
Site	93,808	(60,897)	63.82	(43.39)
Block (site)	—	—	4.35	(3.36)
Family (site)	7	(253)	1.25	(0.68)
Site × rain	745	(1,300)	0.49	(0.72)
Site × ozone	3,081	(2,363)	2.58	(1.47)
Site × ozone × rain	536	(1,266)	—	—
Family × rain(site)	388	(435)	—	—
Blk × ozone × rain (site)	2,187	(1,182)	3.96	(1.15)
Error (site 1)	81,123	(17,782)	21.98	(5.43)
Error (site 2)	2,919	(520)	2.02	(0.34)
Error (site 3)	75,611	(14,765)	37.12	(7.55)
Error (site 4)	151,473	(30,890)	23.04	(2.44)
Error (site 5)	74,386	(11,351)	24.74	(3.87)
Error (site 6)	52,159	(7,941)	20.62	(3.22)

[a]A common response to ozone, acidic rain, and covariates was required , and random effects that gave negative estimates of variances were dropped from the model.

than the average of the error variances; for diameter, the site component is more than twice the average of the error variances. The site component of variance will have a major impact on measures of precision for any inferential statement about the amount of growth expected in different sites. (Recall that "site" differences in this study include pine species differences and management practice differences as well as all the usual environmental and soil factors associated with sites. These differences actually broaden the base of inference.) The other components of variance tend to be much smaller, but there is a meaningful (larger than its standard error) site × ozone interaction component of variance for both variables in both mixed models. This component and the other interaction components of variance involving ozone and/or rain will contribute to the uncertainty of inferences regarding the impact of the pollutants. These comparisons of precision are more easily seen by looking at compara-

Table 10   Parameter Estimates (and Standard Errors) for the Mixed-Effects Weibull Nonlinear Response Model for Total Aboveground Biomass and Incremental Diameter Growth Obtained from Modified Maximum Likelihood Estimation of Variance Components and Estimated Generalized Least-Squares (EGLS) Estimation of Fixed Parameters[a]

Parameter	Biomass		Diameter	
Fixed parameters:				
Intercept	862	(127)	36.87	(3.39)
Acidic rain	−69.97	(19.38)	−1.53	(0.42)
X_a	3.65	(0.71)	1.24	(0.29)
X_b	3.36	(0.56)	1.54	(0.18)
X_d	1,181	(119)	11.67	(1.06)
Omega (ω)	892	(150)	939	(108)
Lambda (λ)	2.42	(0.77)	3.69	(0.99)
Variance components				
Site	93,702	(60,907)	63.44	(43.11)
Block(site)	—	—	4.59	(3.50)
Site × rain	1,028	(1,495)	0.59	(0.78)
Site × ozone	2,660	(2,085)	2.51	(1.47)
Site × rain × ozone	541	(1,306)	—	—
Family(site)	231	(461)	1.26	(0.68)
Family × rain (site)	407	(501)	—	—
Blk × ozone × rain (site)	2,076	(1,256)	4.19	(1.44)
Error (site 1)	81,663	(17,902)	22.02	(5.48)
Error (site 2)	3,490	(857)	2.03	(0.35)
Error (site 3)	76,464	(14,962)	36.67	(7.62)
Error (site 4)	151,429	(30,882)	23.02	(2.46)
Error (site 5)	75,383	(11,539)	24.71	(3.87)
Error (site 6)	51,830	(7,953)	20.67	(3.24)

[a]A common response to ozone, acidic rain, and covariates was required and all random effects giving negative estimates of variances were dropped from the model.

ble predictions and their respective measures of precision based on the three models.

As one would expect, the shape of the fitted response functions obtained from the three models are very similar (Figures 4 and 5 for biomass and diameter, respectively). However, the differences in estimated precision can be large, as illustrated by relative widths of the confidence limits on the estimated mean responses. Figures 4a and 5a show the treatment means for the six sites, and the fitted polynomial responses to ozone and 95% confidence limits (pointwise) on the estimated means for three of the sites as estimated by the fixed-effects model. The responses to ozone are the same for all sites; only the heights of the curves change, depending on the site-specific intercepts; there were no significant site × ozone interactions. Of particular note are the very narrow confidence bands obtained with the fixed-effects model. In contrast, the 95% confidence

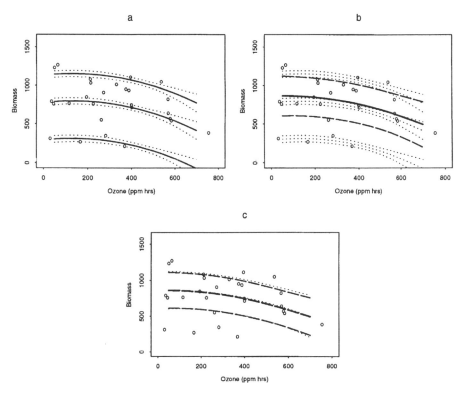

Figure 4. Fitted response equations and 95% pointwise confidence interval estimates of mean response for total aboveground biomass estimated from the three response models. The observed treatment means are shown as small open circles. (*a*) Fitted polynomial response for three of the six sites at vwph = 0 (solid lines) estimated from the fixed model with their 95% confidence interval estimates (dotted lines). (*b*) Fitted polynomial response estimated from the mixed model (dark solid line) and the 95% confidence interval estimates (dark dashed lines) superimposed on the fixed polynomial response. (*c*) Fitted nonlinear response estimated from the mixed model and the 95% confidence interval estimates (dark lines) superimposed on the mixed polynomial response.

limits (pointwise) on the estimated means obtained from the mixed polynomial model (Figures 4*b* and 5*b*) and from the mixed nonlinear model (Figures 4*c* and 5*c*) are much broader. In Figures 4*b* and 5*b*, the polynomial response equations from the mixed model and the 95% pointwise confidence limits have been superimposed on Figures 4*a* and 5*a* for direct comparison. The greater width of the confidence limits for the mixed models reflects the added uncertainty that results from extending the inference on the dose–response relationships to the populations of environmental conditions and genetic material.

Direct comparisons of the results from the two mixed-effects models are shown in Figures 4*c* and 5*c*. (The lighter dotted lines are the results for the polynomial; the darker lines are the results for the Weibull model.) In general, the responses and confidence bands are very similar for the two mixed models

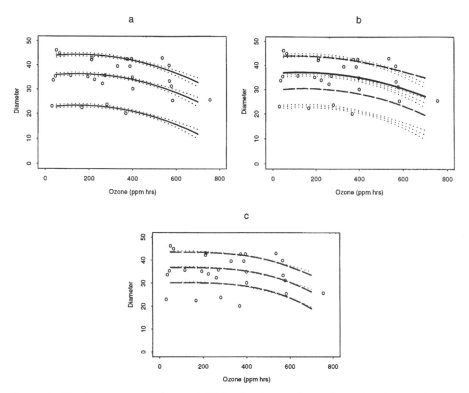

Figure 5. Fitted response equations and 95% pointwise confidence interval estimates of mean response for increment of diameter growth estimated from the three response models. The observed treatment means are shown as small open circles. (*a*) Fitted polynomial response for three of the six sites at vwph = 0 (solid lines) estimated from the fixed model with their 95% confidence interval estimates (dotted lines). (*b*) Fitted polynomial response estimated from the mixed model (dark solid line) and the 95% confidence interval estimates (dark dashed lines) superimposed on the fixed polynomial response. (*c*) Fitted nonlinear response estimated from the mixed model and its 95% confidence interval estimates (dark lines) superimposed on the mixed polynomial response.

with these data. The similarity in the width of the confidence intervals reflects the similarity of the estimates of the dominant variance components (Tables 9 and 10).

The differences in level of precision *for the estimated mean response* differed greatly depending on whether one viewed the model as fixed or mixed. Not all comparisons or estimates will show this degree of change in precision in shifting from a fixed to a mixed model. Statements about mean response for a random environment will include the large site component of variance in its measure of uncertainty. On the other hand, some comparisons of interest will be essentially within-site comparisons and will not involve the site component of variance in the measures of precision. To illustrate this point, the estimated *changes* in response due to increasing ozone from 50 ppm hours to higher levels (200,

Table 11   Estimated Changes (and Standard Errors) in Total Aboveground Biomass and Increment of Diameter Growth for Each of the Three Fitted Responses due to Increasing Ozone Exposure from Ozone = 50 to the Specified Amount

Ozone (ppm hrs)	Polynomial Fixed Model		Polynomial Mixed Model		Weibull Mixed Model	
Total Aboveground Biomass						
200	3	(15)	−18	(30)	−22	(19)
400	−76	(21)	−104	(45)	−115	(41)
600	−251	(42)	−262	(52)	−274	(49)
Incremental Diameter Growth						
200	0.335	(0.251)	0.095	(0.720)	−0.122	(0.144)
400	−1.945	(0.359)	−1.950	(1.076)	−1.550	(0.790)
600	−7.342	(0.667)	−6.477	(1.238)	−6.433	(1.203)

400, and 600 ppm hours), and their standard errors, were computed for each of the three models (Table 11). The estimated changes differ somewhat, but the primary interest, again, is in comparison of the standard errors. The standard crrors cstimatcd from the fixed-effects model, with one exception, are smaller than those obtained from the mixed-effects models, but the relative differences in the standard errors between the fixed and mixed models are much less for estimating change than for estimating mean response.

5   CONCLUSIONS

When the objective of a series of studies is to make inferences over some population of conditions, it is important that the increased uncertainty that naturally accompanies the broader inference be reflected in the associated measures of confidence. Results from classical fixed-effects models are appropriate when the inference is restricted to the conditions of that particular experiment. For the broader inference, however, the level of confidence in the estimates generally will be overstated by the fixed-effects model.

In this study it has been assumed that the intent of the research is to quantify the response of pine seedlings in the southeastern United States to ozone and acidic deposition. Accordingly, the sites, species, and genetic families used are regarded as a random sampling of the southeastern environments and pine material. This case study has demonstrated the degree to which the standard errors of the estimates may be underestimated by the classical fixed-model analyses. The confidence interval estimates of the mean responses estimated from either of the mixed models were several times broader than those from the fixed model. The major component contributing to these broader intervals was the "among-site" component of variance. These broad confidence intervals are consistent with the impression that one would have of a relatively low predictability of *mean response* for another unobserved site simply from observing the large differences in the six individual-site response curves obtained from the fixed model. (The three response curves shown in Figures 4*a* and 5*a* span the range of responses for the six sites.) Unfortunately, the fixed-model measures of precision do not take into account this component of variance.

At the same time, this case study has demonstrated that not all quantities or comparisons of interest automatically suffer low precision from the broader inference. The measures of precision for estimated *changes* in response due to changing levels of ozone were very similar for the fixed and mixed models. This is due to the fact that only those components of variance arising from interactions between random effects and ozone levels (and the random error variance components) enter into these measures of precision, and in this case study these interaction components of variance were relatively minor. Nevertheless, the important point is that mixed model analyses yield estimates of the components of variance, and then appropriately use these to estimate fixed effects and their standard errors.

The validity of the measures of precision obtained from a mixed-model analysis will depend on the adequacy with which the experiments sampled the populations for which inferences are intended. In this case the series of experiments should have randomly sampled the reference populations of environmental conditions and genetic families representing pine production in the southeast. There are certainly problems with this assumption in these studies, as will always be the case when, for example, research sites are chosen for any specific reason, such as convenience or location of the research facilities. Further, random sampling of temporal variation in environments is never possible. Thus, the environments sampled by a series of experiments almost always cannot be regarded as truly random. While one can control to some extent the sampling of locations over a particular geographical region, one must be content with some kind of restricted sampling of locations and simply hope that the environments encountered over the time span of the experiments are reasonably representative. To the extent that the sample of environments is not representative, estimates of variance components will be biased, as will the resulting measures of precision from a mixed-model analysis. Nevertheless, the measures of precision obtained from the mixed-model analysis will be more conservative and probably more realistic for the broader inference. Of course, statements about the degree of certainty of an inference should be tempered by the inadequacies in the sampling of the population of random effects.

ACKNOWLEDGMENTS

These analyses and research were supported by funds provided by the Southeastern Forest Experiment Station, Southern Commercial Forest Research

Cooperative of the Forest Response Program. The Forest Response program, part of the National Acid Precipitation Assessment Program, is jointly sponsored by the U.S. Department of Agriculture Forest Service, U.S. Environmental Protection Agency, and the National Council of the Paper Industry for Air and Stream Improvement. This report has not been subject to Environmental Protection Agency or Forest Service policy review and should not be construed to represent the policies of either agency or of the National Council of the Paper Industry for Air and Stream Improvement.

SOFTWARE NOTES AND REFERENCES

Parameter estimates for the mixed-effects polynomial models were obtained by iterating between modified maximum likelihood estimation of variance components and *estimated generalized least-squares* estimation of the fixed-effects parameters (Giesbrecht, 1984). Estimation for mixed models using the nonlinear Weibull dose–response function required the iterative use of nonlinear estimation of the fixed parameters in the model and modified maximum likelihood estimation of the variance components (Gumpertz, 1991).

Giesbrecht, F. G. 1984. *MIXMOD, a SAS Procedure for Analyzing Mixed Models*, Institute of Statistics Mimeograph Series 1659. Raleigh, NC.: North Carolina State University.

Gumpertz, M. L. 1991. *NLINVC User's Guide*, Institute of Statistics Mimeograph Series 1991. Raleigh, N.C.: North Carolina State University.

QUESTIONS AND PROBLEMS

1. The Box–Cox power family of transformations attempts to find a transformation of the response variable that will satisfy three objectives: make the expectation vector correct [i.e., satisfy $E(Y) = X\beta$ for the defined model] and satisfy the assumptions of normality and homogeneous variance. These multiple objectives are not always compatible. To illustrate this dilemma, generate a set of $n = 40$ observations using the expectation function $E(Y) = 10 + 1.8x - 0.025x$ for $x = 1, \ldots, 40$ and using random normal residuals with $\sigma_i = x_i/10$. Now, regress Y to X assuming a linear model in X and constant variance. Observe the pattern of the residuals. Find the Box–Cox power transformation on Y that minimizes the residual sum of squares. Does the transformation make the variances more homogeneous or linearize the relationship? Is it possible for a power transformation to do both in this case?

2. Assume that you have a balanced randomized complete block design with t treatments and b blocks conducted in sites. Specify the effects model for the combined analysis, including effects for site and site $\times$ treatment inter-

actions. Determine the expectations of the mean squares for a model (a) where all effects are fixed and (b) where treatment effects are fixed but block effects, site effects, and site × treatment interaction effects are considered random. In the derivation of the expectations, assume that the site × interaction random effects are constrained to sum to zero over treatments. Discuss the implications of the expectations on the test of significance of the null hypothesis of no treatment effects for both models, and how these differences relate to the broader inference implied by the assumption of random site effects.

3. For the situation described under Question 2, derive the variance of a treatment mean (averaged over blocks and sites) for each of the two models. Derive the variance of the difference between two treatment means for each of the two models. Pay particular attention to how the components of variance enter into the variances of the treatment mean and of the difference between two treatment means, and how these results relate to the implied inferences.

4. The series of experiments considered in this case study differed in several management factors that would not normally be considered part of the sampling of environments. Discuss the appropriateness of including this variation in management practices as part of the "environmental" sampling in light of the intended inference. What would be the effect of standardizing all management practices to a common procedure on the precision of the estimates? On the generality of the inference?

Geostatistical Estimates of Scallop Abundance

Mark D. Ecker and James F. Heltshe

1 MOTIVATION AND BACKGROUND

Since 1982, the Northeast Fisheries Science Center of the National Marine Fisheries Service (NMFS) has been conducting stratified random surveys on the continental shelf off the northeastern United States to monitor scallop abundance. Many sampling techniques, including stratified random sampling, begin with the assumption that the samples are spatially independent. However, in the biological sciences, data are often positively correlated because points close in space are likely to have similar responses. The geostatistical technique of kriging is attractive for spatial data because it incorporates this spatial correlation into its estimates.

In this chapter, kriging is applied to scallop abundance data. Contour maps of abundance estimates along with their respective variances are produced. The results are compared to estimates based on the standard approach of estimation within preset strata defined by ocean depth. Since kriging works best with approximately normally distributed data, a natural logarithmic transformation of catch (plus one) was employed. The "plus one" transformation, used because of many zero catches, produced biased estimates of the regional means. Because of this bias and the skewed distribution of the scallop data, the median was suggested as a more appropriate measure of central tendency. Since the transformed data were normally distributed, confidence intervals were constructed for the median. Finally, total catch in the New York Bight was examined for three successive years (1989–1991). Year-to-year changes were explored.

Kriging, a computer-intense procedure with a recent history, arises from the regionalized variable theory of Matheron (1963). A regionalized variable, which has both a magnitude and direction, is used to produce estimates for localized

Case Studies in Biometry, Edited by Nicholas Lange, Louise Ryan, Lynne Billard, David Brillinger, Loveday Conquest, and Joel Greenhouse.
ISBN 0-471-58885-7 © 1994 John Wiley & Sons, Inc.

blocks or points rather than the entire region under study. Kriging has been applied in numerous fields. In geology, Starks et al. (1982) used kriging to estimate coal reserves in Greene County, Pennsylvania and also in southwestern Illinois. Krige and Magri (1982) analyzed the Loraine gold mine in South Africa using lognormal kriging and linear kriging (simple and ordinary kriging). In pollution monitoring, Bromenshenk et al. (1985) assessed Puget Sound, Washington with honeybees for such contaminants as arsenic, cadmium, and fluoride. Kriged results showed that the greatest concentrations of these elements were near urbanized areas. Eynon and Switzer (1983) kriged rainfall acidity data over the eastern United States. Their kriged results showed that the lowest pH levels (most acidic) were over northern New England. Gilbert and Simpson (1985) used lognormal kriging to estimate contamination at a nuclear test site in Nevada. As expected, the highest levels of pollutants were near the initial blast (ground zero). In the hydrosciences, Aboufirassi and Mariño (1983) used universal kriging to produce water table estimates at an aquifer in Morocco. Webster (1984) used multistage sampling and kriging to identify components of spatial variation in the soil sciences. Recently, kriging had been applied to remote sensing (Curran, 1988), where it was used to characterize the earth's surface. In the field of ecology, Robertson (1987) applied kriging to *Rhodomonas* data in the epilimnion of a temperate hardwater lake in southwestern Michigan.

2   DATA

The NMFS stratification plan of the Atlantic Ocean resulted in 78 overall strata. The strata were identified primarily by the middle two digits, and all strata numbers begin with the number "6". When the International Court of Justice partitioned the Georges Bank into Canadian and American sections in 1984, the easternmost strata were divided with a fourth digit assigned either a zero or a 1, respectively, to these affected strata.

In each stratum, sample points were chosen in proportion to the area of the strata with the provision that at least two samples were taken to allow a variance computation. These points were randomly selected within each stratum, with approximately 450 sample locations chosen for the entire region. For each sample point, location (latitude and longitude), water depth, bottom temperature, weather, and sea conditions were recorded before the dredge began. However, not all of this information was used in the present analysis.

The scallop data set collected during the 1990 survey cruise by the *R/V Oregon II* was used for this study. For scallops, the five areas of principal concern and their corresponding strata are seen in Figure 1. The U.S. and Canadian sections of the Georges Bank were combined into the Eastern Georges Bank. Also, since the Virginia–North Carolina region had only six samples, they were included with the Delmarva Peninsula data. The NMFS had determined some tows to be inaccurate due to gear malfunctions (flips, breakages, etc.). Hence, these trawls had been eliminated from the database. A display of

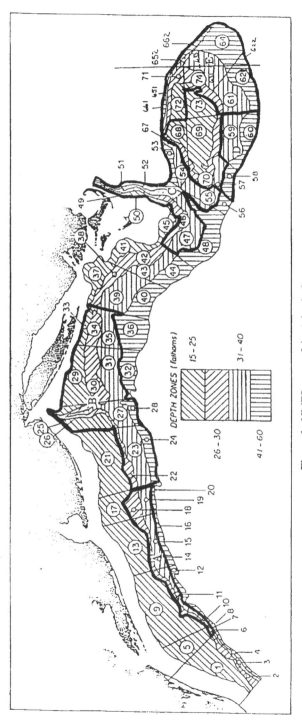

Figure 1. NMFS strata of the Atlantic Ocean.

Region	Strata
A. Delmarva Peninsula	6, 7, 10, 11, 14, 15, 18, 19
B. New York Bight	22–31, 33–35
C. South Channel of GB	46, 47, 49–55
D. Southern Part of GB	58–60
E. Eastern Georges Bank	61, 621, 622, 631, 632, 64, 651, 652, 661, 662, 71, 72, 74

Table 1   1990 New York Bight Data

Strata	Sample	Latitude	Longitude	Total Catch	Prerecruits	Recruits
6350	1	40.55	71.55	0	0	0
6310	10	40.02	72.40	13	6	7
6310	12	39.82	72.48	2750	2278	472
6220	105	38.82	73.70	60	32	28
6230	126	39.38	73.12	264	74	190
6350	211	40.45	71.97	3	3	0

the data diskette contents is shown in Table 1. Each line in the table represents the counts of different-sized scallops collected at different locations in the ocean. Note that a total catch of zero is possible.

Scallop counts were obtained using a standardized New Bedford scallop dredge which was 8 feet (2.44 m) wide and had a 2-inch (5.1-cm) ring bag with a 1.5-inch (3.8-cm) liner to catch smaller scallops. Tows were conducted for 15 minutes at a speed of 3.5 knots. A total of 128,073 scallops were caught in 467 sampling tows. Each scallop shell was measured and classified into a 5-mm interval. Any scallop smaller than 70 mm was termed a prerecruit; while 70 mm or larger was a harvestable-sized or recruit scallop. Thus, total catch was defined to be the sum of prerecruits and recruits at any locale. When scallop hauls were large, the catch was subsampled with the appropriate multiplier used to produce a total for the tow (Azarovitz, 1991).

3   METHODS AND MODELS

Kriging is a spatial interpolation technique that estimates the response of an unsampled point, x_p, from a linear combination of surrounding points. Thus,

$$Z(x_p) = \sum_{i=1}^{n} \lambda_i Z(x_i), \tag{1}$$

where $Z(x_p)$ is the desired response at unsampled location $x_p, Z(x_i)$ are the responses at sampled locations x_i, and λ_i are the weights assigned to the n points with the constraint that $\sum_{i=1}^{n} \lambda_i = 1$. With this restriction, kriging is the best linear unbiased estimator (BLUE) since the λ_i are chosen to minimize the mean-squared difference between the actual and predicted (kriging) values. In general, points closer in distance to x_p are given stronger weight in predicting $Z(x_p)$ than those farther away. Before the weights λ_i in equation (1) can be assigned, however, the spatial variability needs to be modeled. Kriging begins with two basic assumptions which Matheron terms the *intrinsic hypothesis*. These assumptions basically imply that the data are sampled from a homogeneous spatial population with an overall mean μ and spatial variability that is the same in all examined directions. First,

$$E[Z(x_i + h) - Z(x_i)] = 0 \qquad (2)$$

for all points in the region and where h is the distance between points. This directly implies that $E[Z(x_i)] = \mu$ for all locations if μ exists. Second,

$$\text{Var}[Z(x_i + h) - Z(x_i)] = E[Z(x_i + h) - Z(x_i)]^2 = 2\gamma(h), \qquad (3)$$

where $\gamma(h)$ is termed the *semivariogram* and is a function of h. If the spatial variability is the same for any direction examined, the region is defined to be isotropic. Anisotropy is present when the spatial variability differs from one direction to another.

A semivariogram can be estimated from the data as follows:

$$\gamma^*(h) = \frac{1}{2N_h} \sum_{i=1}^{N_h} [Z(x_i + h) - Z(x_i)]^2, \qquad (4)$$

where N_h is the number of pairs of sample points h units apart. Theoretical semivariograms are divided into two classes: those with and those without sills. Related to the sill, the range is the distance at which points no longer exhibit an influence upon each other. Thus the points are independent of each other beyond the range. The sill is the response or $\gamma^*(h)$ at this distance. The nugget is the value of $\gamma^*(h)$ when h is zero. In theory this value should be zero; however, two reasons exist to explain why it might not be so. The first is simple measurement error and the second is a microscale effect which results from trying to estimate $\gamma(h)$ at distances smaller than the minimum h observed in the sample. Since the most important part of the semivariogram is the section near the origin, the nugget needs to be estimated well. Unfortunately, in practice, few points tend to be separated by such short distances.

Once a plausible semivariogram has been selected, a cross-validation technique can assess its fit. Cross-validation is analogous to the jackknife technique (Efron, 1982) in that one point is removed and a predicted value based on nearby samples is obtained for the point removed. Predicted values (kriging estimates) can then be compared to actual values by cross-validating all n points. Cross-validation is an especially useful technique when two or more models are under consideration.

By using the judiciously chosen semivariogram, we solve a system of equations to arrive at the weights that are assigned to estimate the response of one unsampled point. Contour maps of scallop abundance can be produced by estimating many unsampled point responses. For a much more thorough review of kriging, see Cressie (1991, pp. 105–150) or Isaaks and Srivastava (1989, pp. 278–322).

The five regions (Eastern Georges Bank, South Channel of Georges Bank, Southern Part of Georges Bank, New York Bight, and the Delmarva Peninsula) were investigated together with three variables (total catch, prerecruit, and recruit). With the subdivision of the Atlantic Ocean into these five areas of interest, the first assumption of the intrinsic hypothesis (2) was validated using historical information.

The results leading to contour maps for total catch in the New York Bight area only are presented in this section. Figure 2 is a spatial plot showing the distribution of the total catch for the New York Bight. A natural logarithm transformation was employed to transform the data to normality. Because of the large number of zero catches, one was added to each data point before taking the natural logarithm. Although normality is not a prerequisite for kriging, it facilitates this geostatistical procedure. Furthermore, the Matheron estimator of the semivariogram (4) is extremely sensitive to outliers. Figure 3 shows a histogram of the transformed data which supported normality of the transformed nonzero catches. The delta distribution (Pennington, 1983) involves lognormal data plus a spike at zero. It represents an appropriate alternative method for calculating

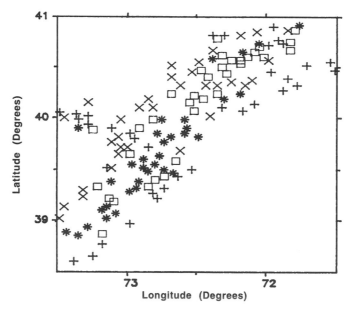

Figure 2. Postplot of 1990 scallop data: total catch in New York Bight.

1st Quartile:	$0.000 \leq + \leq 8.000$
2nd Quartile:	$8.000 < \times \leq 30.000$
3rd Quartile:	$30.000 < \square \leq 114.000$
4th Quartile:	$114.000 < * \leq 7084.000$

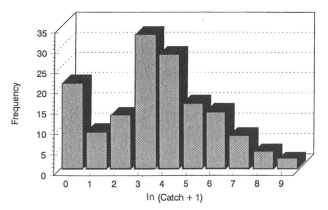

Figure 3. 1990 scallop data for New York Bight.

an unbiased global mean and variance, yet was not pursued here. Figure 4 is a plot of the sample semivariogram as a function of distance. These data suggested an exponential semivariogram with nugget 1.75, sill 5.25, and range of 1.0 degree. Although the nugget was a third of the value of the sill, the model fitted the data accurately. The nugget would most likely be reduced if samples were closer in space.

Next, the second assumption of the kriging process must be assured. Fortunately, an adjustment to counter anisotropy (3) in an area was available. If the region were isotropic, the kriged estimate for an unsampled point x_p would simply be a linear combination of sampled points that were no farther apart than the range. If we construct a circle whose center is the desired point or block to

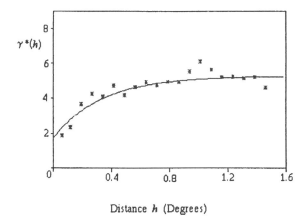

Figure 4. Semivariogram for 1990 scallop data for New York Bight: natural log of total catch. Exponential semivariogram: nugget, 1.75; sill–nugget, 3.5; range, 1.0. Computed from lags: minimum, 0; maximum; 1.45; increment, 0.075.

be kriged while letting the radius of this circle be the range, all sampled points inside this circle would be employed in the construction of $Z(x_p)$. If the region were anisotropic, then instead of a circle we form an ellipse (called the kriging ellipse) whose major radius was oriented in the direction of anisotropy. A diagnostic for anisotropy involves construction of the sample semivariogram for only those pairs of point oriented in the 0, 45, 90, and 135° directions (each ±22.5°). If the region is isotropic, the theoretical omnidirectional semivariogram (cf. Figure 4) would model accurately the semivariogram constructed from any directional subset. After inspection of four bearings (0, 45, 90, and 135°), anisotropy was detected in the 45° direction. Figure 5 shows the results obtained using only points oriented in the 45° direction and clearly illustrates the lack of fit. The spatial plot of the original scaled data (Figure 2) supported less variability among sample points lying along a 45° orientation. Because all semivariogram values in the 45° direction were below the omnidirectional semivariogram in Figure 5, the radius of the kriging ellipse in this direction needed to be longer than the radius of the minor axis (Englund and Sparks, 1991). Thus, the major radius (R major) was 1.0° (approximately 69 miles) and the minor radius (R minor) of the kriging ellipse was 0.8. Finally, a practical rule was employed to save computational time for the scallop database. Since all of the points greater in distance than half of the major and minor radii, respectively, contributed little to $Z(x_p)$, the radii were halved. Figure 6 shows the kriging ellipse used in the calculations, with R major 0.5 and R minor 0.4.

Figures 7 and 8 are the cross-validation results for the chosen semivariogram. Of the 148 standardized residuals (Z = [estimate − ln(catch + 1)]/kriging standard deviation) in Figure 7, none was greater than 3.0 and only three were larger than 2.0. The histogram of these residual z-scores supported normality. The scatter plot in Figure 8 demonstrates that most of the estimates were reasonably close to the actual values, although all of the zero catches were overestimated and most of the higher values were smoothed.

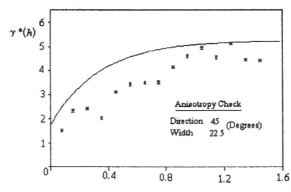

Figure 5. Semivariogram for 1990 scallop data for New York Bight: natural log of total catch.

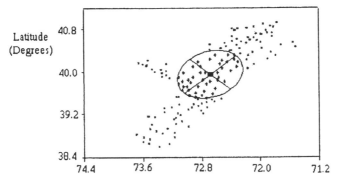

Figure 6. Kriging ellipse for 1990 scallop data for New York Bight.

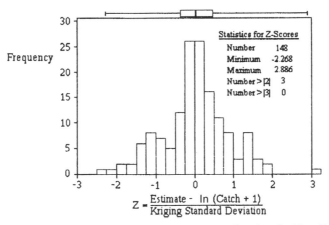

Figure 7. Analysis of cross-validation results for 1990 scallop data for New York Bight.

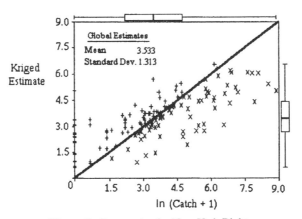

Figure 8. Scatter plot for New York Bight.

A contour map of scallop abundance in the New York Bight is presented in Figure 9. Log-scaled prediction variances could also be attained for any specific locale. Thus, $(1 - \alpha)$ 100% prediction intervals could be constructed using the transformed data for any unsampled point, x_p (Cressie, 1991), according to

$$Z_t(x_p) \pm z_{\alpha/2}\sigma_{K_t}(x_p),$$

where $Z_t(x_p)$ is the kriged estimate (logarithmic scale) and $\sigma_{K_t}(x_p)$ is the prediction standard deviation. The endpoints of this prediction interval could then be back-transformed to the original scale.

Global estimates of the kriging mean, median, and variance for each region were produced by cross-validation. A simple estimate of the back-transformed median can be attained from

$$\text{Median}\,(Y) \;=\; \exp(\bar{x}_t) \,-\, 1,$$

where $\bar{x}_t$ is the mean of the log-transformed data (Bradu and Mundlak, 1970). Since the transformed data are approximately normally distributed, $100(1 - \alpha)\%$ large-sample confidence intervals around the true logscale medians are (Conover, 1971)

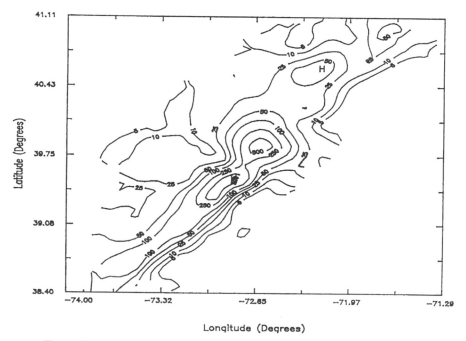

Figure 9. Kriged estimates for 1990 scallop data for New York Bight: total catch.

$$\bar{x}_t \pm z_{\alpha/2} \frac{s_t}{\sqrt{n-1}}.$$

Back-transformed medians with respective confidence intervals can be found in Table 2.

Estimation of the global mean is not quite as simple. The straightforward estimate for μ is

$$E(Y) = \beta \exp(\bar{x}_t + \tfrac{1}{2}s_t^2), \tag{5}$$

where $\bar{x}_t$ and s_t^2 are the sample mean and variance, respectively, of the transformed data and β is calculated as follows to adjust the estimate for bias (Finney, 1941):

$$\beta = 1 - \frac{s_t^2(s_t^2 - 2)}{4n} + \frac{s_t^4(3s_t^4 + 44s_t^2 + 84)}{96n^2}.$$

However, since one was added to each data point, the estimate of the global mean is biased. To assess the degree of this bias, the natural logarithmic scaled

Table 2 NMFS and Kriging Estimates of the Global Median

Variable	Region	N	Kriging Median	95% Confidence Interval for Median by Kriging Lower	Upper	Stratified Random Sampling Median
Catch	East Georges Bank	106	69.0	46.5	102.4	55.4
	New York Bight	148	33.2	26.7	41.4	23.1
	Delmarva Peninsula	68	57.4	46.0	71.7	52.8
	South channel of GB	77	21.8	14.4	32.8	15.7
	South part of GB	32	4.0	2.9	6.3	4.7
Prerecruit	East Georges Bank	106	17.2	11.4	25.8	14.6
	New York Bight	148	12.4	10.9	15.4	9.0
	Delmarva Peninsula	68	7.2	6.2	8.5	6.5
	South channel of GB	77	11.0	7.7	15.4	8.3
	South part of GB	32	0.9	0.7	1.1	0.9
Recruit	East Georges Bank	106	44.7	31.1	64.2	36.6
	New York Bight	148	21.5	17.5	26.4	14.6
	Delmarva Peninsula	68	46.5	38.0	56.8	43.8
	South channel of GB	77	9.5	6.2	14.4	7.8
	South part of GB	32	3.4	2.3	4.8	3.7

estimates of global means and standard deviations are compared in Table 3. NMFS had produced global mean and variance estimates using the same $X = \ln(y+1)$ transformation for comparison. The kriging mean for total catch of the transformed data in the New York Bight is 3.533, compared to 3.183 produced by stratified random sampling.

A $100(1 - \alpha)\%$ large sample confidence interval for μ can be constructed from

$$\bar{x}_t \pm z_{\alpha/2} \frac{s_t}{\sqrt{n}}.$$

This leads to a 95% confidence interval for the transformed global mean of total catch in the New York Bight as 3.321 to 3.745. From equation (5), the back-transformed confidence interval is 65.2 to 99.7. For the transformed data, the estimate for the kriging standard deviation in the New York Bight is 1.317, much lower than is the NMFS estimate of 2.120. Finney (1941) provided the equation to back-transform this standard deviation, but its use was not entirely appropriate, due to the plus one transformation.

Table 3   Comparison of Kriging Estimates to Stratified Random Sampling Estimates in Natural Logarithmic Scale

Variable	Region	N	Kriging Estimates Mean	Std. Dev.	95% Confidence Intervals for μ by Kriging Lower	Upper	Stratified Random Sampling Mean	Std. Dev.
Catch	East Georges Bank	106	4.249	2.035	3.862	4.636	4.032	2.447
	New York Bight	148	3.533	1.317	3.321	3.745	3.183	2.120
	Delmarva Peninsula	68	4.068	0.909	3.852	4.284	3.986	1.451
	South channel of GB	77	3.128	1.749	2.735	3.517	2.816	2.547
	South part of GB	32	1.680	0.889	1.372	1.988	1.745	1.217
Prerecruit	East Georges Bank	106	2.903	2.016	2.519	3.287	2.749	2.422
	New York Bight	148	2.596	1.242	2.340	2.796	2.307	2.053
	Delmarva Peninsula	68	2.110	0.596	1.968	2.252	2.016	1.637
	South Channel of GB	77	2.483	1.407	2.169	2.797	2.231	2.495
	South part of GB	32	0.634	0.252	0.547	0.721	0.665	0.752
Recruit	East Georges Bank	106	3.823	1.852	3.470	4.176	3.628	2.262
	New York Bight	148	3.115	1.214	2.919	3.311	2.745	1.903
	Delmarva Peninsula	68	3.860	0.823	3.664	4.056	3.802	1.350
	South channel of GB	77	2.355	1.684	1.979	2.731	2.170	2.006
	South part of GB	32	1.476	0.814	1.194	1.758	1.539	1.213

4 RESULTS

The first question addressed in this analysis was whether kriging was an appropriate technique for this scallop database. To answer this query, inspection of semivariograms which model spatial variability was required. All theoretical semivariograms for combinations of the five regions and three variables describe the data sufficiently. Thus, kriging was a plausible option. Global kriging estimates for the mean and standard deviation (natural logarithmic scale) for the five regions and three variables are compared to NMFS estimates in Table 3. The 95% confidence intervals for the regional kriging means are also provided. Kriging estimates of global means are reasonably close to NMFS estimates for all variables and regions examined. This closeness further validated kriging as an effective estimation technique for the 1990 scallop database. In all areas, kriging produced lower estimates of the standard deviation than did stratified random sampling. The back-transformed means and confidence intervals are presented in Table 4. Kriging performed extremely well in the Eastern Georges Bank, where 4.249 was the global mean of total catch and 2.035 was the standard deviation. The NMFS mean was 4.032 and standard deviation was 2.447. Back-transformed, the kriging mean was 524.9. Kriging also achieved excellent results in the southern part of Georges Bank. For prerecruits, $\hat{\mu} = 0.634$ and $\hat{\sigma}$ was 0.252, compared to stratified random sampling estimates

Table 4   Back-Transformed Kriging Estimates of Global Means for 1990 Scallop Data

Variable	Region	N	Mean	95% Confidence Intervals for μ	
				Lower	Upper
Catch	East Georges Bank	106	524.9	356.3	773.2
	New York Bight	148	80.6	65.2	99.7
	Delmarva Peninsula	68	87.6	70.6	108.7
	South channel of GB	77	100.3	67.9	148.2
	South part of GB	32	7.8	5.8	10.7
Prerecruit	East Georges Bank	106	131.7	89.7	193.3
	New York Bight	148	28.7	23.5	35.1
	Delmarva Peninsula	68	9.8	8.5	11.3
	South channel of GB	77	31.4	23.0	43.1
	South part of GB	32	1.9	1.8	2.1
Recruit	East Georges Bank	106	243.7	171.3	346.8
	New York Bight	148	46.7	38.4	56.8
	Delmarva Peninsula	68	66.2	54.4	80.5
	South channel of GB	77	41.7	28.6	60 8
	South part of GB	32	6.0	4.5	8.0

of $\hat{\mu} = 0.665$ and $\hat{\sigma} = 0.752$. All kriging estimates for the global mean except in the southern part of Georges Bank are higher than the NMFS estimates.

The strength of kriging lies not only in its ability to produce reliable estimates at a particular location, but also in the production of contour maps of the overall region. Both stratified random sampling and kriging can provide reasonable estimates of global means, medians and variances. However, only kriging can provide prediction intervals at locations different from the specific ones in the original sampling scheme.

Since the original data were highly skewed, perhaps the measure of central tendency utilized should be the median as opposed to the mean. A few large values inflated the mean response; they did not affect the median. Also, the original scaled mean was a function of the transformed variance; cf. equation (5). Thus, when kriging produced lower variance estimates than did stratified

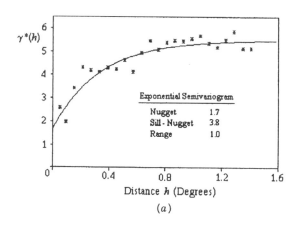

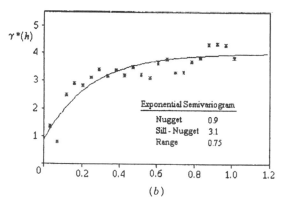

Figure 10. Semivariogram for (a) 1989 and (b) 1991 scallop data for New York Bight: natural log of total catch.

random sampling (cf. Table 3), the back-transformed mean was also smaller. The result was that the kriging global mean was highly affected by a smaller logscale variance. Since confidence intervals could be constructed for the global median, it appeared to be a more appropriate measure of the average response in a region. Table 2 provided estimates of kriging medians with 95% confidence intervals compared with stratified random sample medians for all five regions and three variables.

Another consideration was the applicability of kriging over time. Total catch scallop data in the New York Bight for three consecutive years (1989–1991) were examined. Exponential semivariograms were inferred from samples for each year (Figures 4 and 10). The three years of data were pooled, resulting in a median of 41.5. This value was used to produce a single contour level for each year (Figures 11 to 13) where higher assessments of scallop catches could be found inside the region defined by this median contour. The median was chosen as the arbitrary value to assess year-to-year variability.

Consistent results for the three years were recorded. Exponential theoretical semivariograms best fit the data for each year. The nugget, sill, and the range were all relatively close, respectively, for the three years. A core area of more than 41.5 scallops oriented along a 45° vector was observed for all three years. From the mean and median estimates for the New York Bight in Table 5, the total number of scallops appeared to be decreasing over time. The median estimate fell from 66.1 to 33.2 to 28.5 for the three years; the mean estimate decreased from 176.6 to 80.6 to 63.8 for 1989 to 1991, respectively. This diminishing scallop catch was further evident when directly comparing Figure 11 to Figure 13. The area of 41.5 or more scallops had shrunk from 1989 to 1991.

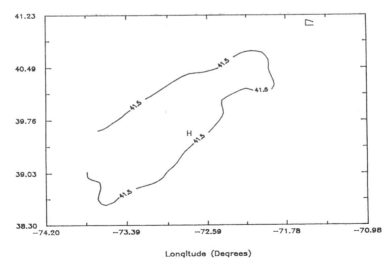

Figure 11. Estimates for 1989 scallop data for New York Bight: total catch.

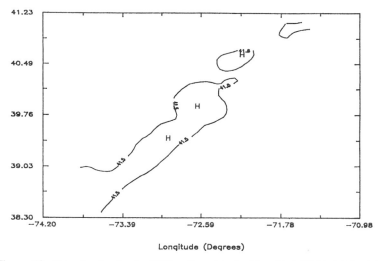

Figure 12. Kriged estimates for 1990 scallop data for New York Bight: total catch.

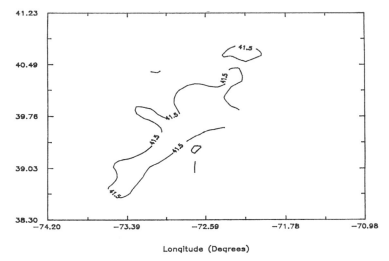

Figure 13. Kriged estimates for 1991 scallop data for New York Bight: total catch.

Table 5 Kriging Estimates for New York Bight 1989–1991

Statistic	1989	1990	1991
Number of samples	161	148	157
Log-scaled data			
Mean	4.191	3.533	3.350
Standard deviation	1.402	1.317	1.270
Original data			
Mean	176.6	80.6	63.8
Median	66.1	33.2	28.5
95% CI for median	(53.2, 82.1)	(26.7, 41.4)	(23.4, 34.8)

5   CONCLUSIONS

Kriging was a plausible technique for analysis of the 1990 scallop database. Semivariograms sufficiently fit the National Marine Fisheries Service data for all five regions and three variables. Contour maps of scallop abundance were produced in these desired regions and global estimates of scallop abundance were developed. In addition to estimates of global means in all areas, kriging produced point estimates for any desired location in a region. Kriging also yielded a lower estimation variance than did the stratified random sampling design. From the mean and median estimates along with contour maps of the median value, scallop abundance in the New York Bight had decreased from 1989 to 1991.

Since the data were approximately lognormally distributed, the median was a better measure of central tendency than was the mean. Valid confidence intervals were constructed for the median response for each variable and region. If only the mean were desired, perhaps stratified random sampling should be retained.

ACKNOWLEDGMENTS

The authors thank everyone at the National Marine Fisheries Service, especially Stephen Clark, Michael Fogarty, Michael Pennington, and Susan Wigley, for their efforts. Also, Michael Pirri's computer expertise was greatly appreciated.

SOFTWARE NOTES AND REFERENCES

The computer package GEO-EAS 1.2.1 (Englund and Sparks, 1991) was employed to produce kriging results. GEO-EAS 1.2.1 is public-domain software compatible with an IBM PC.

Englund, E., and Sparks A. (1991). *GEO-EAS 1.2.1 User's Guide*. Las Vegas, Nev.: United States Environmental Protection Agency.

QUESTIONS AND PROBLEMS

1. Does a symmetric confidence interval make sense for the mean of New York Bight total catch data? Why or why not?

2. If a semivariogram model does not have a sill for some data set, what does that imply about the samples that have been collected?

3. How would the semivariogram look if the data were spatially independent?

4. Construct a 95% interval estimate for the original scaled median if the natural logarithmic mean is 3.725, the log standard deviation is 1.63, and $n = 127$.

5. Produce kriging contour maps of recruit scallop abundance in the New York Bight for 1990.

CHAPTER 7

Survival Analysis for Size Regulation of Atlantic Halibut

Stephen J. Smith, Ken G. Waiwood, and John D. Neilson

1 MOTIVATION AND BACKGROUND

Atlantic halibut (*Hippoglossus hippoglossus*) is the most highly valued ground-fish species on the Atlantic coast of Canada. Landings have peaked at 4031 tons in 1985 but dropped to 1426 tons (provisional landings) in 1991. The landed value in 1991 was approximately 7 million Canadian dollars (personal communication, D. Murphy, Department of Fisheries and Oceans).

A number of conservation measures have been suggested for the bottom trawl and longline fishery, including a minimum size limit for retained halibut. However, a minimum size limit would be effective only if an acceptable proportion of the fish returned to the water survive capture, handling, and release. Neilson et al. (1989) examined the survival of halibut caught by trawls or long-lines, using a live holding facility onboard a research vessel. Commercial practices were simulated during the fishing operations. For halibut less than the proposed limit of 81 cm (32 in), 35% of those caught by otter trawls and 77% of those caught by longline survived on the average more than 48 hours. Significant relationships were found between some of the ancillary factors measured (duration of trawling, maximum depth fished, size of fish, etc.) and the length of time halibut survived in the experiment. The estimates of percent surviving given above would vary according to the conditions present when the fish were brought onboard the vessel. An interim minimum size limit of 81 cm was adopted in 1988 pending the results of an analysis of the effectiveness of the

Case Studies in Biometry, Edited by Nicholas Lange, Louise Ryan, Lynne Billard, David Brillinger, Loveday Conquest, and Joel Greenhouse.
ISBN 0-471-58885-7 © 1994 John Wiley & Sons, Inc.

minimum size limit with respect to enhancing the yield of the halibut fishery (Neilson and Bowering, 1989).

Neilson et al. (1989) used parametric proportional hazards models (Lawless, 1982) to assess the effects of the ancillary factors on the survival times of fish held in onboard tanks. In this chapter we compare parametric and semiparametric proportional hazards models applied to a subset of these data. We also apply diagnostic methods for testing distributional assumptions and proportional hazards assumptions, and to identify influential data points. The conclusions reached by Neilson et al. (1989) under parametric models are compared with those obtained from semiparametric proportional hazards models.

2 DATA

Halibut were collected on 32 bottom trawl sets (422 fish, bottom depth range 83 to 292 m) and on five strings of longline gear (48 fish, bottom depth range was 210 to 300 m) during the experimental fishing operation in the area of Sable Island Gulley (43°56′N, 58°58′W) from June 29 to July 7, 1987. The Western IIA bottom trawl, the standard trawl used in surveys of groundfish species (Halliday and Koeller, 1981), was used with the 20-mm codend liner removed. Standard longline gear was employed, and a fisherman familiar with halibut longlining techniques was contracted to be in charge of this aspect of the fishing operations. Additional details on shipboard procedure may be found in Waiwood (1988) and Neilson et al. (1989).

The measured response for each fish was the elapsed time in hours between placing the fish in the holding tank and death. A common feature of survival studies is that some animals are removed from the experiment before they die and their fate is unknown. Limited holding facilities onboard the research vessel necessitated the occasional removal of live fish after 48 hours from the tanks for disposal or release in order to accommodate more experimental animals. All fish surviving past the 50-day duration for the experiment were assigned the maximum survival time of 1200 hours and treated as right-censored observations. The estimation procedures used here to incorporate both uncensored and censored observations assume that censoring is a random process and independent of the covariates used in the analysis.

Covariates collected during the trawl phase of this study included duration of tow, minimum and maximum depth trawled, handling time on deck, weight of the total catch, and length of each halibut caught. Handling time was defined as the elapsed time between bringing the net on deck and placing the halibut in the holding tanks. Although tow duration and handling time were under experimental control, observations for different combinations of depths, total catch, and lengths of fish were obtained on more of an opportunistic basis. As a consequence, none of the fish in the 30-minute tows was less than 57 cm in length, while fish ranged from 29 to 96 cm in the 100 to 120-minute tows. The maximum depths for 30-minute tows were all shallower than those for

Table 1   Representative Display of the Halibut Survival Data File

Observ. No.	Survival Time (min)	Censoring Indicator[a]	Tow Duration (min)	Diff in Depth	Length of Fish (cm)	Handing Time (min)	Total catch ln(weight)
100	353.0	1	30	15	39	5	5.685
101	377.0	1	30	15	38	5	5.685
107	117.0	1	30	15	36	7	5.685
108	29.5	1	100	5	46	26	8.690
109	111.0	1	100	5	44	29	8.690
113	64.0	0	100	10	53	4	5.323
114	156.0	1	100	10	42	4	5.323
115	64.0	0	100	10	57	4	5.323
116	500.0	1	100	10	44	4	5.323
117	131.0	1	100	10	44	4	5.323
118	59.0	0	100	10	48	4	5.323

[a]0 = censored.

the longer tows. In addition, halibut larger than 57 cm in the longer tows were almost always associated with sets which had longer handling times, larger total catches, and deeper depths. Analysis of the data set as a whole resulted in significant interaction terms due to confounded effects. In the original analyses, the trawl data set was partitioned into subsets based on size ranges ($\leq$57 cm or >57 cm) and tow duration, and each subset was analyzed separately. The analyses in this chapter are confined to subsets containing fish less than or equal to 57 cm fish for the short (107 fish) and long tow durations (187 fish). The covariates *handling time* (measured in minutes), total catch (*catch*) and fish length (*length*) are retained here. However, maximum depth has been replaced with the difference between maximum and minimum depth (Δ *depth*) (see Table 1). This difference in depth often had a wider range in any one tow than the range for maximum depths over the whole experiment. Total catch was expressed as the natural logarithm of the weight of the catch to accommodate its skewed distribution on the original scale.

3   METHODS AND MODELS

3.1   Parametric Models for Hazard Rate

Probability models for survival data are usually specified through the *hazard function* $h(t)$, where t indexes time. The hazard function characterizes the instantaneous rate of death in the small interval, say $(t, t + \delta t)$, given that the individual has survived to time t. Given a specific probability density $f(t)$ defined on the positive real line and its associated cumulative distribution function $F(t)$, the hazard function is

$$h(t) = \frac{f(t)}{1 - F(t)} = \frac{f(t)}{S(t)},$$

where $S(t)$ is the *survivorship function*, giving the probability of surviving until time t. Parametric probability distribution functions commonly used to model survival time data include the exponential, Weibull, extreme value (or Gompertz), gamma, and lognormal distributions (Lawless, 1982). The first four of these distributions yield monotonic hazard functions, while the lognormal hazard function is zero when $t = 0$, increases to a maximum, and then decreases to zero again as t increases; such behavior may make the lognormal an unsuitable model for many applications.

Model identification begins with estimating the empirical cumulative hazard function $\hat{H}(t)$. Plots of $\hat{H}(t)$ against t and $\ln \hat{H}(t)$ against $\ln t$ can be used to ascertain the shape of the hazard function and thus which distribution could be used to model the survival data. A linear trend in the plot of $\hat{H}(t)$ versus t indicates a constant hazard rate and thus an exponential distribution. Curvature in this plot and a linear trend in the plot of the logarithms of $\hat{H}(t)$ and t implies a Weibull distribution. Curvature on the logarithmic plot indicates an extreme-value distribution.

Estimates of the $H(t)$ can be obtained from an estimate of the survivorship function $S(t)$ by using the relationship $H(t) = -\ln S(t)$. A common estimator of the survivorship function is the product-limit or Kaplan–Meier estimate (Lawless, 1982, pp. 71–79), defined as

$$\hat{S}(t) = \prod_{j:t_j < t} \frac{n_j - d_j}{n_j}, \tag{1}$$

where $t_1, \ldots, t_k$ correspond to the set of distinct failure times observed in the study, n_j is the number of individuals alive and uncensored just prior to time t_j, and d_j is the number of deaths at time t_j.

Relationships between covariates and survival time are often modeled through the hazard function. For the proportional hazard models, covariate effects are assumed to be multiplicative and are expressed as

$$h(t|\mathbf{x}) = h_0(t)g(\mathbf{x}), \tag{2}$$

where $h_0(t)$ is the baseline hazard. The covariate vector $\mathbf{x}$ modifies $h_0(t)$ through $g(\mathbf{x})$. Commonly, $g(\mathbf{x}) = \exp(\mathbf{x}\boldsymbol{\beta})$, where $\boldsymbol{\beta}$ is a vector of unknown coefficients. An exponential form ensures that the hazard rate remains positive for all values of $\mathbf{x}$.

Subsequent discussion will emphasize the Weibull distribution, whose density can be written as

$$f(t) = \alpha t^{\alpha-1} \exp(\mathbf{x}\boldsymbol{\beta} - t^{\alpha}e^{\mathbf{x}\boldsymbol{\beta}}), \qquad t \geq 0, \quad \alpha > 0, \tag{3}$$

where α and $\boldsymbol{\beta}$ are unknown parameters. The hazard function for this distribution is decreasing for $\alpha < 1$ and increasing for $\alpha > 1$. When $\alpha = 1$, the model reduces to an exponential distribution. The exponential and Weibull models can be compared through a test of $H_0: \alpha = 1$ versus $H_A: \alpha \neq 1$. Either a Wald or a likelihood ratio test can be used. The latter can be calculated as the difference between the two model *deviances*, defined as -2 times the difference between the log-likelihood for a maximal model, in which the number of parameters equals the number of observations, and the current model.

3.2 Cox Proportional Hazards Model

In contrast to the methods discussed in the preceding paragraphs, Cox (1972) proposed a semiparametric form for the proportional hazards model. The exponential form of equation (2) is retained; yet estimates for $\boldsymbol{\beta}$ are obtained by finding values that maximize a *partial likelihood* that does not involve $h_0(t)$. Once the $\boldsymbol{\beta}$ has been estimated, $S(t)$ and hence $H(t)$ are readily obtained.

3.3 Regression Diagnostics

Certain observations may have a large influence on parameter estimates. Hoaglin and Welsch (1978) discuss influential data identification and model accommodation methods for standard linear models; McCullagh and Nelder (1989, pp. 406–407) address similar issues for generalized linear models. The influence of any one observation is a function of its residual and its *leverage* (i.e., a measure of how far away it is from the center of design or covariate space). In survival analysis, this covariate space changes as subjects leave the experiment through death or censoring. Schoenfeld (1982), Cain and Lange (1984), and Reid and Crepeau (1985) derived residuals and case influences for proportional hazards models. More recently, Therneau et al. (1990) used a time-dependent score residual for individual i defined as $\mathbf{x}_i(t) - \bar{\mathbf{x}}^*(t)$, where $\bar{\mathbf{x}}^*(t)$ is the weighted mean over all subjects present in the experiment at time t with weights $\exp(\mathbf{x}_i\boldsymbol{\beta})$. As pointed out by Cain and Lange (1984), standardizing the score residual by the observed information matrix from the Cox model approximates the change in estimated regression coefficients if observation i were deleted from the analysis.

4 RESULTS

Kaplan–Meier estimates of the survivorship functions for the short (30-minute) and long (100 to 120-minute) tows are plotted in Figure 1. There appear to be marked differences between the survival rates for the two tow durations, espe-

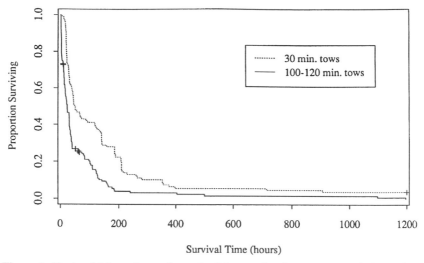

Figure 1. Kaplan–Meier estimates for each of the two durations; +, censored observations.

cially in the first 300 hours after capture. Associated estimates of the cumulative hazard functions $H(t)$ and $\ln H(t)$ for short and long tows are plotted against time and the logarithm of time, respectively, in Figure 2. The curves appear to be more linear in Figure 2b than in Figure 2a, indicating that Weibull models may be appropriate. However, the plots also exhibit a great deal of variation and suggest the presence of significant covariate effects.

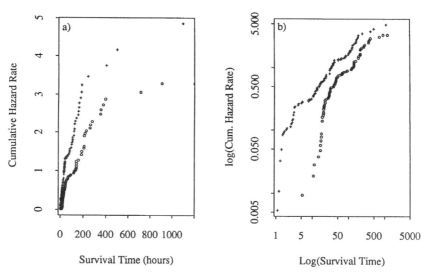

Figure 2. Atlantic halibut survival data: (a) empirical cumulative hazard function vs. time; (b) ln (cumulative hazard function) vs. ln (time). o, 30-minute tows; +, 100 to 120-minute tows.

4.1 Parametric Models

Exponential and Weibull distributions, ignoring covariates for now, were fitted to the data from the two tow durations to assess further the patterns in Figure 2. The deviance approach to constructing the likelihood ratio test is shown in Table 2 and suggests that the Weibull distribution fits the data better than does the exponential distribution, as indicated in Figure 2*b*. The results for fits of all the covariates using Weibull distributions to the combined data and the data from each tow duration are presented in Table 3. The standard errors given in this table have been corrected for the Weibull distribution. The results for the fit of the model to the combined tow durations indicate that survival is enhanced for large fish and associated large catches, while large changes in depth during the tow and long handling times on deck are detrimental to survival. In contrast, the coefficients for the model of the short-tow-duration data only show that large changes in depth during the tow appear to be beneficial to survival. On the other hand, large associated catches of fish are a detrimental effect in the model for the long-tow-duration data.

Note that the estimates for α for the short and long tows are larger than the respective estimates in Table 2. The estimate for the 30-minute tow duration in Table 3 is very close to 1.0. Hypotheses tests for $\alpha = 1$ for the results in Table 3 gives *p*-values of 0.338 and less than 0.001 for short and long tows, respectively, indicating that an exponential distribution may be more appropriate for the data from 30-minute tows once the covariates have been accounted for in the model. These results, along with differences noted above for coefficients from the individual models, support separate analyses for each tow duration.

It may not be necessary to include all of the covariates in each model. Neilson et al. (1989) screened for covariate inclusion using a sequential testing approach. That is, differences between the deviances from simple models and nested sequences of more complex models were evaluated. For instance, the difference between the deviance from a model with a mean term only and a model with a mean term and a ln (*catch*) term would be tested to see if it is large enough relative to a chi-square statistic to warrant the latter's inclusion.

Table 2 Results of Fitting Exponential and Weibull Distributions to the Atlantic Halibut Survival Data[a]

Tow Duration (min.)	Deviance		$\hat{\alpha}$	*p*-Value
	Exponential	Weibull		
30	195.31	176.90	0.7964	< 0.001
100–120	422.79	351.05	0.6672	< 0.001

[a]The *p*-value is for a chi-square distribution with 1 degree of freedom and the null hypothesis is $\alpha = 1$ (exponential distribution) versus the alternative hypothesis $\alpha \neq 1$ (Weibull distribution).

Table 3   Parameter Estimates for All of the Covariates from the Halibut Survival Data[a]

Covariate	Estimated Coefficients (Standard Error)		
	All Data	30-Minute Tows	100 to 120-Minute Tows
$\hat{\alpha}$	0.7521	0.9352	0.7549
	(0.0324)	(0.0659)	(0.0402)
Intercept	−1.4360	0.6912	−2.513
	(0.5007)	(0.7682)	(0.6531)
$\Delta Depth$	0.01526	−0.0462	0.0057
	(0.0072)	(0.0262)	(0.0083)
Length	−0.0342	−0.0872	−0.0377
	(0.0102)	(0.0179)	(0.0134)
Handling Time	0.0690	0.0431	0.0537
	(0.0093)	(0.0248)	(0.0114)
ln(Catch)	−0.2540	−0.3570	0.0912
	(0.0494)	(0.0923)	(0.0811)

[a] A Weibull model was used for data from the combined and separate tow durations.

Neilson et al. (1989) arrive at a final exponential regression model for the short tows with *length* and ln (*catch*) as covariates. The final model for halibut from the long tows was a Weibull model with a decreasing hazard function with *handling time* as the only covariate. These models were reevaluated here using the all-subset approach (Lawless and Singhal, 1978). In the halibut case, this approach was used to evaluate the increase in deviance for all possible models of three, two, and one covariate(s) relative to the deviance from the fit of all four of the covariates used in the study. At each level the combination of covariates which gives the smallest difference in deviance are then tested by using the difference in deviance as a chi-square test statistic with degrees of freedom equal to the difference between the number of parameters in the full and reduced models. Small differences in deviance relative to the chi-square statistic would indicate that the model with fewer terms in the comparison was an adequate description of the data. This approach is quite straightforward when there are only a small number of covariates but can be quite cumbersome for larger numbers of covariates. Lawless and Singhal (1978) discuss computer algorithms for simplifying the screening models with large numbers of covariates.

The final models indentified by the all-subset approach are given for the data from the short-tow duration in Table 4. If an arbitrary type I error rate is set at 0.05, the final model could either be $\beta_0 + \beta_1(length) + \beta_2[\ln(catch)] + \beta_3(handling\ time)$ or $\beta_0 + \beta_1(length) + \beta_2(\ln(catch) + \beta_3(\Delta)depth)$. In either case, the chi-square test for the null hypothesis that $\alpha = 1$ yields p-values greater than 0.2, implying exponential models. Neilson et al. (1989) also chose an exponential model, but only included *length* and ln (*catch*) as covariates. The param-

Table 4   Results of the All-Subset Selection of the Best Exponential
Proportional Hazard Models from the Halibut Survival Data for Tows of
30-Minute Duration

Number of Covariates	Covariate Name	Difference in Deviance	Degrees of Freedom	p-Value
3	Length, ln(catch), Δdepth	3.52	1	0.060
	Length, ln(catch), handling time	3.40	1	0.065
2	Length, ln(catch)	10.15	2	0.017
1	ln(catch)	34.62	3	<0.001
0	Mean only	62.72	4	<0.001

eter estimates for these two three-covariate models are given in Table 5. Note that while the coefficient for *length* is almost identical in the two models, the coefficient for ln(*catch*) differs by a factor of almost 2. The effect of ln(*catch*) appears to be less beneficial when included in the model with Δ*depth* than when associated with *handling time*. Scatterplots (not shown here) of Δ*depth* and *handling time* against ln(*catch*) indicate correlations between these covariates and therefore possible collinearities in the model. In particular, 17 of the largest values of Δ*depth* were associated with the largest values of ln(*catch*). The situation was less serious for *handling time* where only the four largest times were associated with the largest values of ln(*catch*).

From a practical point of view, *handling time* may very well be directly related to the size of the associated catch. In some commercial fishing operations, halibut may be left on deck until all other commercial species have been processed. However, this behavior can be changed to prolong the sur-

Table 5   Parameter Estimates for the Exponential Proportional Hazard
Models of Survival Times of Halibut from 30-Minute Tows[a]

Covariate	Model I[a]		Model II[b]	
	Estimated Coefficients	Standard Error	Estimated Coefficients	Standard Error
$\hat{\alpha}$	1.000	—	1.000	—
Intercept	0.5783	0.8004	0.5784	0.7369
Length	−0.0903	0.0168	−0.0909	0.0158
ln(Catch)	−0.4809	0.0722	−0.2807	0.0724
Handling time	0.0634	0.0229	—	—
ΔDepth	—	—	−0.0619	0.0241

[a]Model I = 1 + *length* + ln(*catch*) + *Handling Time*.
[b]Model II = 1 + *length* + ln(*catch*) + Δ*depth*.

vival of halibut. On the other hand, while the relationship between $\Delta depth$ and $\ln(catch)$ may be due solely to chance, it is impossible to control for the benefit of the halibut being caught in the net. In addition, halibut lack a gas bladder, which may make them less susceptible to damage due to the changes in pressure implied by changes in $\Delta depth$. For these reasons, the model with *length*, $\ln(catch)$ and *handling time* is chosen here for the halibut caught in the 30-minute tows.

The quantiles of the residuals from model I in Table 5 are plotted against the expected quantiles from an exponential model in Figure 3. The residuals should fall on the 45° line given in the figure if the exponential model were appropriate.

The results of all-subset screening of covariates for the data from the 100 to 120-minute tows are presented in Table 6. Again, using a 0.05 type I error rate, the final model chosen is $\beta_0 + \beta_1(length) + \beta_2(handling\,time)$. The parameter estimates for the final model from Table 6 are given in Table 7 with the appropriate standard errors for the Weibull model. The model implies that survival time is prolonged for larger fish experiencing shorter handling times. The estimate of $\hat{\alpha}$ of 0.751 is significantly different from 1.0 with a *p*-value less than 0.001. Note that both $\ln(catch)$ and *handling time* are included in the three covariate model in Table 6.

Neilson et al. (1989) also used a Weibull model for the long-tow-duration data, but only used *handling time* as a covariate. A closer look at Table 3 in their

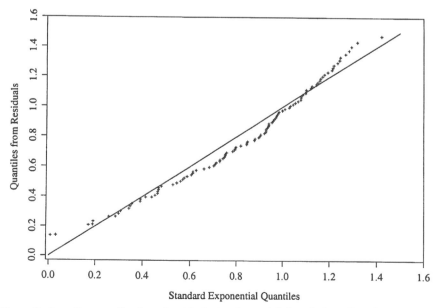

Figure 3. Quantile–quantile plot of residuals for the model $\beta_0 + \beta_1(length) + \beta_2[\ln(catch)] + \beta_3(handling\,time)$ for the survival time of halibut caught in 30-minute tows.

Table 6   Results of the All-Subset Selection of the Best Models from Halibut Survival Data for Tows of 100 to 120-Minute Duration

Number of Covariates	Covariate Name	Difference in Deviance	Degrees of Freedom	p-Value
3	ln(*Catch*), *length, handling time*	0.45	1	0.502
2	*Length, handling time*	2.16	2	0.339
1	*Handling time*	8.13	3	0.043
0	Mean only	48.85	4	<0.001

paper shows that including *length* and *handling time* gave a p-value of 0.05, and therefore could have been included in the model as well. [Note there is a typographical error in Table 6 of Neilson et al. (1989), where the coefficient for *handling time* was erroneously reported as being negative. However, all calculations in that paper were done with a positive coefficient for *handling time*.]

Figure 4 is a quantile–quantile plot of the residuals from the Weibull model in Table 7. It appears to be better behaved than that for the exponential model in Figure 3. Both plots are similar in exhibiting the tendency of the residuals to show heavier than expected upper tails.

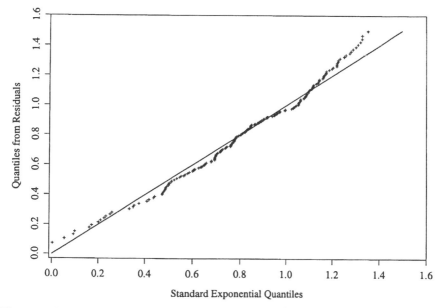

Figure 4. Quantile–quantile plot of residuals for the model $\beta_0 + \beta_1(length) + \beta_2(handling\ time)$ for the survival time of halibut caught in 100 to 120 minutes.

Table 7   Parameter Estimates for the Weibull Proportional Hazards Model of Survival Times of Halibut Tows of 100 to 120-Minute Duration

Covariate	Estimated Coefficients	Standard Error
$\hat{\alpha}$	0.750	0.0399
Intercept	−2.412	0.6115
Length	−0.0302	0.0123
Handling time	0.0619	0.0103

4.2   Cox Model

The parameter estimates from the Cox model for all of the covariates when fitted to the combined data set and the data from each tow duration are given in Table 8. These estimates are comparable to those from the parametric model in Table 3, with the exception of the $\hat{\alpha}$'s and the intercept terms. The parameter estimates given in both tables are within 1 standard error of each other and the differences between standard error estimates from the two tables are small. The only significant covariates for the 30-minute tows were *length* and ln(*catch*). *Length* and *handling time* were significant for the longer tow duration.

The all-subsets regression method was applied to the Cox models. The results for the data from the short tows are given in Table 9. Again, there seems to be a question of whether the best three-covariate model should include *handling time* or Δ*depth* with *length* and ln(*catch*). While a comparison of *p*-values would favor Δ*depth*, the argument used in the section on parametric models to choose *handling time* applies here as well.

Table 8   Parameter Estimates for All of the Covariates Using the Cox Model for the Halibut Survival Data[a]

Covariate	Estimated Coefficients (Standard Error)		
	All Data	30-Minute Tows	100 to 120-Minute Tows
Δ*Depth*	0.0127	−0.0520	0.0037
	(0.0071)	(0.0272)	(0.0084)
Length	−0.0345	−0.0799	−0.0401
	(0.0101)	(0.0179)	(0.0133)
Handling time	0.0663	0.0322	0.0509
	(0.0093)	(0.0236)	(0.0115)
ln(*Catch*)	−0.2302	−0.3101	−0.1077
	(0.0503)	(0.0924)	(0.0817)

[a]The model was fitted to data from the combined tow durations and then separately to each tow duration.

Table 9   Results of the All-Subset Selection of the Best Cox Proportional Hazards Models for Halibut Survival Data for Tows of 30-Minute Duration

Number of Covariates	Covariate Name	Likelihood Ratio Statistic	Degrees of Freedom	p-Value
3	*Length*, ln(*catch*), *handling time*	3.64	1	0.056
	Length, ln(*catch*), Δ*depth*	1.77	1	0.183
2	*Length*, ln(*catch*)	7.47	2	0.024
1	ln(*catch*)	21.891	3	<0.001

The parameter estimates and associated standard errors for Cox model of the short-tow-duration data are presented in the column labelled "All Data" in Table 10. These estimates are very similar to those in Table 5 for the exponential model.

Deviance residuals are plotted against the standardized score residuals for ln (*catch*) in Figure 5 to assess both fit and influence. Observation numbers 19 and 26 are identified as having large standardized score residuals and, in the case of observation 26, a large deviance residual as well. The model for the 30-minute tow implies that survival time is enhanced for larger fish when the total catch of fish in the net is large and *handling time* is short. Neilson et al. (1989) hypothesized that a large total catch in a tow of short duration may provide a cushioning effect for halibut, removing the effect of direct abrasion with the net. However, the fish identified by observations 19 and 26 lived in excess of 200 hours even though they were associated with some of the small-

Table 10   Parameter Estimates for the Cox Proportional Hazards Model of Survival Times of Halibut from 30-Minute Tows and Parameter Estimates When High Leverage Observations with Respect to ln(*catch*) Only Are Removed

Covariate	Estimated Coefficients (Standard Error)	
	All Data	High Leverage Points Removed
Length	−0.0742	−0.0695
	(0.0182)	(0.0180)
ln(*Catch*)	−0.4053	−0.4752
	(0.0790)	(0.0830)
Handling time	0.0464	0.0527
	(0.0227)	(0.0226)

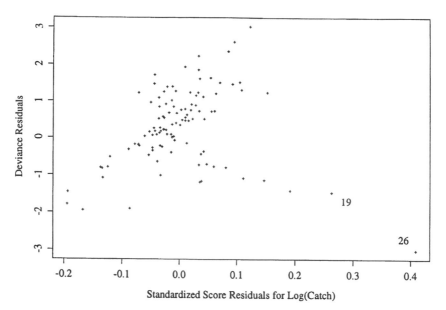

Figure 5. Plot of deviance residuals versus score residuals for the covariant ln (*catch*). Halibut survival data from 30-minute tows.

est total catches. The plot implies that the coefficient for ln (*catch*) will decrease if these two points are removed and this is confirmed in the second column of parameter estimates given in Table 10. Removal of these two points enhances the positive relationship between ln (*catch*) and survival.

The coefficient for *length* was also affected in a small way by the removal of observations 19 and 26. The influence of these two points are marginal compared to some of the other points identified on Figure 6. Observations 22, 30, and 106 are all underestimated because they represent small fish (29 to 35 cm), which survived longer than larger fish under the same conditions. Removal of these observations would result in a stronger relationship between *length* and survival.

Under the assumption of proportional hazards, the relationships between survival and the covariates in the model are assumed to be independent of time, such that the ratio of hazards functions for any two individuals does not vary with time. The *p*-values for the correlation coefficients for the relationship between rank time and the Schoenfeld residuals for *length*, ln (*catch*) and *handling time* were 0.527, 0.359, and 0.519, respectively, indicating that there is insufficient evidence to reject the assumption of proportional hazards.

The results of the all-subset regression method for the data from the 100 to 120-minute tow durations are given in Table 11. *Length* and *handling time* were included in the model, as in Table 6. The estimated covariate effects in

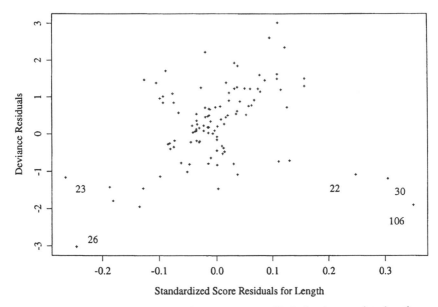

Figure 6. Plot of deviance residuals versus score residuals for the covariate *length.*

the Cox model (Table 12) were very similar to those obtained for the Weibull model in Table 7.

Three influential points are identified for the long-tow-duration data in Figure 7. These points are associated with fish that experienced long handling time but survived longer than expected. The effect of removing these points from estimation of the coefficient for *handling time* is given in the second column of estimates in Table 12. Removal of these points would result in a stronger relationship between enhanced survival times and shorter handling times. Removing high leverage points identified in Figure 8 for *length* results in a stronger relationship between larger fish and longer survival times. As in the previous case, there was insufficient evidence to reject the proportional hazards assumption.

Table 11   Results of the All-Subset Selection of the Best Cox Models from the Halibut Survival Data for Tows of 100 to 120-Minute Duration

Number of Covariates	Covariate Name	Likelihood Ratio Statistic	Degrees of Freedom	*p*-Value
3	ln(*Catch*), *length, handling time*	0.19	1	0.663
2	*Length, handling time*	2.29	2	0.318
1	*Handling time*	9.55	3	0.023

Table 12   Parameter Estimates for the Cox Proportional Hazards Model of Survival Times of Halibut from 100 to 120-Minute Tows and Parameter Estimates When High Leverage Observations with Respect to *Handling Time* Only and *Length* Only Are Removed

Covariate	All Data	Estimated Coefficients (Standard Error)	
		High Leverage Points Removed	
		Handling Time	*Length*
Length	−0.0330	−0.0295	−0.0531
	(0.0122)	(0.0127)	(0.0133)
Handling time	0.0586	0.0700	0.0669
	(0.0104)	(0.0118)	(0.0105)

The estimates of the survivorship function $\hat{S}(t)$ are presented for fixed covariate values of **x** for all the models discussed here. In the case of the 30-minute-tow models, *length*, ln (*catch*), and *handling time* were set to their median values [40 cm, ln (62 kg) and 10 minutes] and the medians of *length* and *handling time* were used for the 100 to 120-minute tow models. Figure 9 is a plot of these estimates against time.

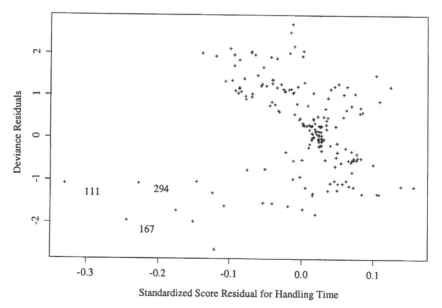

Figure 7. Plot of deviance residuals versus score residuals for the covariate *handling time*. Halibut survival data from 100 to 120-minute tows.

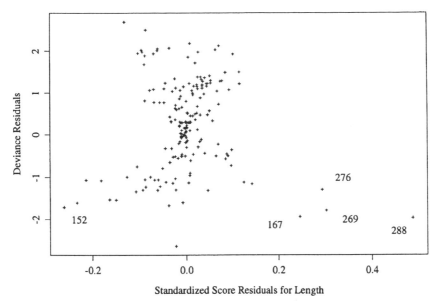

Figure 8. Plot of deviance residuals versus score residuals for the covariate length. Halibut survival data from 100 to 120-minute tows.

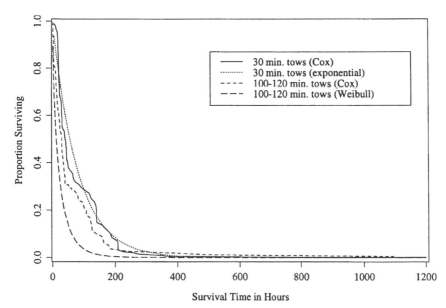

Figure 9. Predicted survival rates for each of the proportional hazards models used in the text. Note that length = 40 cm, ln (*catch*) = ln (62 kg), and handling time = 10 minutes for 30-minute data. Length = 40 cm and *handling time* = 10 minutes for the 100 to 120-minute data.

5 CONCLUSIONS

Parametric and semiparametric proportional hazards models for the halibut data led to similar results in terms of identified covariates and their estimated effects. However, the two approaches differed with respect to the estimated survivorship and hazard functions. For the most part, the exponential model predicted higher survival rates for the data from the 30-minute tows than did the Cox model for the same data (Figure 9). Neilson et al. (1989) used 48 hours as a benchmark time to compare the predictions of the various models used in that study. The predicted proportion of the halibut surviving after 48 hours for the exponential and Cox model are 0.55 and 0.41, respectively, for the 30-minute tow. The assumption of a constant hazard rate implicit in the exponential model appears to give an overly optimistic estimate of survival. On the other hand, the assumption of a constantly decreasing hazard rate implicit in the Weibull model for the 100 to 120-minute tow data results in a more pessimistic view of survival than given by the Cox model for the same data. The 48-hour estimate of the proportion surviving for the Weibull model was less than half (0.15) the estimate from the Cox model (0.31).

The analyses presented here were made with the implicit assumption that the halibut in either tow duration were equally exposed to the same conditions. However, it is not possible to know when the individual halibut entered the trawl during the tow. This may explain the lack of fit of the models as well as the high influence of the observations identified in Figures 5 to 8. At present, this problem will have to be accepted as a shortcoming of this kind of experiment.

SOFTWARE NOTES AND REFERENCES

The GLIM package comes with the macro WEIB which can be used to fit exponential, Weibull, and extreme value distributions and also to fit covariates in a proportional hazards model. The methodology used by this macro is described in Aitken and Clayton (1980) and McCullagh and Nelder (1989, pp. 419–431). This package also provides residual plots, which are available by executing the macro RESP which also comes with GLIM. Software to fit generalized additive models are available in the S-PLUS package.

The standard errors given by WEIB for the exponential model option are correct, but the macro does issue a warning that the standard errors for the Weibull model option are underestimates. The estimation of standard errors for the Weibull case needs to be done outside of WEIB, and the estimating equations are discussed in Aitken and Clayton (1980). Note that the fitted values $\hat{\mu}_i$ discussed in Aitken and Clayton (1980) are available in the GLIM system variable %fv.

Clayton and Cuzick (1985) have provided a series of GLIM macros for fitting the Cox model which uses Breslow's method of dealing with ties. The S-PLUS computer package also supplies the function coxreg, which will fit a Cox model using Breslow's method for ties (also called Peto's method or the Peto–Breslow approximation). The major differences between the output from the two programs is that the GLIM macros provide an intercept term, whereas this term is absorbed into $h_0(t)$ in the S-PLUS macro. Otherwise, the coefficients for the covariates are the same in both cases. The standard errors from the GLIM macros are underestimates of the true standard errors, although in practice these difference are usually small (see Clayton and Cuzick, 1985, for a discussion of this). The standard errors from coxreg are correct.

The S-PLUS function surv.fit has an option to use the results from coxreg to predict $S(t)$ for the Cox model. The product-limit survival estimates for the survival data from the short (30 minutes) and long (100 to 120 minutes) tows were computed using the function surv.fit in the S-PLUS package. The output from the S-PLUS function coxreg provides a test for the null hypothesis $\beta_j = 0$ for each of the coefficients assuming that the ratio of the coefficient to its standard error has a normal distribution. Score, deviance, and Schoenfeld residuals are all available from the S-PLUS function coxreg.

Payne, C. D. (1986). *The GLIM (Generalized Linear Interactive Modelling) System Manual, Release 3.77.* Oxford: Numerical Algorithms Group.

StatSci (1991). *S-PLUS for DOS User's Manual, Version 2.0.* Seattle, Wash.: Statistical Science.

QUESTIONS AND PROBLEMS

1. The halibut survival data were analyzed using the complete duration of the experiment (i.e., 1200 hours). Neilson et al. (1989) suggest that survival in the first 48 hours may be more relevant to the minimum size regulation. Reanalyze the halibut for the maximum duration of 48 hours by setting the censoring indicator for all fish which survived past 48 hours to zero. Compare the results with the analyses of the 1200-hour-duration experiment.

2. The correlation test used in Section 4.2 was used to test for *linear* departures from the proportional hazards assumption. How would one test for other kinds of departures from this assumption? (*Hint:* See Therneau et al., 1990).

3. All the models discussed in this chapter assumed that a model of the form $\exp(\mathbf{x}\boldsymbol{\beta})$ was appropriate for the covariates. Recently, Hastie and Tibshirani (1990a) presented exploratory methods to investigate the nature of the covariate effects in the Cox model. These methods use *generalized additive* proportional hazards models, which are a subset of *generalized additive* models discussed in Hastie and Tibshirani (1990b). Software to fit generalized additive models are available in the S-PLUS package. Apply the techniques given in Hastie and Tibshirani (1990a) to the halibut data to investigate the form of the covariate effects.

4. McCullagh and Nelder (1989), Aitken and Clayton (1980), and the WEIB macro in GLIM present three different ways of calculating the deviance for a Weibull model. Show that the difference in deviance between the exponential and Weibull model is the same for all three deviance calculations. Compare the deviance calculations for the exponential model from each of the three methods to the deviance for a GLIM model with a gamma distribution and a log link for the case where no censoring is present.

CHAPTER 8

Mixture Fraction and Linkage Analysis for Hybrid Onions

Dennis L. Clason, Joe N. Corgan,
Cathy M. Cryder-Wilson, and N. Scott Urquhart

1 MOTIVATION AND BACKGROUND

The Japanese bunching onion (*Allium fistulosum* L.) has many desirable traits, particularly disease resistance, absent in the cultivated bulb onion (*A. cepa* L.). First filial (F_1) interspecific hybrids *A. fistulosum* $\times$ *A. cepa* exhibit a high degree of sterility, but small numbers of backcross (BC_1) and second filial (F_2) progeny have been recovered (Cryder et al., 1991). In 1985, two large populations of F_1 hybrids from different crosses were open pollinated with external pollen sources restricted to *A. cepa*, the recurrent parent. This resulted in two large seed populations and permitted an extensive study of heritable traits expressed by this backcross.

The breeders expected BC_1 individuals to dominate the population, although the possibility for other types of crosses clearly existed. Onions are self-fertile, so seed gathered from an F_1 individual when open pollinated by the recurrent parent can result from self-fertilization ("selfing") as well as the desired backcross. In the sequel, F_2 will be used to denote progeny derived from the selfed part of this mixed population.

Deoxyribose nucleic acid (DNA) is the genetic material in most living organisms. In eukaryotic organisms, the DNA is organized into long strings of genes called chromosomes. A *locus* is a particular location on a chromosome. In a diploid organism, there are two copies of each locus, each occupied by an *allele*. An allele is a specific sequence of DNA coding for one form of a protein. Peffley et al. (1985) showed the existence of alternate alleles in the *A. fistulosum* genome coding for several enzymes. These enzymes include alcohol dehydrogenase (ADH), isocitrate dehydrogenase (IDH), and phosphogluco-

Case Studies in Biometry, Edited by Nicholas Lange, Louise Ryan, Lynne Billard,
David Brillinger, Loveday Conquest, and Joel Greenhouse.
ISBN 0-471-58885-7 © 1994 John Wiley & Sons, Inc.

isomerase (PGI). Analysis of the isozyme patterns can provide an estimate of the F_2 proportion in the seed populations. An appropriate test of independent segregation of these alleles can then be performed.

Parentage can be traced through the isozyme patterns because DNA is transcribed into RNA (ribose nucleic acid). In turn, RNA is transcribed into protein. Proteins serve many roles in living organisms: they may form structural elements, they may serve as messengers, they may be receptors, or they may be catalysts. Catalytic proteins are usually referred to as enzymes. A particular enzyme (for the sake of discussion, we illustrate with ADH) catalyzes a particular reaction, and it (ADH) removes a proton from an alcohol structure. Many organisms have DNA code for ADH, but different species have different ADH enzymes: different not in function, but in structure. Even within a species, several alternative enzyme structures may be found. These alternative structures are called *allozymes.* The particular allozymes produced by an organism are determined by the genetic material (DNA) inherited from its parents.

Allozymes can be classified using a technique called gel electrophoresis. The technique involves digesting the plant material under specific conditions, releasing the enzymes into solution. The enzymes are then placed in a gel with a controlled electric field imposed. Because the allozymes have small areas of positive and negative charges, they migrate through the gel. The rate of migration depends on the size of the enzyme and the amino acid residues involved. The result (when everything works right) is a banding pattern characteristic of the particular allozymes produced. From the banding pattern, one can determine which allozymes an organism produces. In the case of plants with restricted pollen sources, this may identify the pollen parent.

Genes on different chromosomes segregate randomly during gamete formation (*meiosis*). Genes located on the same chromosome tend to segregate together: in genetic terminology they are said to be linked. During meiosis, homologous chromosomes can exchange genetic material by a process called crossing over. The probability of crossover is assumed to be an increasing function of the spatial separation of the loci on the chromosome. The probability of crossover is also referred to as the (raw) *map distance.*

2   DATA

Root tissue samples of the seed population were analyzed electrophoretically for the ADH, IDH, and PGI enzymes. For a particular enzyme, an individual bulb was classified as

> *cepa*: if it produced only *A. cepa* isozyme banding patterns;
>
> *fist*: if it produced only *A. fistulosum* banding patterns; and
>
> *het*: if it produced both *A. cepa* and *A. fistulosum* banding patterns.

Table 1 Data for Population 1034 and 1040[a]

ADH	IDH	PGI Classification		
		cepa	*het*	*fist*
		Population 1034		
cepa	*cepa*	41	15	2
	het	19	15	0
	fist	0	1	1
het	*cepa*	14	22	0
	het	17	24	1
	fist	0	3	0
fist	*cepa*	0	1	0
	het	0	1	0
	fist	0	0	0
		Population 1040		
cepa	*cepa*	52	17	0
	het	8	31	0
	fist	1	1	0
het	*cepa*	13	22	0
	het	14	31	0
	fist	0	1	1
fist	*cepa*	1	0	0
	het	1	2	0
	fist	0	0	0

[a]Population 1034 was derived from *A. fistulosum* variety Heshiko and *A. cepa* variety selection NMSU 792 (accession number 8273). Population 1040 was derived from *A. fistulosum* variety Ishikura and *A. cepa* selection 8020 (accession number 8121). *A. cepa* variety NMSU 8361 was used as the recurrent parent for both backcrosses.

The data collected for the seed populations (accession numbers 1034 and 1040) are shown in Table 1. This is a three-way table giving the cell counts for the 27 combinations of ADH, IDH, and PGI genotypes. In theory, the techniques developed here can be extended to any number of loci, but for simplicity of presentation the loci will be analyzed in pairs.

3 METHODS AND MODELS

3.1 First Analysis: No Linkage

The population is a convex mixture of BC_1 and F_2 subpopulations. (Table 2 gives the multinomial probabilities for the BC_1 and F_2 subpopulations.) Conse-

Table 2 Probability Mass Functions for a Single Randomly Selected Individual from BC_1 and F_2 Populations

Genotype at Locus 1	Genotype at Locus 2		
	cepa	*het*	*fist*
BC₁ Population			
cepa	4/16	4/16	0
het	4/16	4/16	0
fist	0	0	0
F₂ Population			
cepa	1/16	2/16	1/16
het	2/16	4/16	2/16
fist	1/16	2/16	1/16

quently, it should be analyzed by methods addressing the true distribution. If the mixture fraction is ϕ [i.e., $100(1 - \phi)\%$ of the population is BC_1 and $100\phi\%$ is F_2], the population probability parameters are as given in Table 3. These probabilities can be used to derive the likelihood function for the observed data vector $y^T = (y_{11}, y_{12}, y_{13}, y_{21}, \ldots, y_{33})$, $y^T 1 = n$, where 1 denotes a vector of ones. The subscripts 1, 2, 3 refer to the *cepa*, *het*, and *fist* types, respectively. The probability mass function for the counts (which are sufficient statistics for the problem) can be written

$$M_Y(y|\phi) = \left(\frac{n!}{\prod_{i=1}^{3} \prod_{j=1}^{3} y_{ij}!} \right) 16^{-n} (4 - 3\phi)^{y_{11}} (4 - 2\phi)^{y_{12}} \phi^{y_{13}}$$
$$\cdot (4 - 2\phi)^{y_{21}} 4^{y_{22}} (2\phi)^{y_{23}} \phi^{y_{31}} (2\phi)^{y_{32}} \phi^{y_{33}}. \tag{1}$$

If $a = y_{13} + y_{31} + y_{23} + y_{32} + y_{33}$, $b = y_{12} + y_{21}$, and $c = y_{11}$, the mass function

Table 3 Multinomial Probabilities for a Mixed BC_1, F_2 Population[a]

Genotype at Locus 1	Genotype at Locus 2		
	cepa	*het*	*fist*
cepa	$[4(1 - \phi) + \phi]/16$	$[4(1 - \phi) + 2\phi]/16$	ϕ
het	$[4(1 - \phi) + 2\phi]/16$	4	2ϕ
fist	ϕ	2ϕ	ϕ

[a]The mixture proportion is ϕ.

can be rewritten as

$$M_Y(y|\phi) = K\phi^a(2 - \phi)^b(4 - 3\phi)^c, \tag{2}$$

where K is a constant of proportionality involving the combinatorial coefficient and a power of 2. If the log-likelihood $\ln \mathscr{L}(\phi|Y) = \ln M_Y(y|\phi)$ is differentiated with respect to ϕ and the result set equal to zero, the maximum likelihood estimate (MLE) of ϕ must satisfy the following quadratic equation:

$$\left. \frac{\partial \ln \mathscr{L}}{\partial \phi} \right|_{\phi=\hat{\phi}} = 3(a + b + c)\hat{\phi}^2 - 2(5a + 2b + 3c)\hat{\phi} + 8a = 0. \tag{3}$$

The smaller root of this quadratic always lies in the interval [0,1], while the other root lies outside the interval. The root inside [0,1] maximizes $\mathscr{L}$. A chi-square test of model fit (i.e., independent segregation, $H_0: \pi_{ij} = \pi_i\phi_j$) can be based on this distribution and the associated MLE, using asymptotic properties of the log-likelihood [i.e., $-2 \ln \mathscr{L} \sim \chi^2(\nu)$]. Note that this statistic has 7 degrees of freedom, because the unconstrained parameter space has 8 degrees of freedom. The mixture parameter ϕ reduces the degrees of freedom by one.

If the null hypothesis of independent segregation is not rejected, a confidence interval for ϕ can be obtained using likelihood techniques similar to those of Box and Cox (1964), apparently first derived by Wald (1943). Asymptotically,

$$\ln \mathscr{L}(\hat{\phi}|y) - \ln \mathscr{L}(\phi|y) < \tfrac{1}{2}\chi^2_{1-\alpha}(1). \tag{4}$$

Thus, a 95% percent confidence interval consists of all values of ϕ having log-likelihoods within 1.92 units of the maximum.

The same method of analysis can be extended to handle any number of alleles simultaneously. In the general case of k alleles, a kth-degree polynomial must be solved. For the three-allele case, the log-likelihood function is

$$\ln \mathscr{L}(\phi|Y) = K + a \ln(8 - 7\phi) + b \ln(8 - 6\phi)$$
$$+ c \ln(8 - 4\phi) + d \ln(\phi), \tag{5}$$

where $a = y_{111}, b = y_{112} + y_{121} + y_{211}, c = y_{122} + y_{212} + y_{221}$, and $d = n - a - b - c - y_{222}$. When the derivative is taken with respect to ϕ, the resulting cubic can be solved. As in the two-allele case, it can be shown that only one root of the equation is admissible, and that this root maximizes the likelihood function.

3.2   Linked Alleles: A Second Analysis

The preceding models were developed assuming independently segregating alleles. If a pair of alleles fails the test of independence, it may be because the alleles are linked. Other possibilities in this case include a sampling error or fertility barriers in the F_1 parent. Let $0 < \lambda \le 0.5$ be the probability of crossover. When $\lambda = 0.5$, the models reduce to the independent segregation case. Values of λ greater than 0.5 have no biological interpretation, hence the restriction of λ. If random mating is assumed, the probabilities shown in Table 4 are obtained for the multinomial distribution describing the F_2, BC_1, and the mixed population.

A likelihood function can be formed based on the two parameters λ and ϕ, but the result is not easily maximized analytically. Fortunately, it is amenable to numeric maximization using a grid search. Although numerically inefficient compared with Marquardt's algorithm or Newton–Raphson iteration, a grid search works well for this application. The brute-force approach is feasible because the parameter space is bounded and the number of sufficient statistics is small. If a joint confidence region is desired for λ and ϕ, a grid search needs to be performed to generate the likelihood surface. The confidence region is based on the relationship

$$\ln \mathscr{L}(\hat{\phi}, \hat{\lambda}|y) - \ln \mathscr{L}(\phi, \lambda|y) < \tfrac{1}{2} \chi^2_{1-\alpha}(2). \tag{6}$$

Pearson's X^2 statistic

$$X^2 = \sum_{i=1}^{3} \sum_{j=1}^{3} \frac{(y_{ij} - \hat{y}_{ij})^2}{\hat{y}_{ij}}, \qquad \hat{y}_{ij} = n\hat{\pi}_{ij}, \tag{7}$$

can be used as an index of model fit, now with 6 degrees of freedom. Joint confidence regions for (ϕ, λ) are shown as contours in Figure 1.

Table 4   Multinomial Probabilities for a Mixed BC_1, F_2 Population with Linkage among the Alleles[a]

Genotype at Locus 1	Genotype at Locus 2		
	cepa	het	fist
cepa	$\phi(1 - \lambda)^2 + 2(1 - \phi)(1 - \lambda)$	$2\phi\lambda(1 - \lambda) + 2(1 - \phi)\lambda^2$	$\phi\lambda^2$
het	$2\phi\lambda(1 - \lambda) + 2(1 - \phi)\lambda^2$	$2\phi(1 - \lambda)^2 + 2\phi\lambda^2 + 2(1 - \phi)(1 - \lambda)$	$2\phi\lambda(1 - \lambda)$
fist	$\phi\lambda^2$	$2\phi\lambda(1 - \lambda)$	$2\phi(1 - \lambda)^2$

[a]The mixture proportion is ϕ; λ represents the map distance.

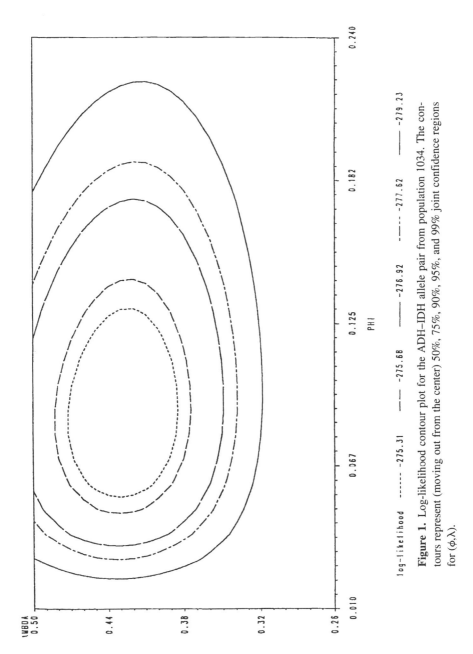

log-likelihood ------ -275.31 ——— -275.68 ——— -276.92 -·—·- -277.62 ——— -279.23

Figure 1. Log-likelihood contour plot for the ADH-IDH allele pair from population 1034. The contours represent (moving out from the center) 50%, 75%, 90%, 95%, and 99% joint confidence regions for (ϕ, λ).

4 RESULTS

4.1 No Linkage Models

The usual procedure would be to derive the expected frequencies from the mass functions given in Tables 1 and 2, and test the goodness of fit using Pearson's X^2 statistic. If it is recognized that the population is a mixture of F_2 and BC_1 individuals, one might try simply testing for independent segregation using the observed marginal frequencies. Pearson's X^2 for this case is 19.7 with 4 degrees of freedom. For the BC_1 population, the test statistic is undefined because the model predicts no individuals showing pure *A. fistulosum* traits for any allele. Finally, for the F_2 population model, X^2 is 337.7 with 8 degrees of freedom. The other pairs of loci give similar results. Superficially, these results suggest that all three loci are linked (i.e., they lie on the same chromosome), a minor coincidence (p-value = $\frac{1}{64}$) in a species with a haploid chromosome number of eight. We are assuming that the genes are randomly dispersed among the eight chromosomes and that each chromosome carries the same number of genes. Hence, the probability that any pair of genes selected a priori lie on the same chromosome is $\frac{1}{8}$ and the probability that three genes selected a priori lie on a single chromosome is $\frac{1}{64}$. This is a first approximation, because the onion

Table 5 Parameter Estimates and Goodness-of-Fit Tests Statistics for Population 1034

| | | | *Unlinked Model* | | 95% Confidence Limits | |
Loci	Criterion	ϕ	X^2	p-Value	Lower	Upper
ADH–PGI	MC	0.10	21.3	0.0033	—	—
	ML	0.08	22.0	0.0025	0.05	0.14
ADH–IDH	MC	0.10	12.4	0.0876	—	—
	ML	0.08	12.8	0.0782	0.03	0.16
IDH–PGI	MC	0.13	11.9	0.1032	—	—
	ML	0.10	13.0	0.0729	0.04	0.18

| | | | *Linked Model* | | |
Loci	Criterion	ϕ	λ	X^2	p-Value
ADH–PGI	MC	0.13	0.39	12.4	0.0539
	ML	0.08	0.38	16.3	0.0124
ADH–IDH	MC	0.11	0.42	8.1	0.2308
	ML	0.09	0.43	8.5	0.2026
IDH–PGI	MC	0.14	0.45	10.1	0.1206
	ML	0.10	0.44	12.0	0.0622

genome is not completely mapped. It is known that the chromosomes are different sizes, so the minor premise is somewhat suspect.

These hypotheses are rejected because the population is neither a BC_1 nor an F_2 population. When the appropriate methods outlined in Section 3 are used, we obtain the estimates given in Table 5. For population 1034, 95% confidence intervals ranged from about 0.05 to 0.15: all three pairs of loci are in agreement. The log-likelihood function for the ADH–PGI allele pair of population 1034 is shown in Figure 2. The available data are rather sparse when expressed as a three-way table, but the data can be analyzed. When all three alleles are used simultaneously, the maximum likelihood estimate is 9.4%; the associated X^2 value is 15.89 with 25 degrees of freedom. A 95% confidence interval for ϕ, based on the three-allele data, is 0.05 to 0.16.

4.2 Linked Alleles: A Second Analysis

Joint confidence contours for the population 1034 ADH–PGI allele pair are shown in Figure 1. Very similar contours were obtained for the other allele pairs. If the model is adequate, it appears that ADH and PGI are linked, with a map distance of about 0.38. The simultaneous confidence contours for ADH and IDH suggest that these loci are not linked.

5 CONCLUSIONS

As Figures 1 and 2 show, the likelihood function is relatively flat near $\hat{\phi}$ for population 1034. This is also true of population 1040 (Cryder et al., 1991). It appears that the mixture is somewhere in the vicinity of 10% F_2 individuals. There is an inferential paradox in these data, however, with 25 degrees of freedom, the X^2 value of 15.9 for the three independent allele model has an observed significance level of 0.918. The model fits quite well. When the alleles are tested in pairs it appears that IDH and PGI are linked, while ADH lies on another chromosome. Neither model fits the IDH and ADH pair very well; the observed significance levels for the goodness of fit statistic is about 1%. It appears that there are some postmeiotic barriers in the F_1 population. Peffley et al. (1985) report independent evidence suggesting that IDH and PGI are linked in *A. fistulosum*. If the breeding barriers are not distorting the results, the linkage models show that the association is not very close. Examination of the cell X^2 contributions to the overall statistic shows that the largest contributions come from the *cepa* × *cepa* and *cepa* × *het* cells. The *cepa* × *cepa* cell is overrepresented and the *cepa* × *het* cell is underrepresented (relative to model expectations). This suggests barriers selecting against seeds heterozygous for these *A. cepa* and *A. fistulosum* chromosomes.

A statistical question opened by these data concerns the choice of estimation criteria. In this study, maximum likelihood is used as the optimality criterion. By

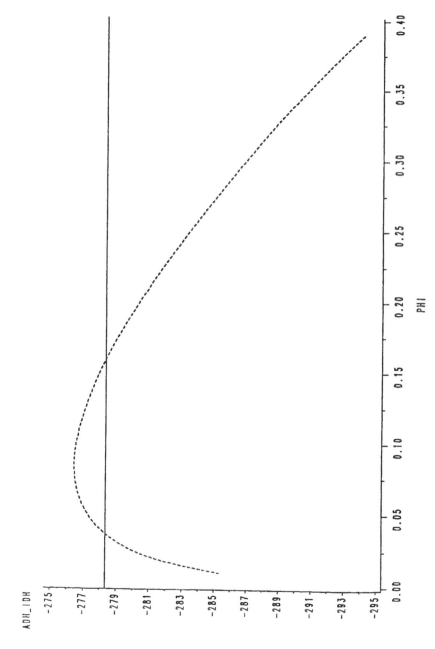

Figure 2. Log-likelihood function for the ADH–IDH allele pair from population 1034 plotted as a function of ϕ. The horizontal reference line indicates the cutoff for a 95% confidence interval.

a simple change of objective function, the same computer code can be used to obtain minimum X^2 estimates. There is a history of debate in the statistical literature between adherents of minimum X^2 estimation and maximum likelihood estimation (e.g., Berkson 1949, 1951, 1980; Neyman, 1949). Rao (1973, Chapters 5 and 6) has an extensive discussion of estimation and testing problems in multinomial distributions. Rao specifically addresses the regularity conditions needed for maximum likelihood estimators and discusses efficiency considerations and other asymptotic properties of maximum likelihood estimators of multinomial probabilities. Note, however, that in these data sets both criteria are in close agreement.

In summary, techniques have been described for simultaneously estimating the mixture fraction and map distance in populations having mixed genetic heritage. The general technique involves deriving the multinomial probabilities for each of the genetic subpopulations, and expressing the population structure as a convex mixture of subpopulation multinomials. The parameters can then be estimated using maximum likelihood or minimum X^2 techniques. When maximum likelihood techniques are used, confidence regions for the mixture parameters are easily obtained.

Similar techniques can be used to estimate self-pollination rates in extant plant populations. The seed parent's genotype must be determined and the allozyme relative frequencies in the subpopulations must be known. Seed recovered from the seed parent can then be typed and the linkage distances and self-pollination rates estimated from the data. This information could be of value to evolutionary geneticists trying to estimate linkage disequilibrium coefficients for plant populations that both self-fertilize and outcross.

As a case study, this experiment has three important features. First, it illustrates why assumptions should be examined when the data disagree wildly with expectations. Second, it shows the development of somewhat novel statistical methods designed to answer specific questions about a breeding system. Finally, it provides a springboard to as-yet-unanswered questions about this breeding system.

QUESTIONS AND PROBLEMS

1. Under the unlinked model, $E\{Y_{13}/n\} = \phi$. Find the variance of this unbiased estimator of ϕ. Find another unbiased estimator of ϕ having smaller variance. [*Hint:* Examine the cell probabilities in (5). A harder way would be to apply the Rao–Blackwell theorem to Y_{13}/n, finding its conditional expectation given the sufficient statistics $A, B,$ and C.]

2. Use the factorization theorem to show that the mass functions—in this case equations (1) and (2)—have the following properties:

   (a) Have the cell counts as sufficient statistics, but the cell counts are not minimally sufficient because a smaller set of sufficient statistics exists in each case.

(b) Are members of an exponential family. Find the natural parameters of the exponential family.

(c) The unlinked loci model [equation (5)] is a subfamily of the linked model.

3. The maximum likelihood estimator is consistent and asymptotically normal (Rao, 1973). Its variance is $1/nF$, where F is Fisher's information measure:

$$F = -E \left\{ \frac{\partial^2 \ln f(y_i|\phi)}{\partial \phi^2} \right\}.$$

Find the asymptotic variance of the MLE. Use these results to give a different confidence interval for ϕ, using the unlinked model of equations (1) and (2). The density $f(y_i|\phi)$ is the density of a *single observation*.

4. Analyze the data for population 1040 using the methods described in this chapter.

PART III

Habitat and Animal Studies

CHAPTER 9

Spatial Association Learning in Hummingbirds

Jinko Graham and A. John Petkau

1 MOTIVATION AND BACKGROUND

The search for a more complete understanding of how organisms relate objects separated in space motivates research on spatial learning in both the biological sciences and psychology. One area of such research is spatial association learning, where organisms learn to associate certain cues (such as colors, lights, or sounds) with reinforcement (such as food, water, or mates) separated in space from the cues. For example, Gori (1989) has shown that bees use the colors of spots on banner petals as cues to select flowers with greater average nectar rewards. The experiment that forms the basis of this case study is concerned with spatial association learning in hummingbirds, as studied by Brown (personal communication, 1991).

Previous experiments, conducted as part of the investigator's ongoing research, show that hummingbirds learn spatial associations very quickly relative to other organisms that have been tested in the laboratory (monkeys, rats, pigeons, and children); see reviews by Mackintosh (1983) and Bowe (1984). One plausible explanation for their success is that, in nature, hummingbirds must frequently learn floral cues in order to extract nectar hidden within flowers efficiently. The fact that many of these floral cues are visibly connected to the nectar of the flower suggests that visible guides may facilitate this learning.

To test this possibility, an experiment was conducted on the feeding behavior of 18 experimentally naive adult rufous hummingbirds (10 females and 8 males). The hummingbirds were assigned randomly by sex to one of three treatments: "no tape" (NT or treatment 1), in which no visible guides connected light cues with the feeders below them; "partial tape" (PT or treatment 2), in which fluorescent orange Dymo type (9 mm wide) provided a discontinuous

Case Studies in Biometry, Edited by Nicholas Lange, Louise Ryan, Lynne Billard, David Brillinger, Loveday Conquest, and Joel Greenhouse.
ISBN 0-471-58885-7 © 1994 John Wiley & Sons, Inc.

(i.e., broken in two places) connection between each light cue and its feeder; and "full tape" (FT or treatment 3), in which the visible guide between each light cue and its feeder (fluorescent orange Dymo tape) was continuous. Figure 1 displays the feeding arrays used in the experiment for each of the three groups. The NT group (treatment 1) had 4 females and 2 males, while the PT (treatment 2) and FT (treatment 3) groups each had 3 males and 3 females.

The investigator expected different learning patterns on each treatment; in particular, she expected hummingbirds in the two treatment groups with visible guides between cues and feeders (2 = PT and 3 = FT) to become aware of the cue–feeder relationship sooner than hummingbirds in the treatment group with no visible guides (1 = NT). From psychological principles of visual perception, she also expected birds in the treatment groups with discontinuous and contin-

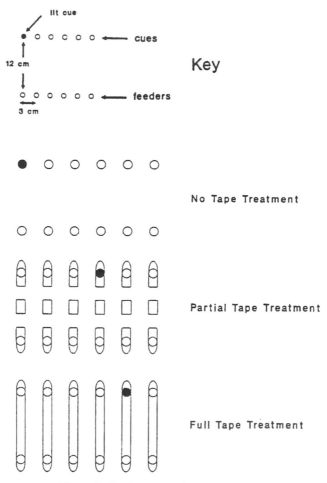

Figure 1. Feeding arrays for the experiment.

uous visible guides to become aware of the cue–feeder relationship at roughly the same time.

2   DATA

On a given day, three birds (one bird from each treatment group) were tested separately in three randomly assigned rooms, $1.3 \times 2.5 \times 2.5$ m high. A portion of one end wall in each room contained a horizontal array of six feeders, spaced 3 cm apart on a thin metal panel and marked by round fluorescent orange Avery labels (see Figure 1). A small red light, 4 mm in diameter, protruded slightly through the metal panel, 12 cm above each feeder. These small lights served as the spatial cues. During each feeding trial, one was lit to signal the feeder below it as the correct or "profitable" one.

Hummingbirds hovered at the feeders and probed their bills into small food reservoirs. If the feeder was the profitable one, 2 μL of sucrose solution was immediately released into the reservoir. Hummingbirds were free to fly and visit feeders at all times during the experiment. Between brief foraging bouts to the feeding array and short nonforaging flights around the room, they spent most of their time on a 1.5 m-high central perch located 1.8 m from the feeding array and designed to place birds at eye level with the feeders. A computer controlled the lights, dispensed the food, and recorded the time and duration of all visits to feeders and perches.

To allow the three hummingbirds to become accustomed to the feeding array used in the experiment, on the morning of the day before testing, the birds were placed in training cages identical to their home cages except that food was available from a wall feeder similar in appearance to the feeding array. The birds quickly learned to feed from these wall feeders. They were moved from their training cages to the experimental rooms that afternoon. Until experimental training began the following morning, the hummingbirds fed from a standard commercial feeder marked with a fluorescent orange Avery label around the access hole. This feeder was hung in front of the central array feeder on which training would start. The other five feeders on the array were covered.

At the beginning of the next day, the standard feeder was removed, exposing the hummingbird to a central feeder on the array. After the birds had fed several times from this feeder, the light above it was lit and training continued. After several more feedings, all other feeders were uncovered and the cue and profitability then reassigned to a different cue–feeder pair. This transfer procedure was repeated until birds had fed several times from each feeder when the light above it was lit. Training lasted approximately 2 hours.

Testing started immediately after training. Each hummingbird was tested for 60 feeding trials on each of three successive days. Birds received initial training on each testing day. Except for the final day, at the end of the day's 60 feeding trials, a commercial feeder was hung in front of a central feeder on the array, the other feeders on the array were covered, and the birds remained in the experimental rooms overnight.

The one profitable feeder and its cue were reassigned randomly among the six feeders for each feeding trial, but the same random sequence was used for all birds. Feeding trials began 2 minutes after preceding trials ended, or as soon as preceding trials ended and the birds perched. Simultaneously, at the beginning of each feeding trial, a buzzer sounded, the cue to the profitable feeder was lit, and the feeder was set to provide 2 μL of solution on each visit. Birds could visit any sequence of feeders and obtain food from the correct feeder up to 11 times, for a total of 22 μL each feeding trial. This quantity provided food at a rate slightly more than average *ad libitum* feeding rates.

No limit was imposed on the time for birds to respond in feeding trials. Feeding trials ended only after birds had probed the correct feeder 11 times, or after they had visited at least one feeder and returned to their perch. When a feeding trial ended, the light cue was turned off and the previously profitable feeder delivered no more food. All feeders remained exposed between trials.

Hummingbird learning was to be evaluated from *first* visits in these feeding trials. If the first visit was to a profitable feeder, the feeding trial was scored as a success; otherwise, it was scored as a failure. The resulting data set is thus comprised of 18 binary series of length 180, corresponding to the successes and failures of each bird on the *first* feeding foray in a trial, for 3 days of 60 consecutive feeding trials.

Associated with each of these binary series are two explanatory variables, or covariates; a label indicating the treatment group (1 = NT, 2 = FT, 3 = FT) and an indicator of the sex of the hummingbird (0 = male, 1 = female). The only other explanatory variables employed in the analyses which follow are related to time through the position of the current feeding trial in the series of 180 trials for each bird. In contrast with the covariates for treatment group and sex, these explanatory variables change over the course of the experiment. The inclusion of these time-dependent covariates will allow examination of the patterns of hummingbird learning over time. Table 1 gives a sample of the data collected in the study.

3 METHODS AND MODELS

3.1 Overview

Three distinct approaches will be employed in the analysis of the binary longitudinal data from this experiment. The first is a classical approach based on analysis of variance (ANOVA) techniques, while the latter two are recently developed, and much more flexible, approaches to the analysis of such binary longitudinal data. The last approach can equally well be applied to count and continuous responses.

A classical approach might be based on the proportion of successes achieved

Table 1   Representative Sample of Data from the Experiment

Bird	Rx[a]	Gender[b]	Results of First 30 (of 180) Trials
1	1	1	0 0 0 0 1 0 0 0 0 0 0 0 0 1 1 0 1 1 1 1 0 1 0 1 0 1 0 1 1 1
2	1	1	0 0 0 0 1 0 0 0 0 0 0 0 1 0 0 0 0 0 0 0 0 0 0 0 0 0 0 0 0 1
3	1	1	0 0 0 0 0 1 0 0 0 0 0 0 1 0 0 0 0 0 0 0 1 0 1 0 0 0 0 0 1 0
4	1	1	0 0 0 0 0 0 1 0 0 0 1 0 0 0 0 0 0 1 0 0 0 0 1 0 0 0 1 0 1 0
5	1	0	0 1 0 0 0 0 1 0 0 0 1 1 0 0 0 0 1 1 1 0 1 1 1 0 0 1 0 0 1 0
6	1	0	0 0 0 0 0 1 1 0 0 0 1 0 0 1 1 0 1 1 1 0 1 0 1 0 0 0 0 0 1 1
7	2	1	0 0 0 0 0 1 0 0 0 0 0 0 1 0 0 0 0 0 0 1 1 0 0 0 0 1 1 0 1 0
8	2	0	0 1 0 1 0 0 0 0 0 0 0 1 0 0 0 0 0 0 1 0 0 0 0 0 0 0 0 0 0 0
9	2	1	1 0 0 0 0 0 0 1 0 0 0 0 1 0 0 0 0 0 0 1 1 0 0 0 0 0 0 0 0 0
10	2	0	0 0 0 0 0 0 1 1 0 0 0 0 0 1 0 1 0 0 0 0 0 0 0 0 0 0 0 0 0 0
11	2	0	1 0 0 0 1 1 0 0 0 0 0 0 1 1 0 1 1 1 1 0 1 0 1 1 0 0 0 1 1 0
12	2	1	0 1 0 0 0 1 0 0 0 0 0 0 0 0 0 0 0 0 0 0 0 0 1 0 0 0 0 0 1 0
13	3	1	0 0 0 1 0 0 0 0 0 1 0 0 0 1 0 0 1 0 0 1 0 1 1 0 0 0 0 0 1 0 1
14	3	1	0 0 0 0 0 0 0 0 0 0 0 1 0 0 0 0 0 0 0 0 0 0 0 0 0 0 0 1 0 0
15	3	0	0 0 0 0 0 0 0 1 0 1 1 0 0 0 0 0 0 1 0 0 0 0 1 0 0 1 0 0 1 1
16	3	0	0 0 0 0 1 0 0 0 0 0 0 0 0 0 0 0 1 0 1 0 0 0 0 0 0 1 0 1 1 0
17	3	0	0 1 0 1 1 1 1 1 1 1 0 1 1 1 0 1 1 0 1 0 1 0 0 0 0 1 0 1 1 1
18	3	1	0 1 0 0 0 1 0 0 0 0 0 0 0 0 0 0 0 0 1 0 1 0 0 0 0 0 1 0 0 1

[a] 1, No-tape (NT) group; 2, partially taped (PT) group; and 3, fully taped (FT) group.
[b] Females are coded as 1; males as 0.

by each bird over blocks of consecutive trials. For example, the binary data for each bird might be summarized as proportions of successful trials on each of the three days in the experiment. These proportions might then be analyzed via multivariate ANOVA or univariate ANOVA for repeated measures, perhaps subsequent to a transformation to improve compliance to ANOVA assumptions. These ANOVA techniques are well known among researchers in the biological sciences and psychology, but they provide a severely limited approach to the analysis of these data. Required distributional assumptions are likely to be violated and this cannot be assessed adequately from the data. Alternative techniques which account for correlation over time within subjects, permit flexible modeling of the success probability as a function of time, and can accommodate covariates readily would be preferable.

The *working likelihood* approach of Zeger et al. (1985) is one such technique. Here, a working likelihood is used to generate estimating equations for regression parameters which model the marginal probability of success as a function of time-independent covariates. The extension of this approach to the case of time-dependent covariates permits success probabilities to be modeled as functions of time while taking into account the correlation between measurements on each bird. Hence, comparisons of the learning trajectories of hummingbirds across treatment groups are more direct than with the classical analysis.

In the *generalized estimating equation* (GEE) approach of Zeger and Liang

(1986) and Liang and Zeger (1986), the marginal distribution of the univariate outcome at each time point is modeled by specifying a known function of the mean as a linear combination of the covariates, and by assuming that the marginal variance is a known function of the mean, up to an unknown constant. This partial specification of the joint distribution gives rise to generalized estimating equations for the regression parameters which incorporate a *working correlation matrix* for the outcome vector for each subject. For the hummingbird data, this approach is more flexible than the working likelihood approach because marginal likelihoods need not be specified and because many possible *working correlations* are available for explicitly modeling correlation in the responses. Moreover, only weak assumptions about the true correlation structure are necessary for valid asymptotic results.

3.2 Classical Approach

One approach to the analysis of binary longitudinal data such as the hummingbird data is to calculate the proportion of correct responses over blocks of an equal number of successive time points for each subject and then "normalize" these proportions via the arcsine square-root or logit transformation (see Draper and Smith, 1981, pp. 238–239). The resulting subject response vectors within the ith treatment group might then be assumed to be approximately normally distributed with mean vector μ_i and covariance matrix Σ_i. If scientific theory suggests that these covariance matrices are the same across treatment groups, or if there is insufficient evidence in the data to conclude otherwise, multivariate analysis of variance (MANOVA) of the response vectors would then be reasonable (see Morrison, 1976, p. 179).

Before proceeding with such a MANOVA, the equality of the covariance matrices across treatment groups should be checked. However, for experiments with small numbers of subjects within treatment groups, there are no satisfactory methods for doing this. Furthermore, when there are few subjects in a treatment group relative to the number of binary responses for each subject, the aggressive blocking of binary responses required to obtain nonsingular estimates of the covariance matrices for the resulting response vectors does not permit a detailed description of how the probability of success changes as a function of time. In particular, the experiment under discussion has only six birds per treatment group, so the length of the response vector must be 4 or less for the estimated covariance matrices to be nonsingular. Clearly, response vectors with only four elements (data blocked over 45 trials) may not provide a sufficiently detailed representation of the learning trajectories. This limitation would be even more pronounced with the more natural blocking over all 60 trials in each day, which leads to response vectors with three proportions of successes, one for each of the three days of experimentation. An alternative method of analysis which is able to provide higher resolution of the learning trajectories would be more desirable.

The obvious way to obtain a more detailed representation of the learning trajectory is to block over fewer trials. However, blocking over fewer than 45 trials precludes estimation of separate covariance matrices within the various treatment groups. If the assumption of equal covariance matrices across treatment groups is justified, the common covariance matrix can be estimated from the binary data blocked over as few as 15 trials. Four elements of the resulting 12-element response vector then describe the learning trajectory within each day of experimentation, and MANOVA allows an assessment of differences in the corresponding mean learning trajectories across treatment groups. Further, univariate ANOVA for repeated measures, a simpler but in some cases less powerful method which is more accessible to subject-area researchers familiar with experimental design, can be used as an alternative to MANOVA (see Morrison 1976, pp. 212–216).

However, the assumption of equal covariance matrices across treatment groups is unlikely to be realistic for such transformed binomial data, where success probabilities are expected to differ across treatment groups. For each treatment group, the entries in these covariance matrices depend upon two distinct sources of variability: that due to estimation of the underlying probabilities of success for each subject by observed proportions, and that due to subject-to-subject variation in these underlying probabilities. While the arcsine square-root transformation could reasonably be expected to stabilize the variances of the observed proportions for each subject, covariances among these observed proportions, resulting from correlation over time in the underlying binary responses, would not be stabilized. Nor would this transformation relate to the distinct issue of homogeneity of subject-to-subject variances and covariances across the different treatment groups; indeed, from previous experience, the experimenter does not anticipate such homogeneity in the data.

Hence, the statistical tests associated with multivariate and univariate ANOVA may not provide valid inferences for such binary longitudinal data. Nevertheless, for the sake of illustration, and to provide a basis for comparison to other approaches, we present the results of a possible analysis using univariate ANOVA for repeated measures. This method is strictly valid only if observations are multinormally distributed with a common covariance structure corresponding to the so-called type-H pattern (Huynh and Feldt, 1970), but conservative tests based on adjusting the degrees of freedom for the univariate tests are available (Greenhouse and Geisser, 1959) and these are used in the analysis presented.

3.3 Working Likelihood Approach

A natural approach to the analysis of binary longitudinal data is to extend logistic regression to the case where the binary outcome variable is observed repeatedly for each subject. Zeger et al. (1985) present the details of such an approach in which, rather than the actual likelihood, a *working likelihood* based on simple assumptions about the dependence over time within each subject's data is used to generate estimating equations which lead to consistent estimators $\hat{\beta}$ of the regression parameters β (i.e., $\hat{\beta}$ converges in probability to β as the number of subjects grows without bound), as well as standard errors for these estimates. Not only does this approach allow for correlation over time within each subject's data, but it also allows flexible modeling of the response, while remaining conceptually simple and easy to interpret.

To establish notation, let $Y_{i,t}, t = 1, \ldots, m_i$, be a stationary binary time series, and let x_i be a row vector of time-independent covariates for the ith subject, $i = 1, \ldots, n$. If $\pi_i = \Pr(Y_{i,t} = 1)$, the probability of success for the ith subject, it is assumed that logit $\pi_i = x_i\beta$. The primary objective is to make inference about the vector β of regression parameters. If, for example, a subset of the covariates are indicator variables for treatment groups, inference for the corresponding regression parameters refers to the assessment of treatment effects.

Zeger et al. (1985) present two estimators of β which arise from maximizing two different working likelihoods. The first, $\hat{\beta}_0$, is obtained from the working assumption that repeated observations for a subject are independent of one another. This estimator is consistent (as $n \to \infty$) for any set of stationary binary time series for which logit $\pi_i = x_i\beta$. The second estimator, $\hat{\beta}_1$ is obtained from the working assumption that each binary time series has a stationary 1-dependent correlation structure (i.e., the correlation between any two observations adjacent in time is constant, with all other correlations being zero). This estimator is consistent (as $n \to \infty$) for any set of stationary binary time series for which both logit $\pi_i = x_i\beta$ and the first lag autocorrelation, $\rho = \text{Cor}(Y_{i,t}, Y_{i,t-1})$, is common to all subjects. Consistent estimates of the asymptotic covariance matrices of both estimators of β are available, thereby enabling inference on the regression parameters.

Note that the covariates x_i in this development are time independent. Hence, the success probabilities π_i do not vary with time. Zeger et al. (1985) were concerned with short binary time series, where there was no need for time-dependent success probabilities. However, the hummingbird feeding trials are long (180 time points), and success probabilities are expected to increase with time, as the birds learn. Indeed, an important objective of the analysis is to model this relationship. To allow the analysis required for this experiment, extension of the Zeger et al. (1985) results to the case of time-dependent covariates is required.

Now let $x_{i,t}$ be a vector of time-dependent covariates for the ith subject, $i = 1, \ldots, n$. If $\pi_{i,t} = \Pr(Y_{i,t} = 1)$, the probability of success for the ith subject at the tth time point, it is assumed that logit $\pi_{i,t} = x_{i,t}\beta$. Besides the vector β of regression parameters there may be additional nuisance parameters in the working likelihood, so let θ denote all the parameters. Let $S(\theta)$ be the score function for the working likelihood [i.e., $S(\theta)$ is the vector of first derivatives of the working log-likelihood]. Then let $H(\theta)$ be the corresponding Hessian matrix [i.e., $H(\theta)$ is the matrix of second derivatives of the working log-likelihood]. Finally, let $\hat{\theta}$ be the estimate of θ obtained by maximizing the working likelihood; in general, we have $S(\hat{\theta}) = 0$. Expressions for elements of the score functions and entries of the Hessian matrices evaluated under the working likelihood are straightforward to derive; details can be found in Graham (1991). Throughout, $E(\cdot)$ denotes the expectation under the true unknown likelihood.

Independence Working Model

Consider first the working assumption that repeated observations for a subject are independent. The estimator $\hat{\beta}_0$ is obtained by maximizing the corresponding independence working log-likelihood, $l_0(\beta) = \sum_{i=1}^{n} l_{0i}(\beta)$, where

$$l_{0i}(\beta) = \sum_{t=1}^{m_i} [y_{i,t}x_{i,t}\beta + \log(1 - \pi_{i,t})],$$

and logit $\pi_{i,t} = x_{i,t}\beta$. Under regularity conditions sufficient to guarantee the consistency of $\hat{\beta}_0$, Proposition 2.1 of Zeger et al. (1985) can be generalized to the case of time-dependent covariates as follows:

PROPOSITION 1. *Let* $Y_{i,t}, t = 1, \ldots, m_i \leq \infty, i = 1, \ldots, n$, *be binary time series such that* $\text{logit } E(Y_{i,t}) = x_{i,t}\beta$. *Then* $\hat{\beta}_0 - \beta$ *is asymptotically multivariate Gaussian with expectation 0 and covariance matrix*

$$V_0(\beta) = E^{-1}[H_0(\beta)]I_0(\beta)E^{-1}[H_0(\beta)],$$

where $I_0(\beta) = E[S(\beta)S(\beta)^{\mathrm{T}}]$.

The asymptotic covariance matrix $V_0(\beta)$ depends on expectations evaluated under the true likelihood, which is unknown. Nevertheless, a consistent estimate is given by

$$\hat{V}_0 = H_0^{-1}(\hat{\beta}_0)\hat{I}_0 H_0^{-1}(\hat{\beta}_0).$$

Here

$$\hat{I}_0 = \sum_{i=1}^{n} S_i(\hat{\beta}_0)S_i(\hat{\beta}_0)^{\mathrm{T}},$$

where $S_i(\cdot)$ is the score function for the ith subject and $H_0(\beta)$ is the Hessian for the independence working likelihood.

First-Order Working Model

The first-order working model assumes that each binary time series has a stationary 1-dependent correlation structure with $\text{Cor}(Y_{i,t}, Y_{i,t-1}) = \rho$. If $p_{i,t} = E(Y_{i,t}|Y_{i,t-1})$, the assumption of a common lag one autocorrelation implies that

$$p_{i,t} = \pi_{i,t} + \rho \left(\frac{\pi_{i,t}\bar{\pi}_{i,t}}{\pi_{i,t-1}\bar{\pi}_{i,t-1}} \right)^{1/2} (y_{i,t-1} - \pi_{i,t-1}), \tag{1}$$

where $\bar{\pi}_{i,t} = 1 - \pi_{i,t}$.

Let $\theta = (\rho, \beta)$. The estimate $\hat{\theta}$ is obtained by maximizing the corresponding first-order working log-likelihood, $l_1(\theta) = \sum_{i=1}^{n} l_{1i}(\theta)$, where

$$l_{1i}(\theta) = y_{i,1}x_{i,1}\beta + \ln(1 - \pi_{i,1})$$
$$+ \sum_{t=2}^{m_i} [y_{i,t} \ln p_{i,t} + (1 - y_{i,t}) \ln(1 - p_{i,t})],$$

$p_{i,t}$ is given at (1), and logit $\pi_{i,t} = x_{i,t}\beta$. Under regularity conditions sufficient to guarantee the consistency of $\hat{\theta}$, Proposition 2.2 of Zeger et al. (1985) can be generalized to the case of time-dependent covariates as follows:

PROPOSITION 2. *Let $Y_{i,t}, t = 1, \ldots, m_i < \infty, i = 1, \ldots, n$ be binary time series such that logit $E(Y_{i,t}) = x_{i,t}\beta$ and Cor $(Y_{i,t}, Y_{i,t-1}) = \rho$. Then, $\hat{\theta} - \theta$ is asymptotically multivariate Gaussian with expectation 0 and covariance matrix*

$$V_1(\theta) = E^{-1}[H_1(\theta)]I_1(\theta)E^{-1}[H_1(\theta)],$$

where $I_1(\theta) = E[S(\theta)S(\theta)^T]$.

A consistent estimate of $V_1(\theta)$, the asymptotic covariance matrix, is given by

$$\hat{V}_1 = H_1^{-1}(\hat{\theta})\hat{I}_1 H_1^{-1}(\hat{\theta}).$$

Here

$$\hat{I}_1 = \sum_{i=1}^{n} S_i(\hat{\theta})S_i(\hat{\theta})^T,$$

where $S_i(\cdot)$ is the score function for the ith subject and $H_1(\hat{\theta})$ is the Hessian matrix for the first-order working likelihood.

3.4 GEE Approach

The generalized estimating equation (GEE) approach described in Liang and Zeger (1986) and Zeger and Liang (1986) provides a unified and flexible approach to the analysis of longitudinal data. For our context of binary longitudinal data, the GEE approach is more flexible than the working likelihood approach because it allows many possible working correlations for modeling correlation over time within subjects. Further, this approach allows the correlation structure to differ not only across treatment groups, but also across individual subjects; this feature is particularly useful when different subjects are observed at different sequences of time points.

Suppose that we are interested in how the outcome variable $Y_{i,t}, i = 1, \ldots, n$ and $t = 1, \ldots, m_i$, depends on the time-dependent covariates $x_{i,t}$. If there were only one time of observation for each subject, a generalized linear model (see McCullagh and Nelder, 1989) could be used to model a variety of continuous and discrete outcome variables. However, for longitudinal data, the possible correlation among the repeated observations for a given subject must be taken into account to obtain efficient estimators of the regression parameters and asymptotically unbiased estimators of their standard errors.

Modeling the correlation directly is often difficult for non-Gaussian longitudinal data because there are few natural models for the joint distribution of the repeated observations. Liang and Zeger (1986) and Zeger and Liang (1986) propose a methodology based on an extension of the quasi-likelihood approach described by Wedderburn (1974). In particular, if $\mu_{i,t}$ and $v_{i,t}$ denote the expectation and variance of $Y_{i,t}$, the expectation is assumed to be a known function of a linear combination of the covariates, that is,

$$\mu_{i,t} = h(x_{i,t}\beta) \quad \text{or} \quad h^{-1}(\mu_{i,t}) = x_{i,t}\beta,$$

where β is a vector of regression parameters. In addition, except for an unknown scale parameter ϕ, the variance is assumed to be a known function of the expectation, that is,

$$v_{i,t} = \frac{g(\mu_{i,t})}{\phi}.$$

For the hummingbird data, the responses are binary, and $\mu_{i,t} = E(Y_{i,t})$ is simply $\pi_{i,t}$, the probability of success of the ith bird at the tth trial. The natural choices of $h(\cdot)$ and $g(\cdot)$ are then the logit link, $h^{-1}(\pi) = \text{logit}(\pi)$, and the Bernoulli mean–variance relationship, $g(\pi) = \pi(1 - \pi)$.

To incorporate the anticipated correlation over time, Zeger and Liang (1986) specify $R_i(\alpha)$, an $m_i \times m_i$ working correlation matrix for the outcome vector, $Y_i = (Y_{i,1}, \ldots, Y_{i,m_i})^{\text{T}}$, of the ith subject. The collection of working correlation matrices is assumed to be fully specified by α, a vector of unknown parameters. The working covariance matrix for Y_i is then

$$V_i = \frac{A_i^{1/2} R_i(\alpha) A_i^{1/2}}{\phi},$$

where A_i is an $m_i \times m_i$ diagonal matrix with $g(\mu_{i,t})$ as the tth diagonal element. Note that observation times and working correlation matrices are allowed to differ across subjects in the GEE approach.

For the estimation of β, Liang and Zeger (1986) propose the generalized estimating equations,

$$\sum_{i=1}^{n} D_i^{\mathrm{T}} V_i^{-1}(y_i - \mu_i) = 0,$$

where $\mu_i = E(Y_i) = (\mu_{i,1}, \ldots, \mu_{i,m_i})^{\mathrm{T}} = [h(x_{i,1}\beta), \ldots, h(x_{i,m_i}\beta)]^{\mathrm{T}}$, and $D_i = \partial\mu_i/\partial\beta$. Since the nuisance parameters α and ϕ enter the GEEs only through V_i and the primary goal is inference for the regression parameters β, an obvious way to proceed is to replace α and ϕ by consistent estimates and solve the altered GEEs for β. The GEE estimate of the regression coefficient, $\tilde{\beta}_G$, is obtained by iterating between solving the GEEs for β and estimating α and ϕ using residuals from the fit based on the current estimate of β. These two steps are repeated until all estimates converge.

Under mild regularity conditions, Liang and Zeger (1986, Theorem 2, p. 16) show that as the number of subjects, n, becomes large, $\sqrt{n}(\tilde{\beta}_G - \beta)$ is asymptotically multivariate normal with zero mean and covariance matrix given by V_G, where

$$V_G = \lim_{n \to \infty} n \left(\sum_{i=1}^{n} D_i^{\mathrm{T}} V_i^{-1} D_i \right)^{-1} \left[\sum_{i=1}^{n} D_i^{\mathrm{T}} V_i^{-1} \mathrm{Var}(Y_i) V_i^{-1} D_i \right]$$
$$\cdot \left(\sum_{i=1}^{n} D_i^{\mathrm{T}} V_i^{-1} D_i \right)^{-1};$$

here $\mathrm{Var}(Y_i)$ is the actual covariance matrix for the response vector of the ith subject. Note that V_G, the asymptotic covariance matrix of $\tilde{\beta}_G$, does not depend on how α and ϕ are estimated, as long as they are consistently estimated. The covariance matrix V_G can be consistently estimated by replacing $\mathrm{Var}(Y_i)$ by $(y_i - \tilde{\mu}_i)(y_i - \tilde{\mu}_i)^{\mathrm{T}}$, where $\tilde{\mu}_i = [h(x_{i,1}\tilde{\beta}_G), \ldots, h(x_{i,m_i}\tilde{\beta}_G)]^{\mathrm{T}}$, β by $\tilde{\beta}_G$, and α and ϕ by their consistent estimates. Further details, particularly on consistent estimation of α and ϕ using the residuals, are provided by Liang and Zeger (1986).

The GEE approach has a strong appeal because it does not require the working correlations to be correctly specified for asymptotically valid results. In practice, the true correlation structure of the response is rarely known. Nevertheless, it is desirable to incorporate whatever knowledge is available about the actual correlation structure present in the data, to obtain more efficient estimators for the regression parameters. The GEE approach allows this through the specification of the working correlation matrices.

4   RESULTS

4.1   Classical Analysis

The analysis is based on the proportion of correct responses for blocks of 15 successive trials, transformed via the arcsine square-root transformation. The averages of the resulting 12-dimensional response vectors within each treatment group are shown in Figure 2. The figure suggests the transformed response grows roughly linearly with time, particularly for birds in treatments 2 (PT) and 3 (FT). The lack of systematic discontinuities in these response curves at measurements corresponding to new days (measurements 5 and 9 in Figure 2) indicates that modeling a day effect is not necessary. Thus, if $\hat{P}_{ijk}$ is the success proportion and ϵ_{ijk} is the noise term for the kth bird within the ith treatment at the jth measurement, a candidate model is

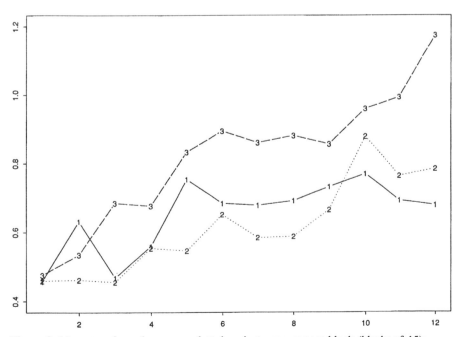

Figure 2. Mean transformed response plotted against measurement block (blocks of 15); ———, treatment one; · · · ·, treatment two; - - - - - -, treatment three.

$$Y_{ijk} = \arcsin\left(\sqrt{\hat{P}_{ijk}}\right)$$

$$= \mu + [treatment]_i + [measurement]_j + [treatment \times measurement]_{ij}$$
$$+ [bird]_{(i)k} + [measurement \times bird]_{(i)jk} + \epsilon_{ijk},$$

for $i = 1, 2, 3$, $j = 1, \ldots, 12$, and $k = 1, \ldots, 6$. Here "treatment" and "measurement" are fixed-effect factors, and "bird" is a random-effect factor nested within "treatment." The assumption that the birds' noise vectors $\epsilon_{ijk}, j = 1, \ldots, 12$, are independent normally distributed random vectors with mean 0 and common covariance matrix Σ justifies a univariate ANOVA using the conservative tests based on the Greenhouse and Geisser (1959) adjustments to the degrees of freedom.

The estimated variances of the transformed responses are plotted against measurement for each treatment group in Figure 3. The plots do not suggest an obvious pattern in the variances over time, but do suggest the variances in treatment 3 are generally largest, while variances in treatment 2 are generally smallest. Off-diagonal elements of the estimated covariance matrices are not presented, but are also clearly different across treatment groups. Although the effects of these possible departures from the assumption of a common covari-

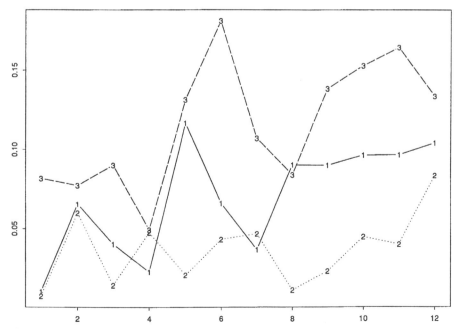

Figure 3. Variance estimates plotted against measurement block (blocks of 15); ———, treatment one; ····, treatment two; ------, treatment three.

Table 2 ANOVA for Blocks of 15 Trials

Source	SS	d.f.	MS	F	Adjusted d.f.	p-Value
Measurement	3.56	11	0.32	8.68	1,15	0.01
Treatment	1.70	2	0.85	1.76		0.21
Bird (within treatment)	7.22	15	0.48			
Measurement × treatment	0.96	22	0.044	1.17	2,15	0.34
Bird × measurement (within treatment)	6.15	165	0.037			
Total	19.59	215				

ance matrix are unclear, certainly conclusions based on statistical tests formulated under this assumption must be considered as tentative.

The ANOVA given in Table 2 confirms one clear indication from Figure 2: "measurement" is an important factor. However, Table 2 provides no strong evidence of "treatment" effects, either through the main effect or through interaction with "measurement." On the other hand, Figure 2 clearly indicates the transformed responses for treatment 3 are generally greater than those in the other treatments. Any treatment main effect seems to be obscured by the relatively large bird-to-bird variability present in the data of the third (FT) treatment group.

A further limitation of this general approach is the difficulty of incorporating the sex of each bird into the analysis because of the unequal number of males and females in the first treatment group (NT). Moreover, the approach models the response as a function of time in an indirect way which lacks intuitive appeal, by including "measurement" main effects and interactions in the model. Multivariate ANOVA, which models changes in response over time through the different elements of the treatment mean response vectors, has the same limitation. Alternative approaches which have the flexibility to model treatment response patterns directly as functions of time while taking into account the correlation of measurements within subjects would be more effective.

4.2 Working Likelihood Analyses

Several plots were first examined to determine appropriate parametric forms to be incorporated into modeling of the learning trajectories. Plots of the average treatment responses on the logit scale $\{\ln[(\bar{y} + c)/(1 - \bar{y} + c)], c = 0.5\}$ for successive blocks of 3, 5, and 10 trials (not included here) suggested no systematic discontinuities at trials corresponding to new days (trials 61 and 121), so as in the classical analysis, modeling of a day effect seemed unnecessary.

To examine how treatment responses changed over time, the averages over birds of the same sex within each treatment were calculated separately at each time point. The logits of these proportions were then smoothed using robust locally weighted linear least squares or "lowess" (Cleveland, 1979); see Figures 4 to 6. These plots suggest that, on average, males have a higher success probability than females in all three treatments throughout the experiment. For treatments 2 (PT) and 3 (FT), the success probabilities increase roughly linearly with time (on the logit scale), whereas for treatment 1 (NT), the success probabilities appear to increase over the first two days but to decrease over at least part of the third day. For all three treatment groups, the figures suggest that a model incorporating an additive (on the logit scale) effect for sex, with males having higher transformed success probabilities than females, may be adequate to explain the patterns in the data. Furthermore, sex-by-treatment interaction may also be present, since the figures indicate that a different additive effect for sex in each treatment group may be necessary.

These exploratory plots suggest the following model for the transformed probability of success on the first feeding foray:

$$\text{logit}\,\pi_{i,t,s} = \mu_i + sex_i + \beta_{lis}T + \beta_{qis}T^2,$$

$$i = 1, 2, 3, \quad s = 1, 2, \quad t = 1, \dots, 180,$$

where $T = (t - \bar{t})/\text{sd}(t), \mu_i$ may be interpreted as an overall effect of the ith treatment group, sex_i is the female-to-male differential sex effect for the ith treatment group, and $s = 1$ refers to the female birds. The explanatory variable

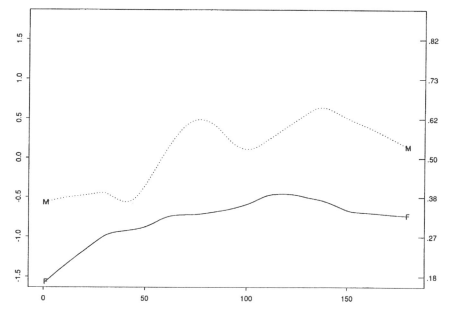

Figure 4. Smoothed logit of average response for treatment one (smoothing window of 60 observations); left-hand axis is logit scale, right hand axis is success probability scale; ———, females; · · · ·, males.

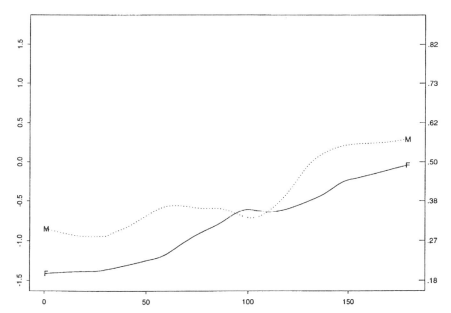

Figure 5. Smoothed logit of average response for treatment 2 (smoothing window of 60 observations); left-hand axis is logit scale, right-hand axis is success probability scale; ——, females; ····, males.

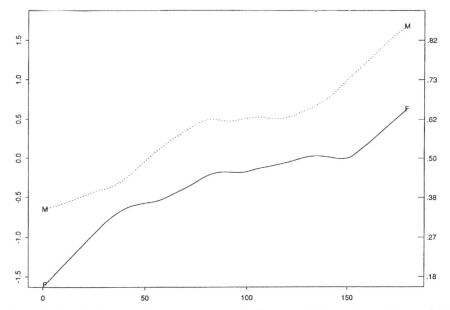

Figure 6. Smoothed logit of average response for treatment 3 (smoothing window of 60 observations); left-hand axis is logit scale, right-hand axis is success probability scale; ——, females; ····, males.

for time has been standardized to orthogonalize the linear and quadratic time covariates which would otherwise be highly collinear (see Draper and Smith, 1981, pp. 260–262).

The primary aim of this analysis is to understand the differences in hummingbird learning across treatment groups. Because birds of different sexes in different treatments may learn in different ways, the initial model allows all possible interactions of time, sex, and treatment. The purpose of subsequent model reductions is to obtain a parsimonious final model which reliably addresses the investigator's questions. To focus the analysis on treatment differences, the reduction procedure eliminates unnecessary terms for negligible interactions first, leaving the examination of overall treatment effects for the final steps. The investigator does not anticipate complicated sex-by-time interactions, so these are checked before the interaction of treatment group and time. In addition, quadratic terms common to males and females within treatments are treated differently from the corresponding linear terms because Figure 4 suggests that birds in treatment 1 may have success probabilities requiring a quadratic component on the logit scale.

All model reductions will be assessed via Wald statistics based on the asymptotic multivariate normal approximation to the distribution of the parameter estimates. (In the usual case of testing whether a vector θ of parameters is equal to 0, the Wald statistic is simply $\hat{\theta}^T \text{Var}^{-1}(\hat{\theta})\hat{\theta}$, where $\text{Var}(\hat{\theta})$ is the asymptotic covariance matrix or, more often, a consistent estimate. Under the hypothesis being assessed, Wald statistics have asymptotic chi-squared distributions with degrees of freedom equal to the number of parameters tested.) In the analyses to follow, a reduction will be considered permissible if the corresponding Wald statistic has a p-value greater than 0.15.

Independence Working Likelihood

Parameter estimates and standard errors for six successively reduced models (M1–M6) are provided in Table 3. The model reduction path is described by the following steps:

1. Check the quadratic terms.
   (a) Can the coefficients for males and females be set equal within each treatment group? Yes; the p-value for this reduction is 0.80.
   (b) Can the quadratic coefficients be eliminated? No; the p-value for simultaneous elimination of all three quadratic coefficients is a marginal 0.12. The z-scores for the three quadratic coefficients are -2.29, 0.35, and -0.70, suggesting the presence of a quadratic trend in the first treatment group only, which is consistent with Figures 4–6.

2. Check the linear terms.
   (a) Can the linear coefficients for males and females be set equal within each treatment group? Yes; the p-value for this reduction is 0.91.

Table 3 Model Reductions with the Independence Working Likelihood

Parameter	M1	M2	M3	M4	M5	M6
			Model[a]			
μ_1	0.36(0.03)	0.36(0.17)	0.36(0.17)	0.39(0.17)	0.18(0.27)	0.18(0.27)
μ_2	−0.59(0.31)	−0.53(0.26)	−0.53(0.24)	−0.53(0.24)	−0.36(0.26)	−0.32(0.20)
μ_3	0.53(0.75)	0.60(0.71)	0.60(0.69)	0.58(0.67)	0.54(0.48)	0.45(0.41)
sex_1	−1.03(0.42)	−1.02(0.42)	−1.03(0.43)	−1.06(0.44)	−0.75(0.28)	−0.75(0.28)
sex_2	−0.25(0.40)	−0.37(0.30)	−0.36(0.30)	−0.36(0.31)	sex_1	sex_1
sex_3	−0.72(0.76)	−0.86(0.66)	−0.86(0.64)	−0.83(0.60)	sex_1	sex_1
β_{l11}	0.21(0.09)	0.21(0.09)	0.29(0.14)	0.48(0.11)	0.47(0.11)	0.48(0.11)
β_{l21}	0.55(0.21)	0.54(0.21)	0.50(0.16)	β_{l11}	β_{l11}	β_{l11}
β_{l31}	0.54(0.38)	0.54(0.38)	0.63(0.24)	β_{l11}	β_{l11}	β_{l11}
β_{l12}	0.41(0.31)	0.41(0.31)	β_{l11}	β_{l11}	β_{l11}	β_{l11}
β_{l22}	0.46(0.23)	0.46(0.24)	β_{l21}	β_{l11}	β_{l11}	β_{l11}
β_{l32}	0.74(0.27)	0.73(0.27)	β_{l31}	β_{l11}	β_{l11}	β_{l11}
β_{q11}	−0.21(0.08)	−0.21(0.09)	−0.22(0.08)	−0.24(0.09)	−0.24(0.10)	−0.24(0.10)
β_{q21}	−0.04(0.05)	0.03(0.10)	0.04(0.10)	0.04(0.10)	0.04(0.11)	—
β_{q31}	−0.16(0.15)	−0.09(0.12)	−0.10(0.15)	−0.10(0.14)	−0.09(0.14)	—
β_{q12}	−0.22(0.21)	β_{q11}	β_{q11}	β_{q11}	β_{q11}	β_{q11}
β_{q22}	0.10(0.18)	β_{q21}	β_{q21}	β_{q21}	β_{q21}	—
β_{q32}	−0.007(0.18)	β_{q31}	β_{q31}	β_{q31}	β_{q31}	—

[a]M1, full model; M2, common quadratic effects for males and females within each treatment; M3, common linear effects for males and females within each treatment; M4, common linear effect for all treatments; M5, common differential sex effect for all treatments; M6, no quadratic effects for treatments 2 and 3.

(b) Can the resulting linear coefficients be set equal for all treatment groups? Yes; the p-value for this reduction is 0.38.

(c) Can this common linear term be eliminated? No; the p-value for this reduction is less than 0.001.

3. Check the differential sex effects.

(a) Can they be set equal for all treatment groups? Yes; the p-value for this reduction is 0.40. (It is perhaps worth noting that this reduction appears possible primarily because the differential sex effects are rather poorly determined; this is a direct consequence of the small numbers of birds in each treatment group.)

(b) Can this additive sex effect be eliminated? No; the p-value for this reduction is 0.007.

4. For interpretability of the final model, consider elimination of the quadratic terms for treatments 2 (PT) and 3 (FT). The p-value for this reduction is 0.74, justifying what is suggested by Figures 5 and 6: these success probabilities can be described adequately by a linear trajectory. The negative quadratic coefficient for treatment 1 (NT) reflects the pattern apparent in Figure 4: the success probabilities appear to increase over the first two days but to decrease over at least part of the third day.

First-Order Working Likelihood

The reduction path with the first-order working likelihood is summarized in Table 4 for six different models (M1–M6), and is similar to the path with the independence working likelihood; the only qualitative difference is the elimination of all quadratic coefficients from model M2, which is permissible here (p-value $= 0.20$). Although not apparent from Table 4, the estimates of ρ increase steadily from 0.127 in model M1 to 0.137 in model M6, paralleling the decreasing complexity in the modeling of time.

Using the first-order working likelihood to fit the final model obtained with the independence working likelihood (see Table 3) yields estimates of 0.17(0.27), $-0.30(0.20)$, 0.46(0.42), $-0.73(0.28)$, 0.47(0.11), and $-0.22(0.10)$ for $\mu_1, \mu_2, \mu_3, sex_1, \beta_{l11}$, and β_{q11}, respectively; these are virtually identical to those obtained with the independence working likelihood. Incidentally, the estimate of ρ in this fit is 0.13(0.03), which agrees with the values in Table 4.

Since Cor $(\hat{\mu}_1, \hat{\mu}_2) \approx 0$, the standard errors for the final model in Table 4 indicate that setting the main effects for treatments 1 and 2 to be equal would be a permissible further reduction of the model. In fact, the p-value for this reduction is 0.35, with the fitted value common to μ_1 and μ_2 being -0.19 ($se =$

Table 4   Model Reductions with the First-Order Working Likelihood

Parameter	Model[a]					
	M1	M2	M3	M4	M5	M6
ρ	0.13(0.03)	0.13(0.03)	0.13(0.03)	0.13(0.03)	0.13(0.03)	0.14(0.03)
μ_1	0.36(0.04)	0.35(0.20)	0.16(0.29)	0.15(0.25)	0.17(0.26)	$-0.04(0.27)$
μ_2	$-0.58(0.30)$	$-0.53(0.24)$	$-0.49(0.19)$	$-0.50(0.18)$	$-0.50(0.17)$	$-0.30(0.20)$
μ_3	0.59(0.87)	0.65(0.81)	0.56(0.76)	0.54(0.69)	0.51(0.64)	0.46(0.42)
sex_1	$-1.03(0.40)$	$-1.02(0.42)$	$-1.02(0.42)$	$-1.02(0.41)$	$-1.06(0.42)$	$-0.73(0.28)$
sex_2	$-0.23(0.37)$	$-0.34(0.27)$	$-0.34(0.27)$	$-0.33(0.27)$	$-0.33(0.27)$	sex_1
sex_3	$-0.79(0.88)$	$-0.89(0.75)$	$-0.89(0.76)$	$-0.87(0.69)$	$-0.84(0.64)$	sex_1
β_{l11}	0.20(0.08)	0.20(0.08)	0.19(0.07)	0.27(0.13)	0.47(0.11)	0.46(0.11)
β_{l21}	0.52(0.20)	0.51(0.20)	0.52(0.20)	0.49(0.15)	β_{l11}	β_{l11}
β_{l31}	0.54(0.38)	0.53(0.38)	0.53(0.38)	0.64(0.26)	β_{l11}	β_{l11}
β_{l12}	0.42(0.35)	0.42(0.34)	0.42(0.36)	β_{l11}	β_{l11}	β_{l11}
β_{l22}	0.46(0.22)	0.46(0.22)	0.47(0.23)	β_{l21}	β_{l11}	β_{l11}
β_{l32}	0.77(0.33)	0.76(0.33)	0.77(0.37)	β_{l31}	β_{l11}	β_{l11}
β_{q11}	$-0.19(0.09)$	$-0.20(0.10)$	—	—	—	—
β_{q21}	$-0.03(0.05)$	0.03(0.10)	—	—	—	—
β_{q31}	$-0.15(0.15)$	$-0.10(0.13)$	—	—	—	—
β_{q12}	$-0.21(0.24)$	β_{q11}	—	—	—	—
β_{q22}	0.09(0.18)	β_{q21}	—	—	—	—
β_{q32}	$-0.04(0.19)$	β_{q31}	—	—	—	—

[a]M1, full model; M2, common quadratic effects for males and females within each treatment; M3, no quadratic effects; M4, common linear effect for males and females within each treatment; M5, common linear effects for all treatments; M6, common differential sex effect for all treatments.

0.21). This reduction could be carried out for interpretability of the final model but is not incorporated into what follows.

The estimated values of ρ throughout Table 4 suggest the presence of a small, though nonnegligible, positive lag 1 correlation over time. In this case, estimates resulting from the first-order working likelihood are expected to be more efficient than those from the independence working likelihood, provided that the additional assumption upon which that analysis is based (a common lag 1 autocorrelation shared by all birds) obtains. Residuals from fitted models permit estimation of a lag 1 autocorrelation for each bird and suggest that a common lag 1 autocorrelation may *not* be shared by all birds. This assumption is required for the validity of the asymptotic results of Proposition 2 concerning parameter estimates obtained from the first-order working likelihood; it ensures that these estimates are asymptotically unbiased. The validity of the corresponding asymptotic results for the independence working likelihood (see Proposition 1) does not require any assumptions about the correlation within each bird's responses, so the fit resulting from the independence working likelihood may be considered the more reliable summary of the experimental results.

Summary

Except for birds in the first treatment group, the final models obtained from the independence and first-order working likelihoods are virtually identical. This can be seen in Tables 3 and 4, and also in Figures 7 and 8, where the fitted female learning trajectories are displayed. Both final models describe the effect of sex as additive only; interactions are not present. Both models describe the success probabilities of males as being about 0.74 (*se* = 0.28) units higher in the logit scale than those for females throughout the experiment; sex is clearly an important covariate. The transformed success probability for birds in treatments 2 (PT) and 3 (FT) appears to increase linearly at about the same rate in both final models, with the transformed success probabilities for birds in treatment 3 being about 0.77 (*se* = 0.35) units higher than those for birds in treatment 2, throughout the experiment.

For birds in the first treatment group, the different working likelihoods lead to different final models. The final model resulting from the independence working likelihood describes the learning trajectory for birds in treatment 1 (NT) by a quadratic trend in the logit scale; the trajectory peaks at about trial 110 (near the end of the second day). The final model resulting from the first-order working likelihood, on the other hand, suggests a steady increase throughout the experiment (see Figures 7 and 8). In fact, on the probability scale, these fits for birds in treatment 1 are not so different; the largest discrepancy occurs at trial 180, where the fitted success probability for females is about 0.38 for the independence working likelihood and about 0.50 for the first-order working likelihood. Collecting data for additional subjects in the first treatment group would presumably clarify the presence or absence of a quadratic effect.

The final model resulting from the independence working likelihood is

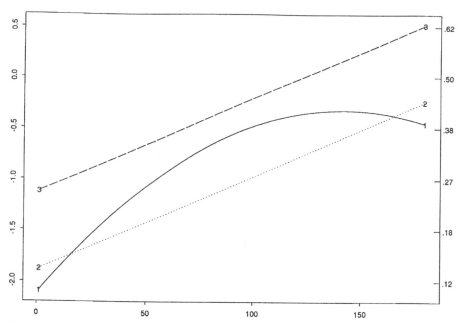

Figure 7. Fitted logits of success probabilities for females from the independence working likelihood model plotted against trial; ——, treatment 1; ····, treatment 2; ------, treatment 3.

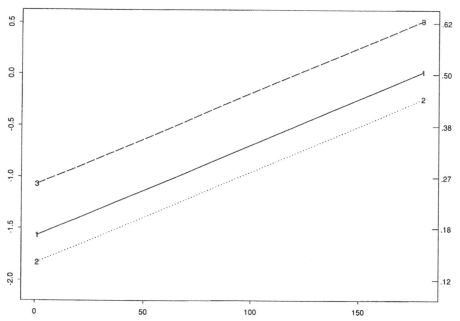

Figure 8. Fitted logits of success probabilities for females from the first-order working likelihood model plotted against trial; ——, treatment 1; ····, treatment 2; ------, treatment 3.

viewed as the more reliable summary of the experimental results because a common lag 1 autocorrelation is required for the validity of the stated asymptotic results for the first-order working likelihood, but the residuals from the first-order fits suggest that a common lag 1 autocorrelation may not be shared by all birds. Note that the patterns in the exploratory plots (see Figures 4–6) provide quite a clear indication of curvature, and this feature is incorporated in the independence fits (see Figure 7).

4.3   GEE Analyses

To correspond to what was done with the working likelihood approach in Section 4.2, the logit link with the Bernoulli mean–variance relationship, up to an unknown scale factor, is used for the GEE analysis of the hummingbird data. All the analyses presented will be based on the specification of a common working correlation matrix for all birds. Little correlation is expected to be present once time has been incorporated into the model, so attention will be restricted to relatively simple working correlation structures.

Specification of an independence working correlation matrix will lead to GEE parameter and standard error estimates identical to those based on the independence working likelihood. In contrast, fits for the first-order working likelihood may differ from the GEE fits based on a stationary 1-dependent working correlation because the working likelihood models the correlation directly, whereas the GEE approach treats the correlation as a nuisance parameter, obtaining a method-of-moments estimator based on the residuals after first estimating the regression parameters at each iteration. To compare these fits, the hummingbird data are analyzed using the GEE approach with a stationary 1-dependent working correlation. To examine the robustness of parameter and standard error estimates across working correlations, the resulting final model is then refit using several other working correlations.

Model Reductions
The same general reduction procedure outlined previously was applied to the initial model for the success probabilities described previously. Table 5 summarizes these model reductions. Interestingly, the reduction path for this GEE analysis with a stationary 1-dependent working correlation matrix matches that for the analysis based on the independence working likelihood rather than that for the first-order working likelihood.

Parameter estimates for the final model fits in Tables 3 and 5 differ noticeably only in the fitted linear coefficient, which is somewhat smaller here. Note, in particular, that the estimated female-to-male differential sex effect is very similar to that obtained from the independence working likelihood. The moment estimates of the lag 1 autocorrelation based on the residuals are 0.123, 0.125, 0.128, 0.129, 0.130, and 0.130 for models 1 through 6, respectively. These are essentially the same as the fitted lag 1 autocorrelations for the first-order working likelihood (see Table 4).

Table 5   Reductions with the Stationary One-Dependent Working Correlation

Parameters	M1	M2	M3	M4	M5	M6
μ_1	0.36(0.03)	0.36(0.17)	0.35(0.16)	0.37(0.16)	0.19(0.26)	0.19(0.26)
μ_2	−0.59(0.31)	−0.52(0.24)	−0.50(0.24)	−0.53(0.24)	−0.35(0.26)	−0.34(0.20)
μ_3	0.53(0.75)	0.60(0.71)	0.60(0.70)	0.57(0.66)	0.55(0.48)	0.46(0.41)
sex_1	−1.03(0.42)	−1.02(0.42)	−1.02(0.41)	−1.05(0.42)	−0.77(0.28)	−0.77(0.28)
sex_2	−0.25(0.40)	−0.37(0.30)	−0.39(0.30)	−0.44(0.30)	sex_1	sex_1
sex_3	−0.72(0.76)	−0.86(0.66)	−0.86(0.64)	−0.81(0.59)	sex_1	sex_1
β_{l11}	0.22(0.09)	0.22(0.09)	0.18(0.11)	0.39(0.10)	0.39(0.10)	0.39(0.10)
β_{l21}	0.55(0.22)	0.54(0.21)	0.42(0.17)	β_{l11}	β_{l11}	β_{l11}
β_{l31}	0.55(0.38)	0.54(0.38)	0.63(0.24)	β_{l11}	β_{l11}	β_{l11}
β_{l12}	0.41(0.31)	0.41(0.31)	β_{l11}	β_{l11}	β_{l11}	β_{l11}
β_{l22}	0.46(0.23)	0.46(0.24)	β_{l21}	β_{l11}	β_{l11}	β_{l11}
β_{l32}	0.74(0.27)	0.73(0.27)	β_{l31}	β_{l11}	β_{l11}	β_{l11}
β_{q11}	−0.21(0.08)	−0.21(0.09)	−0.21(0.09)	−0.23(0.09)	−0.22(0.10)	−0.22(0.10)
β_{q21}	−0.04(0.06)	0.03(0.10)	0.03(0.10)	0.01(0.11)	0.01(0.11)	—
β_{q31}	−0.16(0.15)	−0.09(0.12)	−0.10(0.15)	−0.10(0.14)	−0.09(0.14)	—
β_{q12}	−0.22(0.21)	β_{q11}	β_{q11}	β_{q11}	β_{q11}	β_{q11}
β_{q22}	0.10(0.18)	β_{q21}	β_{q21}	β_{q21}	β_{q21}	—
β_{q32}	−0.008(0.17)	β_{q31}	β_{q31}	β_{q31}	β_{q31}	—

[a]M1, full model; M2, common quadratic effects for males and females within each treatment; M3, common linear effect for males and females within each treatment; M4, common linear effects for all treatments; M5, common sex effect for all treatments; M6, remove quadratic effects for treatments 2 and 3.

Refits with Other Working Correlations

The final model resulting from the use of the stationary 1-dependent working correlation matrix was refit using a variety of working correlation structures; results are summarized in Table 6. Qualitatively, the conclusions obtained with each working correlation are the same; all terms in the final model appear to be important. In general, these robust z-scores indicate a weaker relationship between the response and the covariates than the corresponding naive z-scores (based on the presumption the working correlation matrix correctly specifies the correlation structure, and not presented here), which are up to four times larger in magnitude. Results across working correlation structures are remarkably similar, although the exchangeable working correlation fits a larger female-to-male sex differential and a larger overall effect for treatment 2, as well as larger standard errors for both these estimates. This suggests that parameter and standard error estimates may be reasonably accurate, even with only 18 birds.

Note that among the working correlations represented in Table 6, the exchangeable structure seems scientifically the least plausible because correlations for responses distant in time are modeled to be the same as those for responses adjacent in time. Curiously, of all the working correlations presented, the naive and robust z-scores agree most closely for the exchangeable structure. Although this does not necessarily imply that the true correlation structure is exchangeable, it is interesting to note that when a stationary 8-dependent work-

Table 6   Robust z-Scores (Parameter Estimates) for the Final Model[a]

Working Corr.	μ_1	μ_2	μ_3	sex[b]	β_l[c]	β_q[d]
Independent	0.68(0.18)	−1.54(−0.32)	1.09(0.45)	−2.64(−0.75)	4.31(0.48)	−2.47(−0.24)
Stat. 1-dep.	0.73(0.19)	−1.71(−0.34)	1.12(0.46)	−2.76(−0.77)	3.89(0.39)	−2.27(−0.22)
Stat. 2-dep.	0.73(0.19)	−1.71(−0.34)	1.12(0.46)	−2.75(−0.77)	3.89(0.39)	−2.26(−0.22)
Stat. 5-dep.	0.76(0.20)	−1.74(−0.34)	1.13(0.46)	−2.76(−0.77)	3.98(0.40)	−2.34(−0.23)
Stat. 8-dep.	0.75(0.20)	−1.69(−0.33)	1.14(0.45)	−2.75(−0.76)	4.03(0.40)	−2.40(−0.23)
AR-1	0.73(0.19)	−1.71(−0.34)	1.12(0.46)	−2.76(−0.77)	3.89(0.39)	−2.27(−0.22)
AR-2	0.73(0.19)	−1.71(−0.34)	1.12(0.46)	−2.75(−0.77)	3.90(0.40)	−2.26(−0.23)
AR-5	0.76(0.20)	−1.74(−0.34)	1.13(0.46)	−2.76(−0.77)	4.01(0.40)	−2.38(−0.24)
Exchangeable	0.55(0.16)	−1.83(−0.54)	1.14(0.50)	−2.69(−0.95)	3.51(0.40)	−2.28(−0.23)

[a]Entries are z-score (parameter estimate).
[b]$sex_1 = sex_2 = sex_3 = sex$, the common differential sex effect.
[c]$\beta_{l11} = \beta_{l12} = \beta_{l21} = \beta_{l22} = \beta_{l31} = \beta_{l32} = \beta_l$, the common linear coefficient.
[d]$\beta_{q11} = \beta_{q12} = \beta_q$, the common quadratic coefficient for birds in treatment 1.

ing correlation structure is specified, the lag 1 through 8 correlations are all estimated to be about 0.12 (slightly larger than 0.08, the fitted exchangeable working correlation). This provides some indication that the true correlation may be well approximated by the exchangeable structure.

5 CONCLUSIONS

Steplike changes in learning trajectories associated with sudden awareness of the spatial association between light cue and feeder were expected by the investigator but are not present in exploratory plots of the data for individual birds; see Figure 9 for plots of the smoothed individual learning trajectories of birds in treatment 3 (FT). Instead, the plots suggest a more gradual increase in individual success probabilities over time, with considerable fluctuation throughout the experiment.

The analyses presented have focused on the patterns of increase in the success probabilities over time, but perhaps patterns in the fluctuations of these probabilities are equally important. Plots analogous to Figure 9 for treatments 1 and 2 suggest that the fluctuations are most pronounced for birds on treatment 1 (NT). It is worth noting, in addition, that two of the females on treatment 1 were unsuccessful on almost all of their first feeding forays (a third female on this treatment was almost always unsuccessful until about the 110th trial).

Both the working likelihood and GEE analysis indicate birds in treatment 3 (FT) have the highest success probabilities throughout the experiment. These results differ dramatically from those obtained by the univariate ANOVA for repeated measures, where no important differences in success probabilities across treatment groups was detected.

Unlike the ANOVA approach, both the working likelihood and GEE approaches permit modeling of the response directly as a function of time. The

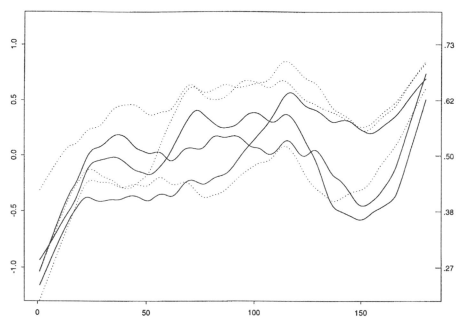

Figure 9. Smoothed logit of response for individual birds from treatment 3 (smoothing window of 60 observations); left-hand axis is logit scale, right-hand axis is success probability scale; ——, females; ····, males.

learning trajectories of birds in treatments 2 (PT) and 3 (FT) appear to improve roughly linearly (in the logit scale) and at about the same rate. However, success probabilities for birds in treatment 2 appear to start out (and remain) lower than those for birds in treatment 3 throughout the experiment. This is contrary to the expectations of the investigator, who used psychological principles of visual perception to predict that birds in the treatment groups with discontinuous (PT) and continuous (FT) visible guides should have similar learning trajectories. The analyses based on the independence working likelihood and the GEE approach indicate that the trajectory for birds in treatment 1 (NT) departs from the linear pattern for birds in treatments 2 and 3. Contrary to the expectations of the investigator, birds in treatment 2 (PT) appear to have lower success probabilities than birds in treatment 1 (except, perhaps, at the very beginning and end of the experiment; see Figure 7). A subsequent explanation, proposed by the investigator, is that the orange Dymo tape for the partially taped feeding array creates three horizontal bands which may interfere with the intended vertical pattern to be perceived by the birds in treatment 2.

Contrary to the accepted wisdom among researchers in hummingbird learning, both the working likelihood and GEE analyses clearly indicate that gender is an important factor in describing success probabilities on the first feeding foray for the hummingbirds in this experiment. The effect of gender appears to be additive, and the fitted models indicate that the odds of success for males are more than twice the odds of success for females. One possible explanation for the importance of gender is the higher body weight/wing span ratio of males; because males must work harder to obtain their food, they may be more likely to succeed.

The investigator clearly devoted a great deal of attention to the careful execution of this experiment. The one obvious recommendation for future experimentation would be to include as many birds as possible in each treatment group. Both the GEE and working likelihood methodologies rely on borrowing strength across subjects for accurate estimation of parameters and their standard errors. Further, the large number of trials in the experiment dictates that more than just six birds are required to obtain an accurate picture of the overall learning trajectory in each treatment group.

Comparison of Methods

Longitudinal data consist of repeated and possibly correlated measurements over time for each of many subjects. If the response vectors are normally distributed with a common covariance matrix, MANOVA permits testing of parallelism and equality of treatment means, provided that the number of subjects is large enough to permit a nonsingular estimate of the common covariance matrix. With fewer subjects, MANOVA can only be carried out if the length of the response vector is reduced, perhaps by blocking over time points. However, this leads to a loss of information.

Modeling of response vectors which are not normally distributed is more difficult. Transformations that stabilize variance for univariate responses do not necessarily stabilize covariance matrices for multivariate responses. Hence, equality of covariance matrices, a necessary assumption for valid tests in any ANOVA approach, may be difficult to approximate.

The working likelihood and GEE approaches to the analysis of binary longitudinal data provide alternatives to the approach based on transforming nonnormal data into forms suitable for ANOVA. The working likelihood approach was originally developed for short binary time series, where detailed models for the change in response over time are unnecessary, and time-independent covariates suffice. Extension to the case of time-dependent covariates, as described previously, allows success probabilities to be modeled as a function of time; such modeling is required for satisfactory analysis of the hummingbird data. One limitation of this approach when correlation is explicitly modeled (to increase efficiency of estimation) is that asymptotic results only hold under certain assumptions on the true correlation structure. The generalized estimating equation (GEE) approach removes this limitation, thereby providing a more general approach to the analysis of binary longitudinal data.

Because both the working likelihood and GEE approaches allow flexible modeling of success probabilities as a function of time and can readily accommodate covariates while taking into account the unknown correlation present in the data, they enable much more information to be extracted from the hummingbird data set than more traditional ANOVA approaches. These methodologies therefore provide useful and powerful tools for researchers in this subject area.

In fact, the GEE approach is applicable to any longitudinal response with univariate marginal distributions for which the quasi-likelihood formulation is sensible. This includes binary, binomial, and count responses as well as a variety of continuous responses. The GEE approach thus provides a unified and very flexible methodology for the analysis of longitudinal data.

ACKNOWLEDGMENTS

The authors thank Gayle Brown of the Department of Zoology at the University of British Columbia for many instructive conversations about hummingbird learning, and, in particular, for Figure 1 of the manuscript. We are also indebted to members of the Biostatistics Research Group at the University of British Columbia for constructive comments throughout the period this work was in progress. Various phases of the research were partially supported by the Multiple Sclerosis Research Group at the University of British Columbia and by the Natural Sciences and Engineering Research Council of Canada.

SOFTWARE NOTES AND REFERENCES

SAS (procedure GLM) was used for the classical ANOVA of Section 4.1; custom-written Splus functions were used for the working likelihood approach of Section 4.2; and a GEE SAS macro written by M. Rezaul Karim of the Department of Biostatistics, Johns Hopkins University, was used for the GEE approach of Section 4.3. The GEE SAS macro permits modeling of the following working correlation matrices: independence, stationary M-dependent, non-stationary M-dependent, AR-M, exchangeable, unspecified, and user specified. Only working correlations which are common to all subjects may be specified. In addition, if observation times are unequally spaced or there are missing data, only the independence, exchangeable, or user-specified working correlations should be used. The Johns Hopkins GEE SAS macro can be obtained upon request via e-mail to: sz@zeger.sph.jhu.edu. Alternatively, an S-plus implementation of the GEE approach can be obtained upon request via e-mail to: statlib@lib.stat.cmu.edu.

QUESTIONS AND PROBLEMS

1. Consider variations on the classical approach to the analysis of these data.

   (a) The factor "measurement" which represents successive blocks of feeding trials could be parametrized, in terms of days and trends within days, for example, thereby providing a simpler description of the pattern of hummingbird learning over time. Would such modifications to the analysis be expected to improve the ability of this approach to detect treatment differences?

(b) The analysis presented was carried out on the arcsine square-root scale. Would the use of another scale be expected to alter the results substantially? Repeat the analysis on the logit scale and compare results.

(c) Carry out a multivariate ANOVA on these data. Is this technique effective in addressing the issue of differences in the patterns over time in the response probabilities?

2. Consider the working likelihood approach to the analysis of these data.

(a) Verify the expression for $p_{i,t} = E(Y_{i,t}|Y_{i,t-1})$ under the assumption of a stationary 1-dependent correlation structure.

(b) Because there are relatively few experimental units, each with a large number of observations, the credibility of the results would be strengthened by residual analyses suggesting that data are not seriously at odds with the assumptions underlying the working likelihoods. What are these assumptions for the independence and first-order working likelihoods? What residual checks are possible for the first-order working likelihood?

3. The model reductions presented for the GEE approach were carried out using a stationary 1-dependent working correlation matrix common to all experimental units. Carry out the model reductions using a different working correlation structure and compare results.

4. Within each of the 180 feeding trials for each hummingbird, the multiple individual feeding forays were each recorded as successful or not. Other response variables, such as the proportion of successful forays or the number of forays until the first successful foray, could therefore also be considered. Discuss the potential utility of these or other possible response variables for describing the pattern of hummingbird learning over time. Which of the approaches employed in this chapter could reasonably be employed for these response variables?

5. The key feature of the GEE approach is that it accounts for correlated data on the experimental units: the successive observations over time on the individual hummingbirds in this case study. Suggest other examples of such "clustered" data for which the GEE approach might be useful. What working correlation matrices might be most plausible in these situations?

CHAPTER 10

Habitat Association Studies of the Northern Spotted Owl, Sage Grouse, and Flammulated Owl

Fred L. Ramsey, Marti McCracken, John A. Crawford,
Martin S. Drut, and William J. Ripple

1 MOTIVATION AND BACKGROUND

In the Pacific Northwest of the United States, conflicting views on the management of federally owned forest lands have dominated local politics, spilled into the courts, and virtually stalled the region's timber industry. The remaining virgin forests—the "old growth"—currently have few legal defenses against the chainsaws. The Endangered Species Act protects habitat for species and distinct populations which are endangered or threatened by human activities. The northern spotted owl (*Strix occidentalis*) therefore finds itself in the center of the storm. The U.S. Fish and Wildlife Service has declared that the northern spotted owl is a threatened species. The law now requires that the owl's survival take priority over other uses of its old growth habitat.

Ensuring survival depends on knowing how much old growth habitat is required by the owl. Studies to answer such questions are called *habitat association* or *habitat preference* studies. This chapter concerns a specific study design for investigating habitat associations. The design was employed by Ripple et al. (1991) in an important study of the northern spotted owl in western Oregon.

Taped vocalizations and whistles were played to locate owl pairs in an intensive three-year search of a 7100-km^2 region of National Forest. The researchers located 37 owl nest sites by following birds which responded. Thirty of the 37 were chosen from the same region at random coordinates, and aerial photographs were examined to determine the percentages of mature forest (over 80 years old) covering seven concentric circles around each site. Thirty other

Case Studies in Biometry, Edited by Nicholas Lange, Louise Ryan, Lynne Billard,
David Brillinger, Loveday Conquest, and Joel Greenhouse.
ISBN 0-471-58885-7 © 1994 John Wiley & Sons, Inc.

sites were chosen from the same region at random coordinates, and aerial photographs were examined to determine the percentages of mature forest in the same seven circles. These control sites were included as indications of what conditions were available to the owls.

Assume that an animal selects a location for nesting, foraging, basking, and so on, based on the habitat characteristics at that location in comparison with the habitat characteristics at other available locations. Thus the animal responds with a Yes (Y = 1) or No (Y = 0) decision to a habitat configuration, denoted by **x**. Because the study design fixes the sample sizes separately for the number of Y = 1 and the number of Y = 0 responses, it has the same structure as case–control retrospective studies that are widely used in epidemiology. The theory and application of case–control retrospective studies in studying risk factors for diseases have developed rapidly in the past decades. Breslow and Day (1980) provide a comprehensive review. By recognizing the retrospective nature of such habitat association studies, much of the development for case–control clinical studies can be applied to wildlife habitat association studies. The principal feature which becomes immediately available is logistic regression, which ties the retrospective study directly to a model for the prospective selection process.

Other analysis strategies include many two-sample tools: t-tests, chi-square analysis, Hotelling's T^2, and discriminant function analysis. Reviews of methods for this and other designs for habitat association study are provided in papers by Alldredge and Ratti (1986, 1992) and Thomas and Taylor (1990). Johnson (1980) also provided a review and suggested rank-based tools which are now widely used. Loglinear models have been applied to habitat association studies by Heisey (1985) and Lunney et al. (1988). Where logistic regression has been applied to habitat association studies (Pereira and Itami, 1991), it has served as a tool for discriminant analysis. This is justifiable on technical grounds alone. Habitat variables are often categorical and have nonnormal distributions. Efron (1975) showed that logistic regression should be preferred to normal-based discriminant analysis in such situations (see also Press and Wilson, 1978).

This chapter is organized as follows. In the next section, the reason for sampling retrospectively is put forward in an example. Section 3 contains the model for habitat selection and a short review of logistic regression. Sections 4 and 5 contain two case studies: one where the design is clear, the other where the design is similar but has important differences. In Section 6 we return to the northern spotted owl study. The discussion in Section 7 reviews issues from the field of medical applications which are relevant to wildlife studies.

2 DATA

A representative sample of our data is given in Table 1. Seven variables contain percentages of mature forest in seven concentric circles surrounding nest sites (N) and random sites (R). Variable names refer to the circle radii.

Table 1 Percentages of Mature Forest in Concentric Rings around Spotted Owl Nest Sites and Randomly Selected Sites in Western Oregon

Site Type	Percent in Ring Diameter (km)						
	0.91	1.18	1.40	1.60	1.77	2.41	3.38
R	26.0	33.3	25.6	19.1	31.4	24.8	17.9
	100.0	92.7	90.1	72.8	51.9	50.6	41.5
	32.0	22.2	38.3	39.9	22.1	20.2	38.2
	43.0	79.7	61.4	81.2	47.7	69.6	54.8
N	80.0	87.3	93.3	81.6	85.0	82.8	63.6
	96.0	74.0	76.7	66.2	69.1	84.5	52.5
	82.0	79.6	91.3	70.7	75.6	73.5	66.8

3 METHODS AND MODELS

The reason for using a case–control retrospective design is to obtain usable information with a feasible sample size. This is illustrated in the following hypothetical example. A forest contains hardwood (H) and softwood (S) trees. A researcher wishes to investigate whether that distinction is involved in the selection of nest trees by a species of woodpecker. Suppose that the forest situation looks like Table 2, in which it is clear that this woodpecker prefers to hammer its nest holes into hardwoods.

The researcher could sample trees in one of three ways: (1) take a simple random sample from all available trees, (2) take separate random samples prospectively from hardwood trees and from softwood trees, or (3) take separate random samples retrospectively from nest trees and from nonnest trees. The consequences of these different sampling options appear in Table 3. For each option, the sampling intensity is that which minimally guarantees that all cells are expected to contain at least 5 trees. With simple random sampling, at least 10% of the entire forest must be sampled in order to expect 5 nests in softwood trees; this means sampling over 1000 trees.

Table 2 Hypothetical Forest Habitat for Nesting Woodpecker Study[a]

	Hardwood (H)	Softwood (S)	Total
Nest tree (N)	500	50	550
Other tree (O)	5,000	6,000	11,000
Total	5,500	6,050	11,550

[a]Probability ratio of H to S = π_H/π_S = (500/5500)/(50/6050) = 11, odds ratio of H to S = ω_H/ω_S = (500/5000)/(50/6000) = 12 (see Section 3.1).

Table 3   Expected Results of Sampling the Hypothetical Forest Using Three Sampling Plans[a]

	Simple Random				Propsective				Retrospective[a]		
	10%				H: 1% S: 10%				N: 10% O: 0.1%		
	H	S			H	S			H	S	
N	50	5	55	N	5	5	10	N	50	5	55
O	500	600	1,100	O	50	600	650	O	5	6	11
	550	605	1,155		55	605	660		55	11	66
	$\pi_H/\pi_S = 11$				$\pi_H/\pi_S = 11$				$\pi_H/\pi_S = 2$		
	$\omega_H/\omega_S = 12$				$\omega_H/\omega_S = 12$				$\omega_H/\omega_S = 12$		

[a]Retrospective sampling has smaller sample size requirements but is unable to provide an estimate of the probability ratio.

If sampling prospectively, only 1% of the hardwoods need be sampled to have expectation of finding 5 nests, but 10% of the softwoods must be sampled. This cuts the total sampling effort down, but only by a factor of 2. Sampling retrospectively, however, the 10% sampling requirement for obtaining 5 nests is applied only to the small number of nest trees, letting the researcher get by with sampling only 0.1% of the nonnest trees. This reduces the total effort to 66 trees. This forest was divided fairly evenly between favored trees and not-favored trees. When animals exhibit preferences for uncommon habitat types, the savings in sampling effort through retrospective sampling are even greater.

These three sampling plans are hardly comparable, and in practice only the retrospective plan would be feasible. With it, biologists may use vocal imitations, bait, trapping, and so on, to locate animals, then follow them directly or indirectly (e.g., with radiotelemetry) to their chosen habitats. This avoids having to know in advance which locations were selected. It does not constitute random sampling from all selected location, so its similarity to random sampling must be assumed (as is frequently done in medical applications).

3.1   Logistic Regression

A traditional chi-square analysis of the woodpecker's habitat selection would focus on the proportions of nest sites among hardwoods and softwoods. This suggests that a habitat preference index might be the ratio π_H/π_S, where π_H and π_S are the proportions of nest sites among hardwood and softwood trees, respectively. The parameters π_H and π_S may also be viewed as probabilities of selection by the woodpeckers. In medical applications the ratio π_H/π_S is called relative risk. In this forest, 1 in 11 hardwoods as opposed to only 1 in 121 softwoods were selected as nest sites. Thus this index shows that hardwoods are preferred 11 to 1 over softwoods. As Table 3 shows, this index may be estimated from simple random samples and from prospective samples. *It cannot be reconstructed from retrospective samples*, however, where the same calculation results in a ratio of 2 to 1.

But define instead a habitat preference ratio (HPR) in terms of the odds on tree selection as

$$\text{HPR} = \frac{\omega_H}{\omega_S},$$

where $\omega_H = \pi_H/(1 - \pi_H)$ and $\omega_S = \pi_S/(1 - \pi_S)$. Then Table 3 shows that HPR may be estimated from all sampling plans including the case–control retrospective design. The odds that a hardwood is selected are 12 times as great as the odds that a softwood is selected. Note that HPR will be very similar to π_H/π_S when selected sites constitute a very small proportion of those available.

Statistical analysis attempts to estimate the logarithm of the odds ratio. When there is a single binary habitat variable, as in the woodpecker example, the variance of the estimate is approximately the sum of the inverses of the expected cell counts. The standard errors for the estimated log odds ratio in the three sampling plans above are 0.48, 0.65, and 0.77, respectively. Thus there is less than a 50% loss in precision associated with the reduced sampling effort available through retrospective sampling. A retrospective sampling of 173 trees apportioned as above would give the same precision as the simple random sampling with 1155 trees; while a retrospective sampling of 92 trees would give the same precision as the prospective sampling of 660.

Let $\mathbf{x}$ denote a habitat configuration [i.e. $\mathbf{x} = (x_1, \ldots, x_p)^T$ is a set of habitat variables measured at some location]. The binary response, Y, indicates whether the location has been selected. Let $\pi(\mathbf{x}) = \Pr\{Y = 1 | \mathbf{x}\}$ be the probability of selection of locations with habitat configuration $\mathbf{x}$. Then let $\omega(\mathbf{x}) = \pi(\mathbf{x})/[1 - \pi(\mathbf{x})]$ be the odds of selection. The logistic regression model for habitat preference is

$$\text{logit}\,[\pi(\mathbf{x})] = \ln\,[\omega(\mathbf{x})] = \beta_0 + \sum_{j=1}^{p} x_j \beta_j.$$

The parameters $(\beta_1, \ldots, \beta_p)^T$ associated with habitat characteristics are most easily interpreted through the parameters $\phi_i = \exp(\beta_i)$ as factors that multiply the odds on selection when the corresponding x_i is changed by a unit amount. These factors represent extensions of the habitat preference ratio. The ability to estimate the odds ratio from retrospective samples in the woodpecker example generalizes to the ability to estimate all these multiplicative factors either from retrospective or from prospective samples. The origin parameter must be different in a retrospective and prospective models and is not informative in the former case [cf. Armitage (1975), Mantel (1973), Seigel and Greenhouse (1973), or Breslow and Day (1980)].

Mechanics of logistic regression analysis are covered in several texts, an excellent reference being Breslow and Day (1980). We shall not repeat them here. Few biologists should find the likelihood-based methods any more mysterious than least-squares technology, so the biostatistician may concentrate on interpreting results with emphasis on explaining those aspects which are different from ordinary multiple linear regression.

One feature that requires explanation in what follows is the *deviance* statistic. The deviance in logistic regression is similar to the residual sum of squares in normal regression, in that it measures the lack of fit of a proposed model to the observed data. Variables that significantly reduce deviance when entered in a logistic regression model are desirable. On the hypothesis of no relationship between the odds of selection and some set of variables, the reduction in deviance for entering the set into a logistic regression model has an approximate chi-square distribution with degrees of freedom equal to the number of variables in the set. This distributional result is used to determine the significance of deviance reduction for variable entry.

3.2   Variable Selection

An advantage of using logistic regression is the availability of sensible variable selection procedures. To illustrate these, we examine a study of nest site selection by flammulated owls (*Otus flammeolus*) in northeastern Oregon. The flammulated owl is a small, relatively unknown nesting species of the ponderosa pine forests in the western United States. It is highly migratory, arriving at its nesting habitat in late May to select a nesting site in a tree cavity. Goggans (1986) used imitations of territorial calls during nightly searches from mid-May to mid-June, 1983 and 1984, to locate cavities of 20 nesting pairs of owls. She located 60 nonnest cavities by taking random coordinates in the study area and searching for the nearest cavity of suitable size.

At each cavity location, 20 factors were measured. All but two were categorical factors, and the categorical factors had up to eight levels. If different levels were considered in the analysis by inclusion of indicator variables, the total number of variables, excluding interactions, is 71, nearly equal to the combined number of cavity locations. Some factors were categorized versions of underlying continuous measurements. For example, *aspect* categorized the orientation of the ground slope into one of eight 45° segments. Other factors had factorial structure. Ground cover type, for example, was categorized into $8 = 2^3$ cells by the presence/absence of grasses, forbs, and shrubs. Still other factors (e.g., the species of the cavity tree) had no particular structure.

With so many possible variables, it was desirable to reduce each factor to a single variable that was both consistent with the factor structure and highly related to selection by the owls. To illustrate the procedure, consider the factor *percent bark cover* on the tree with the nest cavity, which was categorized in four levels: 0%, 0 to 50%, 50 to 100%, or 100%. It is possible to use three separate indicator variables for this factor in a logistic regression, assigning it 3 degrees of freedom. Using only these three variables in a logistic regression lowers the deviance residual by a total of 10.80 from the trivial model with only a constant term. But there are several single-dimensional variables that may accomplish nearly the same deviance reduction.

Seven linear combinations of the indicator variables appear in Table 4. The first six represent ranges of percent bark cover, while the seventh is a linear variable. For example, the variable $bk < 50$ is an indicator that bark cover is in the range from 50% down to and including 0%. That variable alone reduced the deviance by 2.26, leaving $(10.80 - 2.26) = 8.254$ as deviance explained by bark cover, but not by this variable.

The single best variable to represent percent bark cover in a multiple logistic regression analysis is the one that gives the greatest deviance reduction. In this example, it is the indicator of percent bark cover being between 0 and 50%, $bk0–50$, with a deviance reduction of 9.67 and a remainder deviance that is small in relation to its degrees of freedom. So in subsequent analysis, the three-dimensions of back cover percent were reduced to the single variable $BKP = bk0–50$.

Prior to entering all factors in a multiple logistic regression, each factor was summarized by a single variable in this way. We were prepared to include more dimensions for any factor where a single expression could be significantly improved by additional dimensions, but no such situation arose.

Figure 1 illustrates four examples (including bark cover). Note the different levels, the side-by-side histograms of nest and random cavities, and the resulting variable, named by a three-letter acronym. The variable is defined by taking the sum of the products of listed coefficients and level indicator functions. The best ground cover type variable, *GCT*, distinguishes sites with a *mixture* of ground covers from sites with a single ground cover or none. The best mea-

Table 4 Bark Cover Variables as Linear Combinations of Category Indicators, with Deviance Reductions Variable Entry for Including Each Variable and with Deviance Reductions (Remainder) for Subsequent Inclusion of the Remaining Bark Cover Dimensions

Bark Cover Percentage Category	Single Bark Cover Variables (with Coefficients)						
	bk = 0	bk < 50	bk < 100	bk0 – 50	bk0 – 100	bk50 – 100	bkLIN
PCT = 100%	0	0	0	0	0	0	1.00
100% > PCT > 50%	0	0	1	0	1	1	0.75
50% > PCT > 0%	0	1	1	1	1	0	0.25
PCT = 0%	1	1	1	0	0	0	0.00
Deviance reduction (1 d.f.)	2.52	2.26	1.38	9.67	4.98	0.10	0.91
Remainder deviance (2 d.f.)	8.28	8.54	9.42	1.13	5.82	10.70	9.89

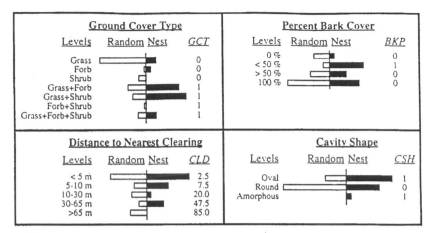

Figure 1. Four habitat factors with factor-level histograms and resulting variables.

sure of distance to nearest clearing, *CLD*, approximates the continuous distance measurement. The best cavity shape variable, *CSH*, distinguishes round cavities (excavated by northern flickers) from oval (excavated by pileated woodpecker) and amorphous (natural) cavities.

After determining single variables to represent each factor, all variables were considered in a forward stepwise variable-selection routine. The results are summarized in Table 5, in which each column shows the 1 degree of freedom chi-square deviance reductions for entering the variables at that step. (The variables are ordered by their chi-square to enter at step 1.)

Table 5 illustrates how the habitat factors are interrelated. Cavity type (which woodpecker made the hole) and cavity shape are strongly related to the percentage of back cover, for example. So when *BKP* enters at step 2, the value of entering either *CSH* or *CVT* is diminished. On the other hand, some variables increase in significance when others are entered: only after the general neighborhood and view are acceptable (*GCT, FTP, CCL*) and the proper house constructed (*BKP, CSH*) does the addition of a deck (*PRD*) appear desirable.

A final check on model validity can be made by expanding the model to include some interactions. Excluding the marginally significant variable *PRD* leaves five main variables. The deviance reduction for adding the 10 interaction terms was 11.10. Although this is far from significant, 6.02 units of the statistic come from the *BKP*-by-*FTP* interaction term, which may be considered as suggestive of an effect.

Table 6 presents a summary of the conclusions. In addition to standard errors for the coefficients of variables in the model, Table 6 gives measures of practical significance in terms of odds ratios. The odds ratios listed are the factors by which the odds on selection increase when the corresponding variable changes from its mean on random cavities to its mean on nest cavities.

Goggans (1986) assessed habitat selection with separate chi-square contin-

Table 5 Forward Variable Selection in Logit Regression[a]

| | | Chi Squares (1 d.f.) for Entry at Step Number | | | | | | |
Variable	TLA	1	2	3	4	5	6	7
Ground cover type	GCT	12.29	—	—	—	—	—	—
Bark cover percentage	BKP	9.67	11.82	—	—	—	—	—
Cavity shape	CSH	7.90	7.21	4.48	6.31	—	—	—
Ground cover percentage	GCP	7.31	6.61	5.55	4.70	4.93	1.88	2.16
Forest type	FTP	6.37	4.91	6.46	4.62	7.54	—	—
Tree height	TRH	5.63	4.56	1.76	3.98	0.98	0.44	1.79
Aspect	ASP	5.07	3.07	3.59	2.72	2.68	3.40	2.52
Tree condition	CND	4.18	2.58	2.00	1.18	0.54	0.01	0.01
Tree species	TSP	4.10	3.49	3.25	2.57	1.44	1.74	1.24
Cavity type	CVT	3.01	3.16	0.46	1.17	1.11	0.18	0.02
Canopy closure	CCL	3.85	2.66	9.26	—	—	—	—
Forest stocking	STK	2.81	2.80	4.41	0.89	1.01	0.16	0.09
Land form	LFM	2.71	3.49	2.40	0.99	0.33	0.23	0.07
Gradient	GRD	2.61	3.45	4.65	4.52	3.04	2.48	1.61
DBH	DBH	2.22	4.49	1.15	0.60	0.01	0.01	0.01
Succession stage	SCC	2.02	5.61	1.75	1.78	0.45	0.40	0.13
Distance to clearing	CLD	1.39	1.40	1.20	0.11	0.20	0.13	0.70
Distance to perch	PRD	0.85	0.86	4.71	3.21	2.83	5.18	—
Clearing perimeter	RPM	0.38	0.67	1.21	0.62	2.07	1.99	1.38
Cavity-to-cover distance	C2C	0.05	0.03	0.07	0.06	0.04	0.00	0.01

[a]Critical chi-square values are 3.84 at $\alpha = 0.05$ and 6.63 at $\alpha = 0.01$.

gency analysis for each factor. She found no relation between selection and cavity type or shape, which appeared in our analysis because we reduced the dimension of cavity shape to the most obvious comparison. She found a significant effect for canopy closure which became nonsignificant when controlled for forest type. Because there was no significant interaction between the canopy closure and forest type ($\chi^2 = 2.10$, $p = 0.15$), we would not come to the same conclusion. Finally, she "believes these data reflect nest placements in mature forest stands where sunlight penetrates through the open canopy to the forest floor stimulating understory growth, rather than selection specifically for ground cover characteristics." In contrast to that statement, ground cover type stands out as a significant factor in the multiple logistic regression analysis above, even after accounting for forest type and canopy cover.

3.3 Continuous Habitat Variables

A technical advantage to logistic regression analysis of habitat association is its ability to incorporate continuous habitat variables. We illustrate this aspect with a portion of a study of sage grouse (*Centrocerus urophasianus*) habitat in the sagebrush steppe of southeastern Oregon, by Drut (1992). Drut attached radio transmitters to hen sage grouse and subsequently determined their locations with broods, at two sites—Hart Mountain and Jackass Creek—during the summers of

Table 6 Logistic Regression Model Parameter Estimates in the Flammulated Owl Study

Variable	Coeff.	se	z-Stat.	p-Value	Odds Ratio	Favorable[a]	Unfavorable[b]
GCT	3.896	1.288	3.025	0.0017	49.2	Mixtures	Pure grass, forbs, or shrub
BKP	4.168	1.287	3.239	0.0009	64.6	0–50%	0% or >50
CCL	3.221	1.231	2.617	0.0054	25.1	<50%	>50%
CSH	2.754	1.125	2.448	0.0084	15.7	Oval or irregular	Round
FTP	2.948	1.306	2.257	0.0135	19.2	Ponderosa pine + Douglas fir or grassland	Pure Ponderosa, no Ponderosa, or presence of grand fir or larch

[a]Marginal: (1) Distance to nearest perch under 3 m favorable ($p = 0.034$); (2) nonadditive effects of bark cover percent and forest type ($p = 0.014$).

198

1989 and 1990. Based on a hierarchical approach to habitat selection (Johnson, 1980), Drut first analyzed selection of general habitat classes and then examined preference for microhabitat features separately within each class.

Microhabitat variables were the percentages of ground cover by forbs (F), grasses (G), shrubs (S), and bare ground (B), measured by the line intercept method at brood locations and at other locations selected randomly to judge availability. An appealing model structure incorporates the possibility of having an optimum configuration surrounded by decreasing desirability as conditions depart further from the ideal. Thus, we began considering a quadratic response surface for logit(π) over the (G,F,S)-simplex, wherein the coefficients might change according to year (Y) and/or site (P).

The single habitat class with the largest number ($n = 57$) of brood sites was low sagebrush. In Table 7 we summarize the elimination of nonsignificant quadratic and interaction terms for the observations from low sagebrush. It was apparent that curvature terms and terms involving interactions of the different vegetation percentages contributed little. Similarly, all variables involving differences between sites were not significant. The only variables that could not be eliminated were the main effect of year, the main effects of all three vegetation variables, and the interactions of grasses and shrubs with year. The resulting model involving these variables is displayed in Figure 2. The story is a simple one: 1989 was a wet year, producing a good crop of forbs, the preferred browse of sage grouse. With forbs available, the grouse frequented sites with high percentages of grasses only moderately more than their availability and were found less frequently at sites with high percentages of sagebrush, the abundant shrub. But 1990 was a dry year, with vegetation of all kinds reduced in availability. The suggested preference for forbs was still as strong, but forbs alone were insufficient to supply the birds' needs. Broods were located more frequently at sites where alternative food sources—grasses and sagebrush—were available. This analysis is supported by samples taken from bird crops, in which sagebrush was found to be a larger component of the diet in 1990 than in 1989.

This analysis must be judged as tentative. First, time of day of the locations

Table 7   Stepwise Variable Elimination, by Blocks of Variables, for Sage Grouse Habitat Association

Variable(s) Eliminated	d.f.	Chi Square
$(F^2, G^2, S^2) \times (1, Y, P, YP)$	12	15.29
$(FG, FS, GS) \times (1, Y, P, YP)$	12	17.35
$(F, G, S) \times Y \times P$	3	2.26
$(F, G, S) \times P$	3	8.03
$Y \times P$	1	0.64
$F \times Y$	1	1.04
P	1	0.18

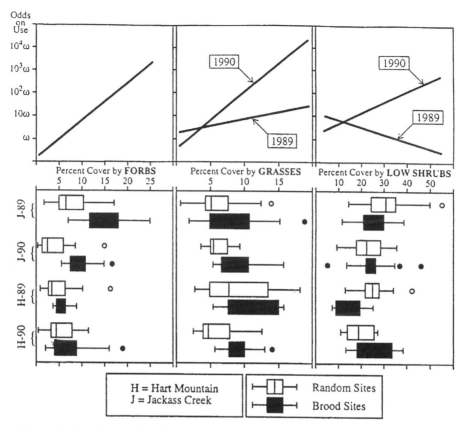

Figure 2. Box plots and logistic regression model, for sage grouse habitat assciation study.

has not been included here, and there probably is some association between time of day and the habitats where broods may be found. Second, as with many studies relying on locations of radio-tagged animals, there were multiple locations of the same brood. These should not be treated as independent in the same sense as would locations for different broods. The expected overdispersion has led Alldredge and Ratti (1992) to suggest that inference be restricted to statements about just those broods that appeared in the sample.

Such problems are more easily tackled within the context of logistic regression, where one is dealing with specific models. We could, for example, construct a mixed regression model with parameters that differ from brood to brood and come from a multivariate normal population (cf. Zeger and Liang, 1986; Breslow and Clayton, 1993). Alternatively, the regression parameters at one location may be allowed to depend on the location of the same brood at the previous occasion. We have not attempted this modeling yet. We include the example in this form as an illustration of how logistic regression can clear up issues of model complexity, allowing researchers to be confident they have not missed significant effects.

There was one outlier initially present in this data set, a random site where over 40% of the ground cover was by grasses. With this outlier in the data set, there were significant curvature effects for grasses and for interactions of the grasses curvature with year and location. With graphical tools associated with logistic regression, the outlier was easily identified. By eliminating it, we restrict inferences to sites where grass cover was no more than 20%.

3.4 Spotted Owl Study

Ripple et al. (1991) compared the percentages of mature timber at nest sites with those at random sites using a series of two-sample t-tests (after transformation). A summary of their analysis is given in Table 8. They concluded that the percentages of mature forest "both adjacent to nests (260-ha plot) and in the surrounding area (3588-ha plot) are important in nest site selection." They also concluded that "we do not know how much fragmentation can be tolerated by spotted owls . . . ." In what follows we attempt to address both issues using logistic regression.

3.5 How Much Mature Forest Area?

Determination of an amount of mature forest area needed to support a nesting pair of owls is a critical issue in the effort to protect sufficient habitat for continued survival of this subspecies. If $C_{ij}, i = 1, 2, \ldots, 7; j = 1, \ldots, 60$, is the percentage of mature forest in the ith circle surrounding the jth site (Table 8), the question may be interpreted as asking which circle is most closely associated with site utilization.

Table 8 Percentages of Area in Mature Forest (>80 yr) near 30 Spotted Owl Nest Sites and 30 Random Sites for Seven Plot Sizes, in the Cascade Mountains of Oregon, 1987–1989

Circle Area (ha)	Nest Sites ($n = 30$)		Random Sites ($n = 30$)		t-Test[a] p-Value
	Mean %	SD	Mean %	SD	
260	78.2	11.8	63.2	20.2	0.0019
440	76.3	11.9	63.5	17.7	0.0026
620	76.5	11.3	63.3	15.7	0.0006
800	75.6	11.1	62.5	15.3	0.0004
980	75.1	11.1	61.6	14.5	0.0003
1826	73.6	9.9	60.8	13.5	0.0001
3588	65.0	8.7	57.3	13.2	0.0101

[a]After arcsine square-root transformation.

Also let R_{ij} be the percentage of mature forest in the *i*th *ring* surrounding the *j*th site. For example, R_{4j} is the percent of mature forest in the outer ring of the fourth circle, which lies outside the third circle. The ring variables are linear combinations of the circle percentage variables, but they represent percentages of mature forest in nonoverlapping regions.

There is a noticeable difference between the distributions of these ring percentages at nest sites and random sites (Figure 3), with the exception of the outermost ring. Correlations among the percentages in different rings range from 25 to 85% (median 59%) at random sites and from 12 to 78% (median 66%) at nest sites. So a second question concerns whether the percentage of mature forest is high in a ring surrounding nest sites because the owls select it that way, or only because it is correlated with the percent of mature forest in circles adjacent to the nest.

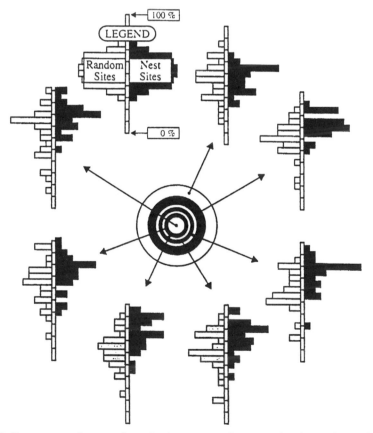

Figure 3. Percentages of mature forest in rings surrounding spotted owl nest sites and random sites in western Oregon, 1987–1989.

For each i, Table 9 shows the results of fitting a one-variable logistic regression using a circle percentage variable and then assessing whether successive rings outside add significantly to the fit. Row 1, for example, shows that the deviance reduction associated with the percentage of mature forest in the innermost circle is highly significant ($p = 0.00051$). Inclusion of the percentage of mature forest in the second ring does not decrease the deviance significantly ($p = 0.86$), but the further inclusion of the third ring percentage gives a highly significant ($p = 0.0009$) deviance reduction; and so on.

The percentage of mature forest in a circle of 1826 ha ($i = 6$) is the single best predictor. It is clear that circles of 260 or 440 ha are significantly improved by high percentages of mature forest in the third ring (440 to 620 ha). After the circle of area 620 ha, addition of variables describing outer rings improve fit marginally. As an example, the addition of R_5 to the model with C_4 results in a reduction of 2.65 in deviance ($p = 0.10$). The difference in mean percentages of mature forest in nest and random sites is 15.1%. The coefficient of R_5 in the model $C_4 + R_5$ is 0.04285. So in terms of practical significance, the observed mean difference would account for about a 90% increase in the odds of selection as a nest site.

3.6 Habitat Fragmentation

If spotted owls tolerated some fragmentation of their habitat, this finding could have considerable implications for our own ability to utilize some of the same habitat without threatening its survival. Is there evidence of an association between site selection and habitat fragmentation? There are three ways that such an association might manifest itself in these data.

1. As *curvature.* If owls selected sites with more than average available mature forest but with less than the maximum available, this would sug-

Table 9 p-Values for Entering the Areas in an Interior Circle, Followed by Entry of Areas in Surrounding Rings

| | Circle Area | p-Values for Entry | | | | | | |
i	(ha)	C_i	R_2	R_3	R_4	R_5	R_6	R_7
1	260	0.00051	0.86	0.0009	0.54	0.058	0.21	0.13
2	440	0.00114		0.016	0.76	0.074	0.28	0.074
3	620	0.00023			0.73	0.070	0.35	0.065
4	800	0.00022				0.100	0.40	0.047
5	980	0.00010					0.21	0.072
6	1826	0.00004						0.089
7	3588	0.00797						

gest a selection for some fragmentation. Such an effect would be recognized in logistic regression models by the presence of quadratic terms in the percentages of mature forest variables.

2. As *interactions*. Consider, as an example, how the odds on a site being a test site increase with increasing percentages of mature forest in the fifth ring. If the increase is weaker when there is a high percentage of mature forest in the inner circle, C_4, than when there is a lower percentage in C_4, that could be interpreted as a condition of tolerance for fragmentation. It would appear as interactions between ring percentages in a logistic regression model.

3. As *negative coefficients*. If there were a definite pattern to a preferred fragmentation which corresponded to the rings chosen by the researchers, the preference could appear as a negative coefficient for some ring variables. In these data the ring variables R_2, R_4, and R_7 did have negative coefficients in all models that used them. None of the three variables contributed significantly to any model, however. We consider the likelihood of this kind of pattern to be negligible. It is more likely that negative coefficients arise because of correlations among the ring percentages.

To assess the possibilities for curvature and interaction terms, we began with a most general quadratic logit expression in the variables $R_1, \ldots, R_6$ and eliminated second-order variables whose coefficients were less than their standard errors. This eliminated all interactions and quadratic terms involving R_4 and R_6. Since their main effect coefficients were also less than their standard errors, we eliminated them entirely. In all, we dropped 17 terms with a combined loss in deviance of 13.53.

4   RESULTS

The final model is summarized in Table 10. The last column of Table 10 is the 1 degree of freedom chi-square (the change in deviance) for dropping the corresponding variable from the model containing all variables listed. Several quadratic and interaction coefficients are borderline significant. As a unit, they are also borderline, with deviance reduction = 14.86 on 6 degrees of freedom ($p = 0.02$). Yet it is instructive to inspect the logit surface for clues. First, the critical point of the sample logit surface occurs where $(R_1, R_2, R_3, R_5) = (0.70, 0.63, 0.57, 0.56)$. The determinant of the second partial matrix is positive, suggesting a minimum, but the second partial for R_1 is negative, so the point is actually a saddle.

As a way of viewing the surface, we constructed four sets of single-variable plots in which the three variables not displayed were taken to be equal, at contour levels of 60%, to 70%, to 80%, and to 90%, giving four separate curves. These are presented as Figure 4. The range of each variable along with the nest

Table 10   Logistic Regression Summary for Ring-Percent, Variables, Allowing for Quadratic and Interaction Terms

Variable	Coefficient	Standard Error	Deviance Reduction
1	−0.984	8.74	—
R_1	0.626	0.347	—
R_2	0.500	0.320	—
R_3	−0.777	0.437	—
R_5	−0.563	0.235	—
$R_1 \times R_1$	−0.00841	0.00356	5.57
$R_2 \times R_2$	0.01251	0.00580	5.33
$R_3 \times R_3$	0.01594	0.00727	4.96
$R_1 \times R_3$	0.00972	0.00469	4.05
$R_2 \times R_3$	−0.03624	0.01521	7.73
$R_3 \times R_5$	0.00984	0.00379	8.54

and random means are also indicated in Figure 4. Even though the observed ranges of the variables span the ranges given in the figure, the full curves represent extrapolations. Sites where ring R_1 had 90% mature forest while all other rings had 60% were not to be found in the data set, because of the strong positive correlations among the ring percentages. Nevertheless, we can examine

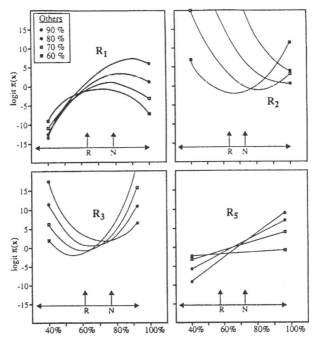

Figure 4. Logit surface cross sections, emphasizing curvature and interactions. Arrows indicate total observation ranges and group means; N = nest; R = random.

the curves for some general indications of whether the kinds of curvature and interactions that were present are consistent with patterns that could have arisen through a tolerance for fragmentation.

In Figure 4 there is a maximum logit for the innermost circle (R_1) which increases as the percentages in the other rings increase but which occurs at a point less than the maximum available. The logit is increasing in R_2 when the other rings have low levels of mature forest, but as the levels increase in the other rings, the logit for R_2 begins to decline. The logit is strongly increasing above the mean of the random sites but increases more rapidly when other sites have lower proportions of mature forest. When all other rings have high proportions of mature forest, the model predicts a positive association of nests, with sites having R_3 below the average at random sites. All these features are consistent with patterns that might arise from a tolerance for fragmentation.

The logit in R_5 is supportive of an association of preference with the *total* of all mature forest. When inner rings all have small proportions of mature forest, the logit is relatively flat in R_5, but when there is more mature forest in the inner rings, response to R_5 is more pronounced.

In summary, there is suggestive but inconclusive evidence of some curvature and interactions among the percentages of mature forest in various rings surrounding sites. Although these features may be related to habitat fragmentation, other explanations are clearly possible. Ripple et al. concluded that "until more data are available" the fragmentation question could not be answered—which is true.

5   CONCLUSIONS

The analyses presented in this paper must be viewed as exploratory, perhaps bordering on data dredging. Case–control studies are observational studies, so cause-and-effect conclusions cannot be inferred. Even the terminology *habitat preference* studies stretches the limits of the study design and should probably be reserved for studies where certain habitat variables are altered deliberately to determine how the animal will respond. The terminology *habitat association* seems more suitable.

The bright side of being exploratory is that considerable latitude may be taken in looking for patterns in the data. Such patterns may reflect biases or the influences of confounding variables, and only further study using a different design can verify their validity. Yet the case–control design is a powerful tool for determining the direction of future research. The potentials for bias and lack of control for confounding variables are discussed in the epidemiological literature on case–control studies. Several of the issues raised there have implications for habitat association studies.

The possibilities for *selection bias* are considerable in wildlife applications, because researchers use a variety of nonrandom search procedures. Target animals may be more detectable in certain habitats than in others. Also, the search technique itself may concentrate effort on certain habitat types, as when night searches for owls are conducted by observers listening from clearings.

Occupation is not the same as selection. The habitat at which an animal is located may not reflect its choice or preference. An animal may return to a traditional breeding site even when the surrounding habitat has degenerated to a condition it would not initially choose. Conversely, some animals may choose not to be located at a site during a study year because they chose that site the previous year. Studies that simply use locations (e.g., via radio tags) are particularly subject to this criticism.

Our review of the use of case–control habitat studies has not found much of a tendency toward overmatching. Although the opportunities for matching are obvious, most researchers have selected control locations randomly within broad habitat classes.

Wildlife applications concentrate on the ensemble of habitat conditions giving rise to animal usage. This is perhaps the largest difference between habitat association studies and clinical case–control studies, where the emphasis is on assessing one or a very few key risk factors in the presence of many confounding variables.

There are many positive aspects to the use of logistic regression in analyzing data from these studies. The format of output from logistic regression analysis is similar to that from multiple regression analysis, which is familiar to most researchers. Instead of F-statistics as measures of variable contributions to explaining response, logistic regression uses chi-square statistics, which may be interpreted in the same way. Logistic regression allows habitat characteristics to be measured on continuous scales. It is not unique in this respect, since discriminant function analysis and rank-based analyses (Johnson, 1980) have been employed with these studies. Yet it is unique in that the researcher need not be overly concerned about mixtures of categorical and continuous habitat variables, nor with nonnormality.

In contrast with Student's t and simple chi-square analyses, the ensemble of habitat characteristics is naturally treated in logistic regression in a multivariable fashion. This seems well suited to habitat analysis, where animals may select sites because the entire habitat configuration is favorable.

The forms of associations may be fully explored using deviance as a criterion. Questions such as these become routine: Are there nonlinearities? Are there interactions among the variables? What is the best way to summarize the influence of each variable? Stepwise and subset selection procedures from multiple linear regression apply. An "analysis of chi-square" table showing deviance changes for model changes is an effective tool for summarization.

Unless habitat variables are few and categorical, the deviance statistic from a fit of a full model does not possess an approximate chi-square distribution and should not be relied upon for goodness of fit. But Landwehr et al. (1984) provided a variety of diagnostic procedures based on residual analysis. That such tools exist and are highly graphical is a boon to the statistician.

ACKNOWLEDGMENTS

Rebecca Goggans, Kitt T. Hershey, David H. Johnson, and E. Charles Meslow supplied us with their original data. Colleagues Daniel Schafer and W. Scott Overton and the CSB review staff provided suggestions that greatly improved the manuscript.

QUESTIONS AND PROBLEMS

1. Using the spotted owl data:

    (a) Construct a variable that measures the percentages of mature forest in the *circles* of radius 2.41 km around the sites. Fit a logistic regression model with this as the single predictor of site usage.

    (b) Expand the model in part (a) to include quadratic and cubic terms. What are the conclusions?

    (c) Construct a matrix of scatterplots for the ring percent variables, first for the random sites and then for the nest sites. Notice the (anticipated) high correlations. What are the implications from this about the analyses performed in the chapter?

    (d) It is possible to check on the random selection mechanism. If selection of the "random" sites was truly random, there should be no consistent differences in the mean percentages of mature forest in the different rings. Discuss how you would go about testing this hypothesis, particularly in view of part (c).

2. A researcher plans to study the influence of an environmental pollutant on den site selections by weasels. Four large study areas have very different levels of pollutant contamination. Each area has a modest population of weasels. The researcher wants to determine if, when pollutants are present, the weasels shift den sites to different soil types.

    (a) Describe how a prospective study could be designed. Also, describe how a retrospective study could be designed.

    (b) What are the relative advantages to the two designs in part (a)?

    (c) If a prospective design is used, will it be possible to attribute any difference in soil type selection to the presence of the pollutant?

3. Suppose, hypothetically, that the flammulated owl study had been prospective; that is, suppose the researchers had randomly selected cavities and then determined which were used by owls and which were not. If the observed data was the same, should the analysis be different? Would the interpretation of the analysis be different from that presented? What would be different?

4. Overmatching in epidemiology occurs when controls are matched too closely to patients on variables such as age, sex, socioeconomic status, geographical region, and so on. The problem arises because some critical risk factor may be correlated with the variables used in the matching, and the matching makes the patients and controls very similar on the risk factor.

(a) Construct a hypothetical example of a habitat association study where overmatching could be a problem.

(b) Describe a wildlife situation where some matching would be advantageous.

(c) In a retrospective study, does matching accomplish the same control that it does in prospective studies?

CHAPTER 11

Time-Series Analyses of Beaver Body Temperatures

Penny S. Reynolds

1 MOTIVATION AND BACKGROUND

Body temperature regulation by animals is a fundamental physiological process, and certainly one of the most studied of all individually based ecological processes (Bartholomew, 1982). Knowledge of thermoregulatory patterns and the factors influencing such patterns is important for determining energy budgets of individual animals, as well as for assessing the general significance of larger-scale patterns of variation and adaptation (Huey, 1982; Garland and Adolph, 1991).

Ideally, body temperature patterns within individuals should be characterized by repeated measurements over extended periods of time (Bennett, 1987; Peterson, 1987). Although isolated or discontinuous body temperature records may provide limited information on body temperature range or the magnitude of fluctuations, body temperature variation within an individual occurs on several different time scales (Avery, 1982). Much empirical attention has been focused on animal response occurring at relatively short time scales (usually within hours). Unfortunately, there are very few studies detailing thermoregulatory variation in individuals over substantially longer periods (e.g., responses occurring on a daily, seasonal, or annual basis). Such longitudinal data are important for adequate and ecologically meaningful comparisons between groups of individuals or populations (Garland and Adolph, 1991).

The paucity of such longitudinal studies may be attributed in part to difficulties associated with past methods of data collection. For vertebrates, the traditional method of obtaining body temperature measurements has been from rectal (or cloacal) measurements of restrained animals, the so-called "grab and stab" technique. In essence, these data comprise single-point estimates of body tem-

Case Studies in Biometry, Edited by Nicholas Lange, Louise Ryan, Lynne Billard, David Brillinger, Loveday Conquest, and Joel Greenhouse.
ISBN 0-471-58885-7 © 1994 John Wiley & Sons, Inc.

perature. However, there are two severe limitations associated with this technique. First, these data are difficult to collect for wild animals. Location, capture, and restraint may involve serious logistic problems, especially if the animal is large and difficult to restrain. Adequate sampling over time may require frequent recaptures, which may become increasingly difficult as the animal becomes more wary. Second, the stress to the animal incurred as a result of handling and restraint will obscure natural variation in temperature patterns (Poole and Stephenson, 1977; Tregust et al., 1979). Thus, time profiles of body temperature obtained from single-point determinations cannot be considered representative of either the animal's true thermoregulatory condition or of the overall thermoregulatory pattern.

The advent of miniaturized radiotelemetry devices has revolutionized the study of wildlife populations (White and Garrott, 1990). In particular, physiological processes such as body temperature can be monitored more or less continuously from unrestrained animals under natural field conditions (MacKay, 1964; Peterson, 1987). Unfortunately, analysis of these data remains a problem for many biologists. Most analytical techniques used in radiotelemetry studies require the assumption of independence between observations (see White and Garrott, 1990). To satisfy statistical demands, sampling intervals have to be widely separated in time. The major drawback with this approach is that much biologically important information is lost, resulting in a completely misleading picture of animal function and behavior (Reynolds and Laundré, 1990). Conversely, even if it is accepted that short sampling intervals are necessary for obtaining biologically relevant information, the problem remains of finding an appropriate analytical technique. Analytical methods for time-dependent auto-correlated data are not presented in many statistical textbooks used by biologists.

What potential problems are associated with the analysis of sequential observations? When data are collected as a time-dependent series, observations are highly correlated and ordered in structure (Box and Tiao, 1975; Neter et al., 1989). Although estimates of the mean are usually robust with respect to these violations (but see Samarov and Taqqu, 1988), the variance is underestimated severely. As a result, the mean does not have the minimum variance property and is inefficient, and confidence intervals and statistical tests are invalid (Box and Tiao, 1975; Neter et al., 1989).

Apart from purely statistical concerns, ignoring lack of independence between observations will also have serious consequences for data interpretation. This is because certain statistics are frequently given biological meaning. For example, the mean is the most commonly used measure of the central tendency of body temperature measurements. The variance (or standard error) has been used in many studies (those concerned with reptile thermal biology in particular) as a measure of "thermoregulatory precision" (Bowker, 1984; Sievert, 1989). Obviously, incorrect assumptions regarding these statistics will comprise or invalidate further biological interpretation.

Autocorrelation in sequential biological observations may be accounted for by statistical time-series models. Time-series analysis is a powerful statistical technique that has been used for evaluating a wide variety of dynamic, time-dependent systems. In ecology, time-series models are used most often to describe population phenomena (Finerty, 1980; Turchin, 1990; Turchin and Taylor, 1992). Recently, these models have been applied to descriptions of process dynamics for entire ecosystems (Carpenter, 1990; Jassby and Powell, 1990). However, time-series models have been underutilized in studies of ecological processes occurring at the level of the individual.

A second potential problem for body temperature studies results from the confounding of temperature patterns with individual activity patterns. The relative level and intensity of activity exhibited by an animal varies nonuniformly over time; both daily and seasonal changes in activity patterns are well documented for many species. Considerable individual variation also exists. Activity generates metabolic heat, which in turn alters body temperature (Bartholomew, 1982). Changes in the relative intensity of activity will therefore affect the magnitude of the temperature change. In mammals, for example, high-intensity activities (such as sustained locomotion), will result in an increase in metabolic expenditure by a factor of 3 to 7 times that of resting levels; body temperature changes may be pronounced. In contrast, low-intensity activities (such as sleeping, resting, standing, grooming, etc.) incur relatively little metabolic cost (usually in the range of 1.7 to 2 times resting levels), with concomitantly smaller effects on body temperature (Karasov, 1992). Therefore, differing activity states are likely to have separate deterministic effects on body temperature. These effects may be controlled statistically by incorporating dummy variables into the model (Draper and Smith, 1981).

In this chapter we extend the principles of Box–Jenkins univariate time-series models as a method of quantifying autocorrelated body temperature data. Several types of body temperature patterns are presented, together with problems associated with the conventional statistical estimators commonly used to describe these data. Box–Jenkins autoregressive–moving average models (Box and Jenkins, 1976) are presented as an alternative method of analysis. It is shown how the confounding effects of activity may be controlled for by the inclusion of a dichotomous dummy variable scheme into the model. Finally, practical suggestions are made regarding the design and implementation of field studies when autocorrelated data must be obtained.

2 DATA

2.1 Study Animals and Field Techniques

The data presented in this chapter are part of a study on the long-term body temperature dynamics of beaver (*Castor canadensis*) in north-central Wisconsin. Beaver are large, semiaquatic, herbivorous rodents common over most of North America. Beaver are of considerable ecological importance in that they are considered to be a "keystone" species, that is, a species which, through its activities, causes considerable alteration of ecosystem dynamics and structure (Naiman et al., 1986). This is one of the few longitudinal studies of a wild species examining natural seasonal variation in a physiological trait (Garland and Adolph, 1991).

Four female beaver were live-trapped and surgically implanted with temperature-sensitive radiotransmitters (Model S4 transmitter, Telonics Inc. Mesa, Arizona). Animals were relocated weekly between 1000 and 1300 hours (during the inactive period), using a hand-held directional antenna and a portable digitizer (TDP-2 Digital Data Processor) and receiver (Telonics Inc., Mesa, Arizona). Individuals were monitored continuously for 24 to 30 hours for a minimum of three sampling periods each season. Beaver were tracked on foot, and by canoe during the open water period (late March to November). Body temperature and location data were recorded every 10 minutes. Beaver activity was described as a two-state phenomenon; activity was scored as either 0 (presence within the retreat) or 1 (presence outside the retreat). This dichotomy was justified on the biological grounds that low-intensity activities occur within the retreat, whereas high-intensity activities (swimming, terrestrial locomotion) can occur only outside the retreat.

2.2 Examples of Body Temperature Patterns

Figure 1a shows field body temperature data for a 15-kg female beaver in early winter, just after complete freeze-up of water. Winter body temperatures for all four beaver typically followed an essentially "random" pattern of body temperature fluctuation over the monitoring period. Because of extensive ice cover, activity outside the resting site was infrequent in winter, and restricted to the immediate vicinity of the retreat.

In contrast, a "plateau" body temperature pattern (Peterson, 1987) was typical for all four beaver in the ice-free seasons, when animals were active outside the retreat site from dusk to dawn. Representative data (Figure 1b) were obtained for a 10-kg female beaver in late autumn. During the rest period, body temperatures of all four beaver usually varied by less than 1°C (36.3 to 37.2°C). At dusk, when beaver emerged from their retreat (the beginning of the active phase), body temperatures rose by approximately 1.0°C in 100 minutes. When beaver returned to their retreat at dawn, body temperatures declined to resting levels by approximately 1°C in 40 minutes.

3 METHODS AND MODELS

3.1 Working Models and Abused Assumptions

Suppose that we have a series of body temperature measurements Y_t observed at equal time intervals $t = 1, 2, \ldots, T$. Conventional estimates for the mean and

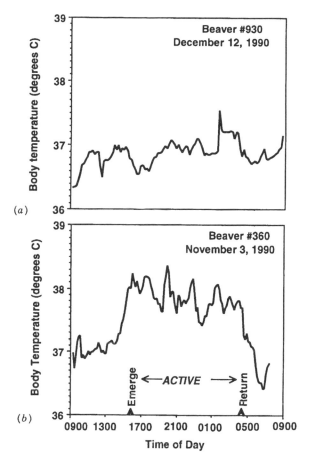

Figure 1. Representative body temperature patterns of free-ranging female beaver *Castor canadensis*. (*a*) Body temperature pattern of an adult female in early winter (freeze-up). There was little or no activity outside the lodge during the monitoring period. (*b*) Body temperature pattern of a subadult female during late autumn (ice-free period). The animal remained in its retreat during the day (rest phase), and emerged at dusk to feed; it remained outside the retreat until dawn (active phase).

variance assume that the series consists of *T independent* observations, such that the series average is estimated by

$$\overline{Y} = \frac{1}{T} \sum_{t=1}^{T} Y_t,$$

and the variance σ^2 is estimated by

$$\hat{\sigma}^2 = \frac{\sum_{t=1}^{T}(Y_t - \overline{Y})^2}{T - 1}. \tag{1}$$

The standard deviation is $\sqrt{\hat{\sigma}^2}$, and the standard error of the mean is $\sqrt{\hat{\sigma}^2/T}$.

Frequently, ordinary least-squares regression (OLS) is used to describe a body temperature series, especially if a trend is observed or suspected. The general representation is

$$Y_t = f(\mathbf{X}_t, \boldsymbol{\beta}) + \epsilon_t. \tag{2}$$

In other words, body temperature at time t depends on the independent variable matrix $\mathbf{X}_t$ (chronological time, age, etc.) through some specified functional relationship f, involving a vector of unknown parameters $\boldsymbol{\beta}$. The simple linear form

$$Y_t = \beta_0 + \beta_1 X_t + \epsilon_t$$

is commonly used. Here β_0 is assumed to represent some constant body temperature, and β_1 is the overall rate of temperature change (heating or cooling). If no time trend in body temperature occurs, equation (2) reduces to

$$Y_t = \beta_0 + \epsilon_t$$

(with $\hat{\beta}_0 = \overline{Y}$), and the variance reduces to equation (1). This model assumes that the residuals ϵ_t are normally distributed with mean 0 and variance σ^2, and are uncorrelated over time.

When temperature data are analyzed by the foregoing models and correlation is ignored, variance will be underestimated. The magnitude of such underestimation can be shown by a simple example. Suppose that correlation $0 < |\rho| < 1$ is present between each successive observation in a stationary series (i.e., the statistical properties do not change with time). Then the body temperature series may be described by

$$Y_t = \rho Y_{t-1} + \epsilon_t.$$

It is assumed that the residuals ϵ_t are normally distributed with mean 0 and variance σ^2 equal to 1. Then the variance of the series Y_t is $\sigma^2/(1 - \rho^2)$; the variance of the series mean $\overline{Y}$ is

$$\mathrm{Var}(\overline{Y}) \approx \frac{\sigma^2}{T(1 - \rho)^2}.$$

Thus, even moderate correlation between observations, say $\rho = 0.5$, will result in the actual variance being many times larger than the value calculated under the assumption of no correlation. Cochrane and Orcutt (1949) derived a similar result for the variance of regression parameters β.

These results can be extended to examine the effects of autocorrelation on estimating the variance of a shift in body temperature averages. Suppose that a continuous temperature series Y_t exhibits a shift in average temperature at time t_0, from $\overline{Y}_A$ to $\overline{Y}_B$. The null hypothesis of no significant difference between mean levels is evaluated with respect to the variance of the difference:

$$\text{Var}(\overline{Y}_B - \overline{Y}_A) = \text{Var}(\overline{Y}_A) + \text{Var}(\overline{Y}_B) - 2\,\text{Cov}(\overline{Y}_A, \overline{Y}_B).$$

Given autocorrelation ρ occurring between consecutive observations (i.e., ρ at lag $s = 1$, and $\rho = 0$ for $s \neq 1$), and $\rho(s) = \text{Cov}(Y_t, Y_{t+s})/\text{Var}(Y_t)$, it has been shown that

$$\text{Var}(\overline{Y}) = \frac{\sigma^2}{T}\left[1 + \frac{2(T-1)}{T}\rho\right] \quad \text{and} \quad \text{Cov}(\overline{Y}_A, \overline{Y}_B) = \frac{\sigma^2}{T^2}\rho$$

(Box et al., 1978). Consequently, the variance of a difference between the means of two consecutive series is

$$\text{Var}(\overline{Y}_B - \overline{Y}_A) = 2\frac{\sigma^2}{T}\left(1 + \frac{2T-3}{T}\rho\right). \tag{3}$$

This contrasts to the "usual" estimate of $2\sigma^2/T$, which assumes independence of observations (i.e., $\rho = 0$ for all s). Clearly, error increases enormously with correlation between observations, as well as (less intuitively) with the number of observations in the series.

3.2 An Alternative: Application of Time-Series Models

A series of consecutive body temperature measurements may conveniently be described as a series consisting of two additive components: a *structural* component, containing the biologically relevant parameters to be estimated (temperature average, temperature change, activity level, etc.); and a *residual* component, which accounts for the confounding effects of autocorrelation and time ordering. These two components may be described relatively simply by combining an OLS regression model with a time-series model. Here a regression function captures the biologically relevant details of the response as a function of time; activity level is incorporated as a dummy variable. A low-order *autoregressive–moving average* (ARMA) process describes the autocorrelation between consecutive observations (Tsay, 1984; Ware, 1985). The formal representation of this model is

$$Y_t = f(\mathbf{X}_t, \boldsymbol{\beta}) + Z_t. \tag{4}$$

Here the "residuals" Z_t are assumed to be correlated over time but uncorrelated with the input $\mathbf{X}_t$. Z_t takes the form of an ARMA process:

$$Z_t = \sum_{i=1}^{p} \phi_i Z_{t-i} + \epsilon_i - \sum_{i=1}^{q} \theta_i \epsilon_{t-1}, \tag{5}$$

where ϕ_i are the autoregressive parameters, of order p, and θ_i are the moving-average parameters, of order q.

In this chapter, model fitting follows a two-step procedure adapted from Tsay (1984) and Ware (1985). First, preliminary *model identification* is performed; this step consists of four parts: (1) specification of the time profile, (2) fitting of the OLS model, (3) estimation of the order p and q of Z_t, and (4) model diagnostics to confirm or reject the suitability of the hypothesized model. Several preliminary models may have to be tried and rejected before an acceptable candidate is found; criteria for acceptance will be discussed briefly in a later section. The second step is formal *model estimation*: all parameters ($\boldsymbol{\beta}, \phi_i, \theta_i$) are estimated simultaneously by maximum likelihood (Tsay, 1984; Jones, 1980).

3.3 Specification of the Time Covariate

The potentially confounding effects of different activities and their temporal patterning can be accounted for by judicious selection of the time covariates. In certain cases, the series itself is of primary interest and the time dimension may be considered as an ordering phenomenon only; activity may or may not correlate strongly with observed variation in body temperature. Then the values of interest will be some measure of average body temperature and its variation over a given time period (Figure 2a). The series can be described by the equation $Y_t = \beta_0 + \beta_1 X_t + Z_t$. Here X_t is a dummy variable consisting of a string of values representing different activity levels. For example, in the simple two-state case, $X_t = 0$ for observations made during the animal's rest period, and $X_t = 1$ for observations made during activity. The regression coefficients β_0 and β_1 represent the average resting body temperature and the average difference between resting and active body temperature, respectively. If β_1 is not significantly different from 0, the temperature profile may be described in terms of a mean and residual term, $Y_t = \beta_0 + Z_t$, where β_0 is the average body temperature. If the series appears to show a linear trend, the model form is again $Y_t = \beta_0 + \beta_1 X_t + Z_t$. However, in this case, β_1 describes the overall rate of temperature change (heating or cooling) over X_t, and $X_t = 1, 2, \ldots, T$, for $t = 1, 2, \ldots, T$. [To ensure orthogonality, it may be necessary to center X_t such that $X = X_t - \overline{X}$; see Draper and Smith (1981) for details.] It must be emphasized that the usual tests of the hypothesis for the significance of the regression coefficients (i.e., $H_0: \beta_1 = 0$) are invalid when consecutive observations are correlated and independence is assumed, because the test statistic $t = (\hat{\beta} - 0)/(\hat{se}(\hat{\beta})$ no longer has a t-distribution (Neter et al., 1989).

More complex models may be generated by intervention, or linear systems, analysis (Box and Tiao, 1975; Chatfield, 1980). Suppose that the investiga-

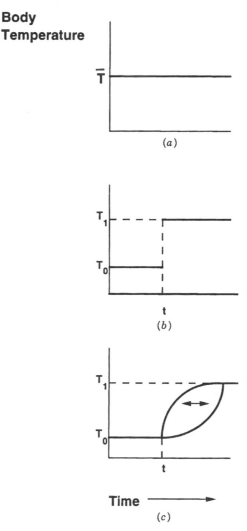

Figure 2. General patterns of animal body temperature over time. (*a*) Model $Y_t = \beta_0 + Z_t$. Of interest is the estimation of the long-term average body temperature $\overline{T}$ and some measure of variation. (*b* and *c*) Linear transfer model incorporating a state change in input at time t. Possible responses in body temperature are (*b*) a step function and (*c*) an exponential increase.

tor wishes to compare the change in body temperature response between some "baseline" time period and a subsequent time period (Figure 2b and c). Examples include the body temperature change that occurs when an animal switches from a resting to a prolonged active state, or moves from one habitat type to another. These cases exemplify the problem set out in equation (3); that is, the estimation of the variance of a difference between two consecutive, autocorrelated series. Again, X_t may be specified as a dummy variable describing activity state. For a two-state condition, X_t takes on the values 0 and 1, as before; however, these values are distributed over the total time period T such that T is partitioned into two subsets:

$$X_t = \begin{cases} 0, & t < t_0 \\ 1, & t \geq t_0, \end{cases}$$

where $t < t_0$ is the time period before the state change (e.g., no activity), and $t \geq t_0$ is the time after the state change (e.g., activity). If average body temperature exhibits an immediate shift, the response approximates a step function (Figure 2b). Here $\hat{\beta}_0$ estimates average "baseline" temperature, and $\hat{\beta}_1$ estimates the change between the baseline average and the average temperature of the alternative state.

More realistically, body temperature is likely to change gradually with the onset of the active phase until it reaches a new equilibrium level (Figure 2c). Modeling this type of response may require incorporation of a dynamic transfer term, such as that described by Box and Tiao (1975):

$$Y_t = \frac{\omega B}{1 - \delta B} X_t + Z_t.$$

Here B is the backshift operator, such that $BX_t = X_{t-1}$. The unknowns ω and δ are estimated from the data, and define the timing and magnitude of the change in body temperature averages. Specifically, the shape of the response changes from exponential to linear as δ approaches 1. The difference between baseline and the new body temperature average may be estimated by $\omega/(1 - \delta)$, and the time constant (the time to achieve 63.2% of the final equilibrium body temperature) by $1/(-\ln \delta)$ (Box and Tiao, 1975). The time constant is another biologically useful value in thermoregulatory studies (e.g., Kingsolver and Watt, 1983).

3.4   Fitting of the OLS Model

Once the time profile has been specified, the preliminary model is fitted by least squares and the residuals ϵ_t calculated. The residuals are used as the first approximation of the time series Z_t (Tsay, 1984), such that $Z_t \approx Y_t - \mathbf{X}_t\boldsymbol{\beta}$.

3.5 Estimation of the ACF and Diagnostics

The third feature of the analysis is the estimation of the order of the process Z_t. In general, Z_t will be of the form described by equation (5). In practice, the data are often described adequately by a low-order autoregressive process AR$[p]$. In an AR$[p]$ series, p is a measure of the "memory" of the series, since p is the maximum time lag beyond which a past value of the observed response has no direct effect on current values. In the simplest case, there is correlation between consecutive observations only; thus the model is an AR$[1]$ process and the autoregression parameter ϕ equals the correlation ρ between observations (Box and Jenkins, 1976). Of course, the form of the ARMA process should not be assumed a priori without careful diagnostic checking.

The diagnostic process involves fitting a tentative ARMA model, the form of which is based on patterns exhibited by the correlation coefficients calculated for each pair of residual observations derived from the initial model. The sample *autocorrelation function* (ACF) is estimated by calculating the correlation coefficients ρ_τ between pairs of observations Y_t and $Y_{t-\tau}$ separated by lag $\tau, \tau = 1, 2, \ldots, k$. The sample *partial autocorrelation function* (PACF) measures the correlation at lag τ not accounted for by an AR$[\tau - 1]$ model. A useful diagnostic property is that the sample ACF for a stationary AR$[p]$ series will tend to decrease, either exponentially or as a damped sinusoidal pattern, as lag τ increases, whereas the sample PACF "cuts off" (i.e., $\phi_{\tau\tau} = 0$) for all lags $\tau > p$ (Box and Jenkins, 1976; Chatfield, 1980). In contrast, a series consisting only of moving-average components of order MA$[q]$ will show a reversal of these patterns, with the sample ACF exhibiting a cutoff at $\tau = q$ and sample PACF decaying gradually with increasing τ. In cases where the series exhibits nonstationarity (i.e., the statistical properties change with time), the sample ACF will exhibit very slow decay with increasing τ. This will be observed if the series approximates a random walk ($\hat{\rho} \rightarrow 1$). The sample *inverse autocorrelation function* (IACF) is also a useful diagnostic tool; it is especially advantageous in diagnosing subset or seasonal effects (Chatfield, 1979).

Model fit is assessed by residual checks; one of the criteria for an acceptable model fit is that residuals should behave as a white noise process (i.e., $\hat{\rho} = 0$ for all time lags). The large-sample standard error ($\pm 2/\sqrt{N}$) is used to test for significance of the correlation coefficients (Box and Jenkins, 1976; Chatfield, 1980). Alternative procedures for selecting the appropriate order of the postulated model include the *Akaike information criterion* (AIC), and the *Bayesian information criterion* (BIC). Katz (1981) discusses the relative performance of each procedure. No one method will be best in all circumstances; information criteria in particular should be regarded as a guide rather than a hard-and-fast rule (Chatfield, 1980). Other criteria include simplicity (the model should not be overly complicated with unnecessary parameters) and goodness of fit (Ljung and Box, 1978).

4   RESULTS

4.1   Body Temperature Series with No Change of State

Data obtained for an adult female beaver in winter (Table 1) consisted of 114 serial observations; receiver failure due to extreme cold terminated data collection before the end of the complete 24-hour monitoring period. The subject made seven short (<5 minutes) excursions outside the retreat during the monitoring period. There was no statistical difference between body temperature observed for each activity state. Therefore, the final model describing this series was estimated by $Y_t = \beta_0 + Z_t$.

If independence between observations is assumed, the estimated mean and standard error are 36.87°C with standard error 0.02°C. However, examination of the sample ACF and PACF of the residuals shows considerable correlation between consecutive observations (Figure 3a). On the basis of these diagnostics, an AR(1) model was indicated. The autoregressive term, estimated by maximum likelihood, is $\hat{\phi} = \hat{\rho} = -0.898$ with standard error 0.042. Sample ACF and

Table 1   Sample Body Temperature Data (First 20 Observations) for an Adult Female Beaver (*Castor canadensis*) in Early Winter

Obs. No.	Julian Day	Time[a]	Body Temperature (°C)	Activity[b]
1	346	0840	36.33	0
2	346	0850	36.34	0
3	346	0900	36.35	0
4	346	0910	36.42	0
5	346	0920	36.55	0
6	346	0930	36.69	0
7	346	0940	36.71	0
8	346	0950	36.75	0
9	346	1000	36.81	0
10	346	1010	36.88	0
11	346	1020	36.89	0
12	346	1030	36.91	0
13	346	1040	36.85	0
14	346	1050	36.89	0
15	346	1100	36.89	0
16	346	1110	36.67	0
17	346	1120	36.50	0
18	346	1130	36.74	0
19	346	1140	36.77	0
20	346	1150	36.76	0

[a]The time code is formatted as hour-min.

[b]Activity is scored as either 0 (no activity outside retreat) or 1 (outside retreat).

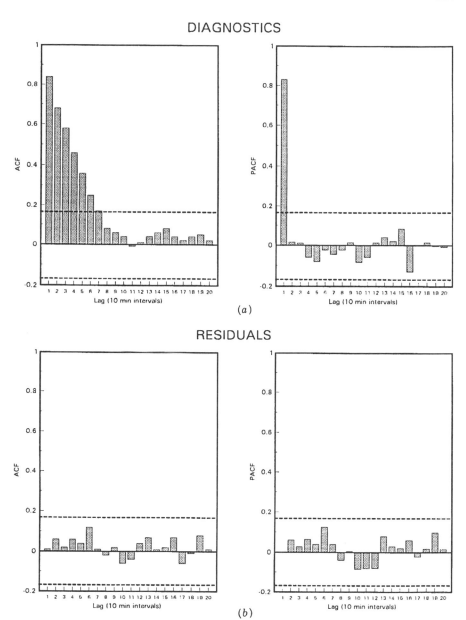

Figure 3. Diagnostics and residual plots for body temperature data from a female beaver in early winter. (*a*) Diagnostics show the ACF and PACF patterns obtained for the series Z_t: ACF "decays" and PACF "cuts off" at lag 1, indicating an AR[1] model. (*b*) Residuals for the fitted model $Y_t = \beta_0 + Z_t, Z_t = \text{AR}[1]$ process follow a white noise pattern; dotted lines are the large-sample confidence intervals $2/\sqrt{N}$.

PACF for the residuals were less than the estimated large-sample standard error, indicating that all correlation between observations was accounted for (Figure 3*b*). The final model is thus

$$Y_t = 36.85°C + Z_t; \qquad (1 - 0.898B)Z_t = \epsilon_t;$$

where the estimated standard error of $\hat{\beta}_0$ is 0.08°C and $\sigma_\epsilon^2 = 0.009$. Violating the assumption of independent observations had no effect on the estimate of the average body temperature; however, estimates of standard error differed by a factor of 4.

4.2   Body Temperature Profile with a Prolonged State Change

Data presented for a subadult female beaver (Figure 1*b*) in late autumn show a plateau pattern typically observed for beaver during all ice-free seasons. For simplicity, only the first 100 out of a total 245 observations were analyzed. Assuming no serial correlation between observations, resting body temperature was estimated to be 37.02°C with standard error 0.03°C, and active temperature as 37.80°C with standard error of 0.02°C. The average rate of body temperature change during the transition from rest to activity was estimated to be 0.89°C over 100 minutes. By contrast, the linear transfer model with autocorrelated errors resulted in estimates of resting body temperature of 37.05°C with standard error of 0.09°C, and active temperatures of 38.02°C with standard error 0.12°C. The errors followed an AR[1] process, with $\hat{\phi} = \hat{\rho} = 0.791$. The estimate for δ was 0.783, a value significantly different from 1.0; this suggested that the body temperature pattern during the warm-up phase was an exponential increase. The total body temperature change during the warm-up phase was estimated to be 0.81°C, with a time constant of 41 min. Again series means were approximately the same, regardless of assumption violation, but standard errors differed by a factor of 4 to 5.

5   CONCLUSIONS

Animal thermoregulatory processes are time dependent, a feature shared with many other physiological phenomena. However, the inclusion of time as a biologically significant covariate has been neglected in many physiological studies. Part of this neglect may be attributed to lack of awareness of analytical tools required to handle autocorrelated data. In this chapter we describe a methodology for empirical modeling of animal body temperature. The key features of body temperature data are that consecutive observations are correlated and time ordered rather than independent and random. Lack of independence invalidates many commonly performed statistical tests, and consequently, affects biological interpretation. As an example, two sets of body temperature data for beaver were analyzed, both with and without the assumption of independence. In each case, there was significant correlation between observations ($0.79 < \hat{\phi} < 0.90$). Standard errors were affected substantially by inappropriate assumptions of independence. Because standard error may be interpreted as a measure of thermoregulatory precision, the consequences of violating these assumptions are faulty assessment of the extent of animal thermoregulatory response.

The time-series models described here represent a general class of models that should be broadly applicable to other types of individually based longitudinal data. A number of statistical packages are available for time-series analyses and deal adequately with the sequence of model identification, parameter estimation, and diagnostic stages involved in the statistical model-building process.

Regardless of the actual statistical model employed, careful consideration of study design is a critical first step in the model-building process. Essential design features include *definition* of biologically meaningful variables, identification of the *experimental unit*, choice of an appropriate *sample size* (or number of experimental units), selection of an appropriate *sampling interval* (time between observations), and choice of sampling *period length* (total number of observations).

Most working *definitions* of thermoregulatory patterns are vague. For example, several textbooks describe a "heterothermic" animal as one in which thermoregulatory patterns "vary widely" over time (Bartholomew, 1982; Eckert, 1988). These definitions do not make it clear whether this "variation" refers to fluctuation around some constant level or whether there are shifts in the temperature average itself. Many reptiles and mammals exhibit both patterns of variation on either a daily or a seasonal basis (Dill, 1972; Peterson, 1987; Poole and Stephenson, 1977). Thus, the first part of the modeling exercise is to establish practical working definitions of the response to be modeled in terms of relevant statistical entities.

In many studies, the individual animal will be the *experimental unit*. Animals must therefore be independent of each other [but see White and Garrott (1990) for exceptions]. One of the more common errors in physiological studies is the pooling of observations for a number of individuals (Mather and Silver, 1980). This results in the artificial inflation of the degrees of freedom (leading to false rejection of the null hypothesis) and the confounding of series (within-individual) variation with between-individual variation. Unfortunately, there are no hard-and fast rules for determining appropriate sample sizes. In many instances the investigator is constrained by expense and logistics; it may be too costly to outfit, and too labor intensive to monitor, the number of animals required for adequate statistical power. As a result, sample sizes may be so small that the use of extensive statistical analyses is unwarranted.

Selection of the appropriate *sampling interval* requires knowledge of the biology of the system. In general, methods of data analysis for radiotelemetry studies require statistical independence between observations (White and Garrott, 1990). In contrast, physiological studies require closely spaced sampling intervals to capture the time-dependent features of the data. A major problem in selecting an appropriate sampling interval is that reduction of interval length beyond a certain threshold increases the number of observations without contributing additional information. Additionally, very short sample intervals add greatly to the costs and inconvenience of data collection (White and Garrott, 1990). The appropriate sampling interval should be roughly proportional to the animal's expected time constant, such that the amount of change occurring within each interval is small relative to the overall fluctuation in the system (Box and Jenkins, 1976). Statistically, the effect of reducing the sampling interval is a concomitant reduction in variance; the appropriate sampling interval minimizes the residual mean square error of the series.

The *sampling period length* must be long enough to capture the biologically important features of the data. For example, a total period of 1 hour will be inadequate if the investigator wishes to examine daily amplitudes of temperature fluctuation. Criteria for deciding on the appropriate length of both sampling interval and total sampling period include information on the response time of the animal as well as the measuring device itself. Animal response is a function of the amplitude and lag inherent in body temperature patterns. Amplitude influences the detectability of change (alteration in response with respect to inherent fluctuations in the data), whereas lag indicates time from a given input until response. Body size will be an important determinant of amplitude and lag; very large animals usually exhibit greater thermal stability (small amplitude) and longer lags than do small animals. The response time and precision of the detecting device (transmitter and receiving package) may differ independently from that of the animal; such measurement error must be accounted for before the study is begun (White and Garrott, 1990). Obviously, pilot studies are indispensable for determining both statistical and biological aspects of the experimental design.

Missing data frequently become an issue during the data collection stage and are almost inevitable in a field situation. If large chunks of data are missing, rigorous statistical modeling will not be an option. However, if the missing data comprise only a few observations in a long series, these may be estimated by the average body temperature for a stationary series or by linear interpolation for a trended series. Interpolation of data missing at random intervals may be performed by Kalman filtering (Jones, 1980). Finally, analysis of specific subsets of data with few or no missing observations may be considered.

Time-series models such as those described here may be used when it is desired to compare responses for two or more groups of individuals. Yang and Carter (1983) showed that one-way ANOVA is an appropriate method of assessing differences between groups when data consist of a number of serially correlated observations on each individual. The usual ANOVA F-test is an efficient test of the null hypothesis of equality of group means. Sample sizes should consist of $n \geq 8$ individuals with $N \geq 30$ observations per individual (Yang and Carter, 1983).

Ultimately, the characterization of a body temperature series depends on both the hypotheses to be tested and assumptions of the underlying mechanistic model. For example, in reptile thermal studies, use of the mean of a series of body temperature observations has been criticized for its implicit assumption of a single setpoint control. If alternative mechanistic models are postulated (e.g., the dual-limit control model; Barber and Crawford, 1977), the mean will not be an appropriate description of the data (Huey, 1982). However, it must be emphasized that for many animal species the necessary physical/physiological knowledge may be absent or insufficient to allow the form of the functional relationship to be specified. Therefore, statistical models of the type described in this chapter will provide a useful first approximation to observed phenomena. Of course, highly sophisticated models are not always necessary. Certain simple statistics (e.g., the mean and variance) provide useful and readily interpretable summaries of extensive and complex data. Visual inspection of time plots of the raw data is extremely valuable as a diagnostic tool and for deciding on reasonable candidates for descriptive models. The bottom line is that both sensible statistics and sensible biology will prescribe the final form of the quantitative model. Underlying assumptions of any model must be carefully checked; if violations occur, the biological significance of the information provided by such models will be greatly reduced. However, the best quantitative model is equally useless if it has little relevance to the biological processes it was meant to describe. In the final analysis, the selection of an appropriate statistical model will be iterative: both biological and statistical principles (plus a good measure of common sense) must be called upon both to define and refine the quantitative models used to describe ecological processes.

ACKNOWLEDGMENTS

The author thanks S. C. Adolph, N. R. Draper, R. Johnson, W. H. Karasov, R. M. Lee III, and especially B. S. Yandell for advice and reading the manuscript in its various formative stages. Several anonymous reviewers made excellent suggestions. M. Zechmeister (Superintendent, Sandhill Wildlife Demonstration Area) and J. Haug (Department of Natural Resources, Wisconsin Rapids) gave permission to work at the study site. P. Thorsen and S. Hubbard-van Stelle performed the surgeries, and J. Augustine and L. Tate provided excellent field assistance. The financial support of the Theodore Roosevelt Memorial Fund (American Museum of Natural History), the American Society of Mammalogists, and the Lois Almon Grant-in-Aid of Field Research (Wisconsin Academy of Arts, Science and Letters) is gratefully acknowledged; additional funding was provided by DOE grant DE-FG0288-ER60633 to W. P. Porter.

SOFTWARE NOTES

Modeling procedures in this chapter were performed with SAS/ETS (Version 6) software (SAS Institute, 1988).

QUESTIONS AND PROBLEMS

1. It has been hypothesized that core temperatures of small fish will show a closer correspondence with the surrounding water temperature than will those of large fish. However, large fish are also expected to show larger time constants (time lag before temperature stabilizes). Design an experiment to test these hypotheses. Questions that should be addressed include: What constitutes an adequate body size range? What time frame is required to evaluate response? What constitutes an appropriate sampling scheme? What is an appropriate sample size? How many replicates should be performed?

2. Frequently, correlations exist between several time-dependent physiological traits (such as body temperature and metabolic rate), or between a physiological trait and a behavioral trait. How appropriate are cross-correlations for evaluating these phenomena? What problems may arise if the investigator wishes to analyze continuous data in conjunction with categorical data?

3. Statistical power is—or should be—a real concern. Unfortunately, transmitter equipment is extremely expensive, thus limiting the total number of subjects available per study. Locating subjects and collecting data may be extremely arduous and time consuming. What statistical strategies should be implemented to identify both the optimal field effort and the maximum usefulness of the resulting data for a given biological question?

4. Sampling variation is inherent in both the experimental units and with respect to the measuring device (in this case, the transmitter). What statistical strategies should be recommended for the evaluation of measurement error in each component?

PART IV

Health Care and Public Health Policy

CHAPTER 12

Parametric Duration Analysis of Nursing Home Usage

Carl N. Morris, Edward C. Norton, and Xiao H. Zhou

1 MOTIVATION AND BACKGROUND

Although one and a half million people in the United States are residents of nursing homes, and over $40 billion is spent annually on nursing home care, relatively little is known about how long people stay in these facilities. Researchers have not modeled adequately the length of stay distribution, nor is it known how different patient characteristics affect the length of stay. Previous analyses have used nonrepresentative samples (Garber and MaCurdy, 1989), or have used data in which the length of stay is measured only to the nearest month (Liu et al. 1991), or have reported the length of stay in tabular form only.

The first goal of this chapter is to model and to estimate nursing home duration times, measured in days, as a function of patient characteristics. These parametric probability models are then used to predict durations and to determine the accuracy of these predictions. A second goal is to determine how economic incentives, offered in a social experiment, affect lengths of stay.

The data are from a controlled experiment that gave monetary incentives to selected nursing homes, encouraging them to provide more appropriate care to their Medicaid residents. The expected net effect of these incentives was to produce shorter lengths of stay for Medicaid patients in treatment nursing homes than for similar patients in control nursing homes. The results here indicate, instead, that treatment nursing home residents actually had slightly longer (but statistically insignificant) lengths of stay than those in control nursing homes.

Several parametric models and one semiparametric model are explored and compared; Kalbfleisch and Prentice (1980), Lawless (1982), and Lancaster (1990), are general references on the topics studied here. Each models the length

Case Studies in Biometry, Edited by Nicholas Lange, Louise Ryan, Lynne Billard, David Brillinger, Loveday Conquest, and Joel Greenhouse.
ISBN 0-471-58885-7 © 1994 John Wiley & Sons, Inc.

of stay as a function of a few explanatory variables. We discuss censored data modeling, proportional hazards models, and graphical methods.

2   DATA

We analyze data from an experiment sponsored by the National Center for Health Services Research in 1980–1982, involving 36 for-profit nursing homes in San Diego, California. The experiment was designed to assess the effects of differing financial incentives on the admission of nursing home patients, on their subsequent care, and on the durations of stay. The 18 treatment nursing homes received higher per diem payments for accepting more disabled Medicaid patients. They also received bonuses for improving a patient's health status and for discharging patients to their homes within 90 days. These incentives were not offered to the 18 control nursing homes. The variable *treatment* is coded 1 for treatment nursing homes and 0 for control nursing homes. Despite the random assignment of nursing homes to the control and treatment groups, the percentage of Medicaid patients was much higher in the control group (70% of admissions) than in the treatment group (45% of admissions), a potentially confounding problem not addressed here.

Personal characteristics such as marital status, gender, health, and age significantly affect the length of stay. Married patients are more likely to be admitted in poor health, and also more likely to return home earlier because they more often have an alternative caregiver at home. *Married* is coded 1 for married patients, and 0 otherwise.

Women and men also differ in their lengths of stay. Men have poorer functional status at admission because elderly men are much more likely to be married than elderly women. The variable *male* is coded 1 for men, and 0 for women.

Health status strongly affects length of stay. The variable *health* is coded on a scale from 2 (second best) to 5 (worst). Those with the best health, *health* = 1, were excluded from this analysis because the economic incentives did not apply to them. Patients with zero to four dependencies in activities of daily living (i.e., $ADL \leq 4$) are classified as *health* = 2 (Katz and Akpon, 1976). *Health* = 3 and *health* = 4 correspond to $ADL = 5$ and $ADL = 6$. Patients with complications requiring additional care (such as comatose care, tube feeding, or decubitus ulcer treatment) were assigned *health* = 5. Separate indicator variables are included for each health status, with *health* = 3 the omitted group.

Age affects the duration time because older patients are less likely to have surviving spouses, and their frailty makes them less able to return home. However, older patients also are more likely to die sooner. The variable *age spline* is specified as linear from ages 65 through 90, and constant thereafter. Thus, *age spline* = min (age, 90). This specification was justified through early exploration with the data.

All patients in the data set are age 65 or older. Summary statistics for the variables used in the analysis are shown in Table 1. They correspond to a sub-sample of 1601 residents from the original sample of 10,928, selected as follows. Residents in the sample had to be age 65 or above (the vast majority) to concentrate on the elderly. They also had to be covered by Medicaid and to have health status 2 through 5, because the economic incentives were directed only at this less healthy Medicaid population. Finally, only those admitted to a participating nursing home between May 1, 1981 and April 30, 1982 are included. All residents admitted prior to May 1, 1981 would either be subject to "length bias" or could not have been subjected to the incentives, even in treatment nursing homes, in the initial portion of their stay. Table 2 shows 10 observations selected at random from the full sample of 1601. The length of stay (LOS) is the number of days in the nursing home. Ten residents in the sample have LOS equal to zero.

Some residents were censored, meaning that their time of discharge was not observed and is not known. Rather, the value reported is a lower bound for the actual LOS corresponding to the number of days the resident was known to be in the nursing home. Such values are designated by introducing the indicator variable *censored*, which equals zero whenever LOS is the actual length of stay. See the eighth row of Table 2 for an example of a censored observation, coded *censored* = 1, which has LOS equal to 970 days. Residents never were censored until they had stayed in the nursing home for at least one year. The censoring

Table 1   Summary Statistics for the 1601 Observations in the Nursing Home Data

Continuous Variables	Minimum	Median	Mean	Maximum
LOS (days)	0	115	241.2	1092
Age (years)	65	83	82.6	104

Dichotomous Variables	Frequency		Mean
	0	1	Mean
Treatment	889	712	0.44
Male	1178	423	0.26
Married	1326	275	0.17
Censored	1279	322	0.20

Categorical Variable	Frequency			
	2	3	4	5
Health	343	576	513	169

Table 2   Ten Observations Chosen at Random from the Nursing Home Data

LOS	Treatment	Age	Male	Married	Health	Censored
12	0	85	1	1	5	0
412	1	65	1	0	2	0
144	1	82	0	0	2	0
7	0	65	0	0	4	0
120	0	86	0	0	2	0
0	1	82	1	1	4	0
53	0	66	0	0	4	0
970	1	86	0	0	3	1
25	0	85	0	0	4	0
110	0	74	0	1	3	0

rule, which determined when the resident no longer would be observed, was as follows. Residents in treatment nursing homes were censored after April 30, 1984; those in control nursing homes were censored after April 30, 1983.

3   METHODS AND MODELS

3.1   Review of Existing Models

The models considered here specify a continuous, positive distribution for LOS, with the natural logarithm of LOS linearly predicted by the explanatory variables of Table 1. That is,

$$\ln(LOS) = \mathbf{x}\boldsymbol{\beta} + \sigma U, \tag{1}$$

$$LOS = e^{\mathbf{x}\boldsymbol{\beta}} W^{\sigma}, \qquad \text{where} \quad W = e^{U}, \tag{2}$$

where $\boldsymbol{\beta}$ is a location vector, σ is a scale constant, $\mathbf{x}$ is a vector of known covariates, and U has a specified univariate distribution. Both $\boldsymbol{\beta}$ and σ are unknown and to be estimated. The three baseline distributions used here for $W = \exp(U)$ are: exponential (unit mean), lognormal [i.e., $U = \ln(W) \sim N(0, 1)$] and gamma(α), $\alpha > 0$. The baseline gamma distribution has an additional *shape parameter* α, which corresponds to the exponential for $\alpha = 1$ and to the normal for very large α. Thus, with the introduction of the *scale parameter* σ and the regression parameter vector $\boldsymbol{\beta}$ of dimension k, there are $k + 1$ unknown parameters $(\boldsymbol{\beta}, \sigma)$ to be estimated for the Weibull and lognormal models, and $k + 2$ for the generalized gamma model.

Table 3 provides specific formulas for the densities and survival functions. In each of the three cases, the baseline distribution for W at $W = t$ is given as exponential, lognormal, and gamma. The Weibull and other "generalized" distributions have survival functions obtained by substituting $t^{\gamma}\exp(-\gamma\mathbf{x}\boldsymbol{\beta})$ for

Table 3 Density and Survival Functions for Three Parametric Models[a]

Duration Distribution	Density $= f(t)$	Survival $= S(t)$
Weibull	$\dfrac{\gamma t^{\gamma-1} \exp\left[-t^{\gamma}\exp(-\gamma\mathbf{x}\boldsymbol{\beta})\right]}{\exp(\gamma\mathbf{x}\beta)}$	$\exp\left[-t^{\gamma}\exp(-\gamma\mathbf{x}\boldsymbol{\beta})\right]$
Exponential	$\exp(-t)$	$\exp(-t)$
Generalized log normal	$\dfrac{\gamma}{t}\,\phi\{\gamma\ln(t\exp(-\mathbf{x}\boldsymbol{\beta})]\}$	$\Phi\{-\gamma\ln[t\exp(-\mathbf{x}\boldsymbol{\beta})]\}$
Lognormal	$\dfrac{1}{t}\,\phi[\ln(t)]$	$\Phi[-\ln(t)]$
Generalized gamma	$\dfrac{\gamma[t\exp(-\mathbf{x}\boldsymbol{\beta})]^{\alpha\gamma}\exp\left[-t^{\gamma}\exp(-\gamma\mathbf{x}\boldsymbol{\beta})\right]}{t\Gamma(\alpha)}$	$1 - \mathrm{I}[\alpha, t^{\gamma}\exp(-\gamma\mathbf{x}\boldsymbol{\beta})]$
Gamma	$\dfrac{t^{\alpha-1}\exp(-t)}{\Gamma(\alpha)}$	$1 - \mathrm{I}(\alpha, t)$
Defining	$\mathrm{I}(\alpha, x) = \dfrac{1}{\Gamma(\alpha)}\displaystyle\int_{0}^{x} u^{\alpha-1}\exp(-u)\,du$	

[a]Both the general case and the baseline case, where $\gamma = 1$ and $\boldsymbol{\beta} = \mathbf{0}$, are listed. Note that $\gamma = 1/\sigma$. The hazard function, $h(t) = f(t)/S(t)$, is unlisted.

t in the baseline survival function. The densities are obtained by differentiating the negative survival functions. Throughout, $\gamma = 1/\sigma$.

The Weibull and lognormal models are limiting cases of the generalized gamma: the Weibull for $\alpha = 1$, because gamma(1) is the exponential; and the lognormal for $\alpha = \infty$, because $\sqrt{\alpha}\ln(1/\alpha G_{\alpha})$, with $G_{\alpha} \sim$ gamma(α), has an asymptotic $N(0, 1)$ distribution as $\alpha \to \infty$. These relationships permit tests within the generalized gamma model for the validity of the Weibull ($1/\alpha = 1$) or lognormal ($1/\alpha = 0$) models.

The baseline survival functions for the three cases are $S_{o}(t) = \Pr(\exp(U) > t)$, and the hazard functions are $h_{o}(t) = -d\ln S_{o}(t)/dt = f_{o}(t)/S_{o}(t)$. The survival function for *LOS* is therefore, from (2),

$$S(t) = \Pr(LOS > t) = \Pr[W > t^{\gamma}\exp(-\gamma\mathbf{x}\boldsymbol{\beta})] \qquad (3)$$
$$= S_{o}[t^{\gamma}\exp(-\gamma\mathbf{x}\boldsymbol{\beta})], \qquad \gamma = 1/\sigma. \qquad (4)$$

It follows that the hazard function $h(t; \mathbf{x}) = -d\ln S(t)/dt$ satisfies

$$h(t; \mathbf{x}) = \gamma t^{\gamma-1}\exp(-\gamma\mathbf{x}\boldsymbol{\beta})h_{o}[t^{\gamma}\exp(-\gamma\mathbf{x}\boldsymbol{\beta})]. \qquad (5)$$

3.2 Proportional Hazards

An alternative to the three models above is to make the "proportional hazards" assumption (Cox, 1972). This assumption requires that the ratio of the hazard functions for any two individuals does not depend on time. That is, if two individuals have covariate vectors x_1 and x_2, respectively, the ratio $h(t; x_2)/h(t; x_1)$ may not depend on t, although it may depend on x_1 and x_2.

For location-scale models in the form of (1) and (2), the hazard ratio is

$$\frac{h(t; x_2)}{h(t; x_1)} = \exp\left[\gamma(x_1 - x_2)\beta\right] \times \frac{h_o[t^\gamma \exp(-\gamma x_2 \beta)]}{h_o[t^\gamma \exp(-\gamma x_1 \beta)]}. \tag{6}$$

The proportional hazards model postulates that the ratio in (6) is independent of t. It can be shown that (6) is independent of t if and only if h_0 is a monomial, $h_0(t) = at^b$ for some constants a, b. The Weibull hazard is monomial. It follows that the Weibull model is the only proportional hazards model in the form of (1) and (2) [i.e., where $\ln(LOS)$ is a location-scale family (meaning that $U = [\ln(LOS) - x\beta]/\sigma$ has a distribution not depending on β or σ]. Note that the lognormal and generalized gamma are not proportional hazards models.

An equivalent requirement of the proportional hazards assumption in models of the form (1)–(2) is that for all x, the following ratio should not depend on x:

$$\frac{h(t_2; x)}{h(t_1; x)} = \left(\frac{t_2}{t_1}\right)^{\gamma-1} \frac{h_o[t_2^\gamma \exp(-\gamma x\beta)]}{h_o[t_1^\gamma \exp(-\gamma x\beta)]}. \tag{7}$$

Equation (7) is independent of x if and only if $h_o(t) = at^b$, and then (7) depends only on the ratio t_1/t_2. Note that when (7) is independent of x, if the hazard function of one individual changes by a certain factor between t_1 and t_2, the hazard function of all other individuals changes by that same factor over the interval.

3.3 Adding a Constant to LOS

A model that is expressed in additive form for logarithmic time, as in (1), has two potential problems. First, taking the logarithm of LOS causes difficulties because $\ln(LOS)$ cannot be computed in the 10 cases in which LOS equals zero. Second, the use of logarithms puts heavy emphasis on the short stayers (e.g., the logarithmic difference between 1 and 3 days is the same as between 1 and 3 months or between 1 and 3 years). The interests of public policy, however, focus on the longer times.

These problems are reduced by including a constant $c > 0$, to be added to LOS before taking the logarithm (Mosteller and Tukey, 1977). Thus we choose an appropriate c and use $\ln(LOS + c)$ in (1) and (2) instead of $\log(LOS)$.

After experimentation with several values of c, including 0.1, 1, 2, 3, the value $c = 2$ was chosen for its ability to produce a relatively short tail on the left side of the $\ln(LOS + c)$ distribution (see Figure 1). A small value such as $c = 2$ reduces the effect of the short LOS values. Equation (1) now is replaced by

$$\ln(LOS + 2) = \mathbf{x}\boldsymbol{\beta} + \sigma U. \tag{8}$$

3.4 Censored Data

In the nursing home data set, the actual LOS is not observed in 322 of the 1601 cases (i.e., 20% of the observations are censored). For these censored observations, the actual LOS is known only to exceed the observed value. In this data set, the minimum censoring time is one year, so no observations under 365 days are censored. After three years, all observations are censored, the largest censored value being 1092 days (2.99 years). In fact, only 126 (28%) of the 448 observations for 365 days or more are not censored. The censoring cannot be ignored without risk of substantial bias. If the 322 censored observations are removed from the data set, the length of stay will be estimated to be too small. The same is true if the censored observations are included but are treated as the actual LOS. Instead, one must either model the survival distribution completely, or make the proportional hazards assumption. Both approaches are considered here. The likelihood function for censored data uses the $m = 1279$ uncensored values $t_1, \ldots, t_m$, the $n = 322$ censored values $t_{m+1}, \ldots, t_N$, where $N = m + n = 1601$, and the observed censoring indicators $C_i = 1$ if censored, or $C_i = 0$ if

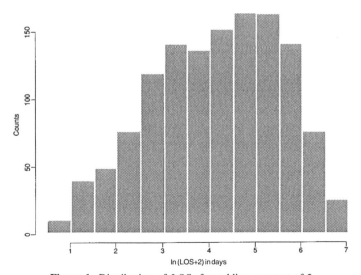

Figure 1. Distribution of LOS after adding constant of 2.

uncensored, $i = 1, \ldots, N$. For any chosen distribution,

$$\mathscr{L}(\boldsymbol{\beta}, \sigma, \alpha) = \prod_{1}^{N} [S_i(t_i)]^{C_i} [f_i(t_i)]^{1-C_i}$$

$$= \prod_{1}^{m} f_i(t_i) \prod_{m+1}^{N} S_i(t_i). \tag{9}$$

The parameters $\boldsymbol{\beta}$, σ and α in the likelihood function index the unknowns in the three distributions introduced earlier, α being necessary only for the generalized gamma.

The proportional hazards estimation method does not use the full likelihood function in (9) but instead uses the partial likelihood function (Cox, 1972). Because β_0 is not estimated, the Cox proportional hazards model cannot be used to make forecasts. It has been shown that the maximum partial likelihood estimate of $\boldsymbol{\beta}$ has the same asymptotic properties as the maximum full likelihood estimate (Fleming and Harrington, 1991).

3.5 Computing

The computer program used for this analysis specifies the generalized gamma distribution in the following manner. The program reparameterizes α in the gamma distribution as $\alpha = \lambda^{-2}$ with $-\infty < \lambda < \infty$. The baseline model then is

$$W \sim \{\lambda^2 \, \mathrm{Gam}\,(\lambda^{-2}, 1)\}^{1/\lambda}. \tag{10}$$

In view of (2),

$$LOS \sim \exp(\mathbf{x}\boldsymbol{\beta})[\lambda^2 \, \mathrm{Gam}\,(\lambda^{-2}, 1)]^{\sigma/\lambda} \tag{11}$$

is the full model specification. Allowing $\lambda < 0$ in this way permits negative powers of LOS also to be fitted, as following a gamma distribution. The Weibull model is $\lambda = 1$, and the lognormal is $\lambda = 0$ [$\alpha = \lambda^{-2} = \infty$ is a limiting case of (11)]. Many individuals in the nursing home data set have tied values of LOS. Breslow's method for handling ties was used in our calculations.

4 RESULTS

4.1 Fitting the Models

In Table 4 we list the estimates of the parameters with their standard errors in parentheses obtained from the SAS program. The ratios of the parameters

Table 4 Censored Survival Regressions for ln(LOS + 2)

	Weibull	Log-normal	Generalized Gamma	Prop. Hazard[a]	Adjusted Prop. Hazard[b]
Intercept	5.777	5.036	4.635	c	c
	(0.149)	(0.155)	(0.173)		
Treatment	0.209	0.153	0.1497	0.0621	0.0964
	(0.0884)	(0.0938)	(0.0933)	(0.0575)	(0.0894)
Age spline	0.00717	0.01099	0.01032	0.00440	0.00684
	(0.00656)	(0.00691)	(0.00691)	(0.00421)	(0.00654)
Male	−0.550	−0.567	−0.519	−0.340	−0.529
	(0.104)	(0.111)	(0.111)	(0.067)	(0.104)
Married	−0.251	−0.216	−0.169	−0.1554	−0.241
	(0.121)	(0.131)	(0.131)	(0.0778)	(0.121)
Health 2	0.041	−0.107	0.154	−0.0342	−0.053
	(0.121)	(0.127)	(0.127)	(0.0780)	(0.121)
Health 4	−0.401	−0.526	−0.556	−0.254	−0.395
	(0.106)	(0.113)	(0.112)	(0.0682)	(0.106)
Health 5	−0.887	−0.959	−0.905	−0.550	−0.855
	(0.148)	(0.161)	(0.162)	(0.0953)	(0.148)
Scale (= σ)	1.5538	1.8059	1.8287	c	c
	(0.0357)	(0.0375)	(0.0376)		
Shape (= λ)	1[d]	0[d]	−0.501	c	c
			(0.0991)		
Log likelihood	−2995.5	−2897.9	−2885.4	−8587.9	—
Number of Observ.	1601	1601	1601	1601	1601
Median *LOS*[e]	180.6	151.9	139.0	c	c

[a] Signs reversed from computer printout to correspond to other models.
[b] Not available in Cox model.
[c] Values are $\hat{\beta} \times 1.554$, where 1.554 equals the scale parameter (σ) for the Weibull model.
[d] Theoretical value, not estimated.
[e] The predicted median length of stay for a 65-year-old unmarried woman with health status 3 in a control nursing home (only the intercept).

to their standard errors, the z-score, are approximately $N(0, 1)$ under the null hypothesis of no effect and can be used to determine statistical significance. Each model follows

$$\ln(LOS + 2) = \beta_0 + \beta_1(treatment) + \beta_2(age\ spline) + \beta_3(male)$$
$$+ \beta_4(married) + \beta_5(health\ 2)$$
$$+ \beta_6(health\ 4) + \beta_7(health\ 5) + \sigma U. \quad (12)$$

Here, LOS = days in the nursing home; *treatment* = 1 if treatment nursing home and 0 if control; *age spline* = min(*age*, 90) − 65; *male* = 1 if male and 0 if female; *married* = 1 if married and 0 otherwise. The health variable is expanded into four categorical variables: *health* 2 = 1 if health status = 2 and 0 otherwise; *health* 3 is the omitted group; *health* 4 = 1 if health status = 4 and 0 otherwise; and, *health* 5 = 1 if health status = 5 and 0 otherwise. See Section 2 for a description of health status.

Table 4 shows that the results are sensitive to the choice of model. For example, the treatment effect is $\hat{\beta}_1 = 0.2093$ with the Weibull model, with the z-score of 2.37 (strongly significant). It is 0.1497 with a z-score of 1.60 for the generalized gamma model (not statistically significant). It is 0.0621 with a z-score of 1.08 (not statistically significant) for the proportional hazards model.

The Weibull model predicts that the distribution of LOS for a married male age 80 (= 15 years above 65), with health status 3 in a treatment nursing home is

$$LOS = \exp(5.777 + 0.00717(15) - 0.550 - 0.251$$
$$+ 0.2093)W^{1.5538} - 2$$
$$= (198.91)W^{1.5538} - 2,$$

with W a unit exponential random variable. The median of W is $\ln(2) = 0.6931$, so the median LOS is predicted by the Weibull model to be 110.5 days.

The lognormal model gives the prediction

$$LOS = \exp(5.036 + 0.01099(15) - 0.567 - 0.216 + 0.153)W^{1.8059} - 2$$
$$= (96.63)W^{1.8059} - 2,$$

where $\ln(W)$ is standard normal. Since W has a median of 1, the median of LOS for the lognormal model is 94.6 days.

The generalized gamma model provides the prediction

$$LOS = \exp(4.635 + 0.01032(15) - 0.519 - 0.169 + 0.1497)W^{1.8287} - 2$$
$$= (70.21)W^{1.8287} - 2,$$

where W now has the distribution given in (10). Substitute $\hat{\lambda} = -0.5008$, and $\hat{\alpha} = \lambda^{-2} = 3.987$ into (10) and use 3.660 as the approximate median of this gamma to give

$$LOS = (70.21)(0.2508\,G)^{(1.8287/-0.5008)} - 2$$
$$= 10,959\,G^{-3.65616} - 2,$$

with G following the Gam(3.987,1) distribution.

The median (LOS) is found by substituting the median of Gam(3.987,1) into the formula above. We approximate the median of Gam(3.987,1) as the median of Gam(4,1) times (3.987/4). Since 2 Gam(α, 1) is the same distribution as $\chi^2(\nu)$, with $\nu = 2\alpha$, 2 Gam(4,1) is $\chi^2(8)$. The median of $\chi^2(8)$ is found in a standard chi-square table to be 7.34412, so the median of G is approximated by $(0.5)(7.34412)(3.987/4) = 3.660$. This gives median$(G) = 3.660$, so median$(LOS) = 94.0$.

The estimated gamma model specifies an inverse relation of LOS to the gamma distribution because $\lambda < 0$. A consequence of this fact is that $E(LOS) = \infty$, clearly impossible. In general, $E^r(LOS)$ is finite for the generalized gamma model with $\lambda < 0$ only when $r < 1/(\sigma|\lambda|)$. Given the estimated values above, $r < 0.7575$ is required for finiteness. Thus, the mean LOS ($r = 1$) does not exist for the distribution estimated here. The example of the 80-year-old male predicts median LOS values of 135.9, 94.6, and 94.0 days, depending on the model choice. Predictions for quantiles other than the median are available in the same way, although some difficulty can occur for small quantiles because the final subtraction of two days can lead to a negative prediction. Table 4 also lists the median LOS for a 65-year-old unmarried woman with health status 3 in a control nursing home (all covariates equal to zero), again showing that predictions depend on the model selected, thereby showing that we must do more to choose among these models. The Cox proportional hazards model cannot be used to make predictions for specific individuals because it does not assume a baseline hazard function.

Among the three parametric models, only the Weibull is a proportional hazards model. It follows from (6) that $\gamma\beta$ in the Weibull model is the vector of regression coefficients being estimated by proportional hazards. Thus, dividing the Cox proportional hazards coefficients by γ, or equivalently by multiplying the scale parameter $\sigma = 1/\gamma = 1.5538$ (for the Weibull) adjusts the Cox model for direct comparisons with the Weibull model; this is done in the final column of Table 4. The standard errors change similarly, leaving the z-scores unaffected. The treatment coefficients are 0.2093 and 0.0964 for the Weibull and proportional hazards models, a substantial difference of more than one standard error.

4.2 Model Checking and Model Choice

A criterion for choosing one model over another is to choose the model with the largest value of the estimated log likelihood, the logarithm of (9) evaluated at the maximum likelihood estimates. The generalized gamma model dominates the lognormal model, which further dominates the Weibull model in this regard. The shape parameter estimate for the generalized gamma is $\hat{\lambda} = -0.5008$, with standard error 0.0991. This value is not close to the theoretical value $\lambda = 0$ for the lognormal, and is even further from $\lambda = 1$ for the Weibull model. This information supports the generalized gamma as the preferred distribution. Other evidence for this conclusion is considered below. However, this fit is preferred *only* within the range of the observed data ($LOS < 3$ years), and the gamma will be seen to overpredict length of stay for longer stays, while the lognormal is somewhat better in that way.

Estimates like those of Table 4 were obtained with similar results for other values of c, including $c = 0.01$, 1, and 3, each time making the generalized gamma the preferred distribution. The value of the log-likelihood increases for each of these distributions, with increasing c through a large range. However, this is not indicative of better choices for c because the variable being predicted changes with c. The magnitude and significance of *treatment* and of Medicaid diminishes dramatically as c increases for the generalized gamma, but the significance of *treatment* actually increases with c for the lognormal model. The Cox proportional hazards model, however, is invariant to the value of c. That is, the regression estimates for the Cox model do not change for any monotone transformation of the dependent variable.

Figure 2 helps further to visualize and to understand the fit of these models. The discrete hazard functions are plotted for each of four homogeneous subsets of the data, all with $70 \leq age \leq 90$ (the median age is 83 years), and separately for male–female and for two grouped health levels. The horizontal axis is $\ln(LOS + 2)$, and this logarithm scale distorts visual perceptions. For example, one month is $\ln(30 + 2)$, at the middle of the graph, one year is at $\ln(365 + 2)$, and three years is at $\ln(1095 + 2)$. Two-thirds of the time scale is compressed by the logarithmic transformation into the last one-sixth of the horizontal axis.

The computations in Figure 1 break each data set into 13 bins, equally spaced on the logarithmic scale. The empirical hazard function for each interval i is calculated as

$$\text{hazard}_i = \frac{\text{number who leave in interval } i}{\text{person-days observed in interval } i}, \qquad (13)$$

where

$$\begin{aligned}
\text{person-days}_i = \ & (\text{number not censored or discharged}) \times (\text{days in interval } i) \\
& + (\text{number censored}) \\
& \times (\text{average number of days until censoring}) \\
& + (\text{number discharged}) \\
& \times (\text{average number of days until discharge}). \qquad (14)
\end{aligned}$$

The denominator of (13) is defined more explicitly in (14). Note that people who are censored or discharged are treated similarly in the denominator—the number of days between the beginning of the interval and the time of censoring or discharge is summed for all those people.

An example of the use of formula (13) is given for one of the graphs in Figure 2, that of women with health status 4 or 5. The sixth interval is from day 21 to day 33. At the beginning of the sixth interval there were 317 residents,

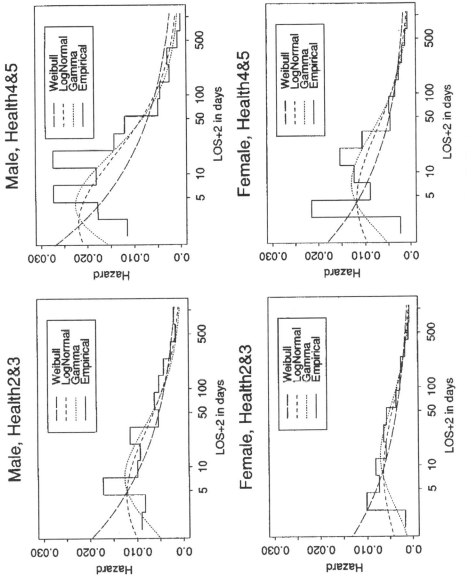

Figure 2. Empirical hazard function plotted against three distributions.

243

of whom 41 were discharged, 0 were censored, and 276 remained at the end of the interval. The numerator is therefore 41. The denominator is the sum of $276 \times 13 = 3588$ days and $41 \times (6.463) = 265$ days, where 6.463 is the average number of days observed from the beginning of the interval until discharge. This gives an empirical hazard for the sixth interval of $41/(3588 + 265) = 0.0106$ discharge per day, or about 1% per day. The empirical hazard is calculated for other intervals in an analogous way. Note that all empirical hazard functions in Figure 2 diminish strongly after a couple of weeks. A patient not leaving within two weeks has a rapidly, and monotonically, diminishing chance of leaving in each successive week.

The theoretical hazard functions from the three models of Table 4 are plotted in Figure 2, together with the discrete hazard estimates, for each of the four cases. All four theoretical curves specify the age as 80 years with health status and gender specified for each graph. The hazard functions follow formula (5) with constants from Table 4. The generalized gamma appears to give the best fit in these plots, especially in the left two-thirds (first three months) of Figure 2.

Differences in Figure 2 are harder to see in the rightmost portion because relative heights are low, compressing years 1 to 3 together. However, these long stays are the most policy-relevant portions, long stays being most costly. We therefore use a different plot to emphasize the fit for longer stays.

The *weighted hazard* plot, introduced in Figure 3, is especially useful for plots that decline on a logarithmic scale. It is designed as a visual aid to emphasize better the right-hand side of the hazard function. For the data under consideration, $h(t)$ declines at a certain rate, but the weighted hazard function $h^*(t) = t^p h(t)$, $p = \frac{2}{3}$, is larger for large t than for smaller t, (see Figure 3). In other applications, a different power of t might be used to weight the hazard function, but $p = \frac{2}{3}$ was chosen, after experimentation, as a good value for this example. Figure 3 graphs $h^*(t)$ for the three fitted distributions together. Also graphed is an *empirical weighted hazard*, obtained by multiplying the empirical hazard (13) in each interval by t^p. The graphs of Figure 3 show that the generalized gamma fits better than the other two models for longer lengths of stay, as well as for shorter lengths, as seen in Figure 2.

The ratio of empirical hazards in Figure 2 can be used as a guide to the validity of the proportional hazards assumption. Figure 4 shows the empirical ratio of these two empirical hazard functions. For example, the ratio of the hazard for (*male, health* 4–5) to (*female, health* 4–5) moves from high to low as times increases, violating the proportional hazards assumption. The fact that the empirical ratio is not nearly constant is visual evidence of the failure of the proportional hazards model for these data. This nonconstancy sheds doubt on the Cox model and also on the Weibull model for this case. Although not attempted here, formal tests of the proportional hazards hypothesis can be based on time-dependent covariate methods (Cox and Oakes, 1990). Furthermore, both the lognormal and generalized gamma models assume implicitly that the ratio of

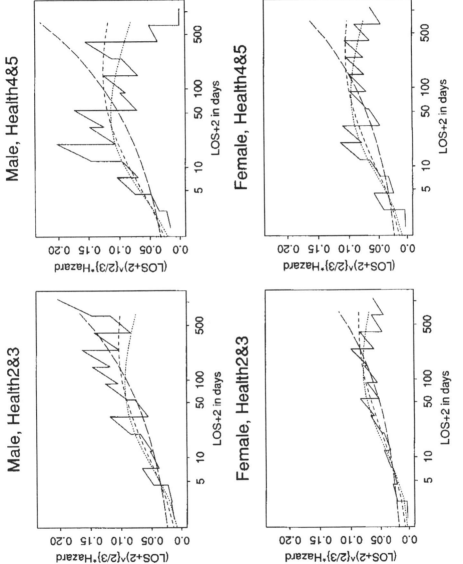

Figure 3. Empirical weighted hazard function plotted against three distributions.

245

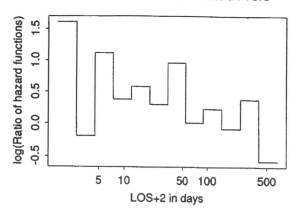

Figure 4. Ratio of empirical hazard functions, to check proportional hazard assumption.

hazards is not constant but shrinks asymptotically to 1. This is consistent with the results in Figure 4.

This section has provided evidence favoring the generalized gamma model among the three given. The generalized gamma for these data has the following advantages:

1. It has the largest log likelihood.
2. The estimated value $\hat{\lambda} = -0.5008$ (with standard error 0.0991) is not close to $\lambda = 0$ for the lognormal and it is very far from $\lambda = 1$ for the Weibull model.
3. It fits both the empirical hazard function and the empirical weighted hazard function best. Those graphs suggest that the lognormal and Weibull models tend to overstate the probability of exit between one and three years.
4. The empirical hazard ratios vary with time, contrary to the proportion hazard assumption in the Weibull and proportional hazard models.

Based on this evidence, we adopt the generalized gamma model as the best of the four models considered for the nursing home data, in the range of the observations. However, no data are available for the period exceeding three years, and the true hazard curve, unlike any of those considered, must rise eventually to reflect human lifespan limitations.

4.3 Other Results

The policy-relevant variable *treatment* has an unexpected sign, although it is not statistically significant in the gamma model. The median length of stay for a 65-year-old unmarried woman is 141.0 days in a control nursing home, compared to 163.8 days in a treatment nursing home, according to the gamma model. Only the Weibull model estimates a statistically significant difference. These results support the belief that the experiment did not achieve one of its stated goals, that of reducing the length of stay.

The other covariates generally have their expected signs and are statistically significant. Length of stay increases with age linearly until age 90. Further increases in age do not significantly affect the length of stay, although the data are limited in that range. Men stay for a shorter time than women, probably because men tend to be admitted in a worse state of health, and because they are more likely than women to have a spouse at home to serve as an alternative caregiver. A 65-year-old unmarried woman has a median length of stay of 141.0 days in a control nursing home compared to only 83.9 days for a man, according to the gamma model. Future work must distinguish whether men are more likely to be discharged as a result of death, or to return home. As with the gender effect, the sign of the marital status effect is negative, although it is not significant in the gamma model. Health status has a clear effect on the hazard. The hazard decreases as health worsens, implying that the relatively healthy people are discharged home, while those who are sicker stay longer and die in the nursing home.

5 CONCLUSIONS

This chapter provides a case study of applying duration (survival) analysis to nursing home data. The generalized gamma regression model fits the data best, as judged by formal tests and graphical techniques, when compared to the Weibull, lognormal, and Cox proportional hazard models. The median length of stay is close to five months; longer if the resident is older, female, in a treatment nursing home, or in better health.

The effect of the experimental incentives in the treatment nursing homes increases the length of stay, relative to control nursing homes, but this is not a statistically significant difference. Future work with these data must separate further the reasons for leaving the nursing home into positive outcomes, such as going home, and into negative outcomes, such as dying or hospitalization.

ACKNOWLEDGMENTS

We are grateful to Cindy Christiansen, Sarah Like, Martin McIntosh, and Carolyn H. Norton for their comments and help. This research was supported by the Agency for Health Care Policy Research, grant HS-07306-01.

SOFTWARE NOTES AND REFERENCES

The maximum likelihood model in (9) was estimated using SAS (Statistical Analysis System) software and its LIFEREG procedures for the Weibull, lognormal, and generalized gamma distributions. The Cox model was also estimated using SAS software, using the PHREG procedure.

SAS Institute, Inc. (1985). The LIFEREG procedure, in *SAS User's Guide: Statistics.*, Cary, N.C.: SAS Institute.

SAS Institute, Inc. (1990). The PHREG procedure, in *SAS User's Guide: Statistics.* Cary, N.C.: SAS Institute.

QUESTIONS AND PROBLEMS

1. Estimate the generalized gamma model using interactions between *treatment* and the four health variables. This introduces three new regression coefficients. Show that the effect of *treatment* is diminished when the interactions are included. Subtract the mean of the variables before multiplying them to form the interaction terms.

2. Evaluate the three survival functions at *LOS* equals zero (with c equal to 2), using the results in Table 4. Do this for married men, age 82, in *treatment* nursing homes, in the health status 4. Compare the prediction with the actual number of residents who remain in the nursing home until the first day.

3. The Weibull and lognormal models are both special cases of the generalized gamma model. Use the results in Table 4 to test whether the shape parameter λ is equal to either 0 or 1. Then do a chi-square test of this difference using the difference of log likelihoods. Show that the results are comparable.

4. Verify that the following two models yield exactly the same regression coefficients. First, use ordinary least squares to regress $\log(LOS+2)$ on the treatment, age, male, married, and health variables, while *ignoring* the censoring variable. Second, use maximum likelihood to estimate the lognormal model, but treat all variables as uncensored.

5. Split the data set into two groups, one for married people and the other for unmarried people. Estimate the generalized gamma model for each group. Compare the coefficients and shape parameters for these two groups and with the full-sample results listed in Table 4.

CHAPTER 13

Analysis of Attitudes toward Workplace Smoking Restrictions

Shelley Bull

1 MOTIVATION AND BACKGROUND

This chapter arises from a health promotion survey in the area of prevention of exposure to environmental tobacco smoke. Two population-based surveys of a large metropolitan area were conducted to determine the impact of a municipal bylaw regulating smoking in the workplace: one immediately before implementation and a second, eight to nine months later. The primary analysis considered associations between implementation of the bylaw and a variety of measures of attitudes, knowledge, and behavior. In this chapter we describe a secondary analysis that focused in greater depth on one measure of attitudes toward restrictions in the workplace and included individual characteristics as covariates. It provides a detailed description of the general approach that was used in the primary analysis and illustrates the usefulness of polychotomous logistic regression in modeling health survey data with categorical outcomes.

Background
A bylaw regulating smoking in all workplaces in the city of Toronto was implemented in March 1988. The city of Toronto itself is surrounded by five jurisdictions that were not covered by the bylaw. However, many residents of these areas were personally affected by the bylaw because their workplaces were in the city. The method used to evaluate the workplace bylaw was a population telephone survey targeting adult residents (aged 18 years and older) of metropolitan Toronto, including the city of Toronto and the other five jurisdictions. It therefore included those who worked in the city of Toronto, as well as those working outside the city of Toronto in other jurisdictions and those not working outside the home. The latter two groups served as natural control

Case Studies in Biometry, Edited by Nicholas Lange, Louise Ryan, Lynne Billard, David Brillinger, Loveday Conquest, and Joel Greenhouse.
ISBN 0-471-58885-7 © 1994 John Wiley & Sons, Inc.

groups for comparison to the city workers in that they were expected to exhibit similar general societal changes occurring in the perceptions of and responses to environmental tobacco smoke. They differed, however, in having no direct personal experience with the bylaw in their own place of work. Two population surveys were conducted to determine the impact of the legislation on knowledge, attitudes, and behavior: one in January–February 1988, immediately before the bylaw came into effect, and a second, eight to nine months after its implementation (November–December 1988).

Sampling was carried out independently for each survey. The sample survey design was simple random sampling of households by random-digit dialing, with one respondent per household selected for a telephone interview (i.e., a two-stage design). A random sample of telephone numbers was generated from a list of working three-digit exchanges in metropolitan Toronto. At least six callbacks were made at prespecified times during the day, in the evening, and on weekends, before a number was classified as unanswered. Once an eligible household was reached, a respondent was selected using the most recent birthday method (O'Rourke and Blair, 1983). Responses to a pretested interview schedule were collected during a 25- to 30-minute interview, using a computer-assisted telephone interviewing (CATI) system. In the pre-bylaw survey, 1543 respondents completed the interview, and in the post-bylaw survey, 1430 completed the interview. Estimated response rates were 68.4 and 62.5%, respectively.

The primary analysis evaluating the impact of the bylaw on measures of knowledge found that larger changes occurred in city of Toronto workers in awareness of the bylaw's existence, its requirements, and implementation and enforcement provisions than in either of the other two groups (Pederson et al., 1993). After implementation, city of Toronto workers reported more frequently than other workers that there had been changes in workplace smoking policy and that they were satisfied with existing smoking policies. There were changes in some but not all measures of attitudes toward restrictions on smoking in the workplace among all three groups. Although there were some changes in patterns of smoking behavior in the workplace among city of Toronto workers, there was no change in the overall prevalence of smoking (Pederson et al., 1993).

This case study focuses on one measure of attitudes toward restrictions in the workplace in which respondents were asked: Do you think smoking ... should *not be permitted* at all?, should be *permitted in restricted* areas?, or should *not be restricted* at all? This item was one of a series asking about support for restrictions in a variety of locations, including airplanes, hospitals, movie theaters, and restaurants (Pederson et al., 1993). It was hypothesized a priori that changes in attitudes toward restrictions on smoking in the workplace associated with implementation of the bylaw in the city of Toronto would be greater among workers in workplaces within the city than among workers outside the city, and/or greater than among those not working outside the home: that is, that the impact of the bylaw would depend on place of work. The objectives of the analysis were to test this hypothesis, to control for the influence of other potential determinants of attitude, to estimate the magnitude of changes in attitude, and to estimate and describe the associations between attitude and characteristics of the respondents.

2 DATA

The primary outcome of interest, attitude toward restrictions on smoking in the workplace, had three possible responses: preference for not permitted at all (prohibited), permitted in restricted areas only (restricted), or not restricted at all (unrestricted). The number of responses of "don't know" or "refused" was quite small in both the pre- and post-implementation surveys (1 and 3%, respectively), and these were therefore eliminated. The category of preference for restricted smoking, which had a frequency of 68%, was chosen as the reference category for the logistic model, primarily for ease of interpretation, although it was also advantageous to use the largest category as the reference.

Each observation in the survey data set was assigned a weight according to the respondent's probability of selection from the household and according to the frequency of the respondent's age–sex category relative to the 1986 census distribution for metropolitan Toronto. [See Cox and Cohen (1985, Chapter 7) concerning selection and post-stratification weighting.] This procedure ensured that the two independent surveys had the same age–sex distribution. As a consequence, weighted frequencies include fractional numbers of respondents.

There were three bylaw-related determinants of attitudes that were relevant to the hypothesis of interest: *time of survey* (pre- versus postimplementation), *place of work* (in the city of Toronto, outside the city, not outside the home), and *place of residence* (city of Toronto versus other metropolitan Toronto jurisdictions). For *smoking status*, which has been associated with attitudes previously (Pederson et al., 1987), each respondent was categorized as a current smoker, a smoker who had recently quit (within 6 months), a former smoker of short duration (6 to 12 months since quitting), a former smoker of long duration (over 12 months), or a nonsmoker who had never smoked regularly. The breakpoint at 12 months in duration of quitting was chosen to capture a window around the time of bylaw implementation for the postimplementation respondents, and the 6-month breakpoint was used to distinguish those who had not met the usual criterion for successful cessation (Schwartz, 1987). Other known determinants of attitudes (Pederson et al., 1989) included a score of the respondent's *knowledge* of the health effects of environmental tobacco smoke that combined six items concerning eye irritation, lung cancer, chest problems in children, heart attack, irritability or annoyance, and headaches; and the sociodemographic characteristics *sex*, *age*, and *level of education*.

A representative display of the data set, along with variable definitions and coding, is included in Table 1. The weighted frequency distributions of the

Table 1 Display of Six Representative Observations from the Data Set of 2855 Observations[a]

ID No.	y	w	x_1	x_2	x_3	z_1	z_2	z_3	z_4	z_5	z_6	z_7	z_8	z_9
10314	0	0.899	0	0	1	0	1	0	0	0	0	0	2.5	0
10338	2	1.502	0	0	0	1	0	0	1	1	8	1	−2.4	1
14563	2	1.976	0	0	1	0	0	1	0	0	6	1	1.9	1
14595	1	0.395	0	0	0	1	0	0	0	0	7	0	−2.2	0
22102	2	0.458	1	1	0	1	1	0	0	0	10	0	−1.5	1
29447	1	0.458	1	0	0	0	1	0	0	0	10	0	−1.2	1

[a]Definition and coding of variables in the data set:

Outcome

Smoking in the workplace should be:	y	(prohibited = 1, restricted = 2, unrestricted = 0)
Sampling weight	w	(ranges from 0.305 to 4.494)

Bylaw-related covariates

Time of survey	x_1	(post = 1, pre = 0)
Place of work	x_2	(outside city of Toronto = 1, otherwise = 0)
	x_3	(not outside the home = 1, otherwise = 0)
Place of residence	z_1	(city of Toronto = 1, other metropolitan Toronto = 0)

Smoking-related covariates

Smoking status	z_2	(current smoker = 1, never smoked or quit = 0)
	z_3	(quit <= 6 months ago = 1, otherwise = 0)
	z_4	(quit > 6 months ago = 1, otherwise = 0)
	z_5	(quit 6–12 months = 1, otherwise = 0)
Knowledge of health effects of environmental tobacco smoke	z_6	(score, ranges from 0 to 12)

Sociodemographic covariates

Sex of respondent	z_7	(male = 1, female = 0)
Age of respondent	z_8	[(age in years − 50)/10]
Level of education	z_9	(elementary = −2, some high school = −1, high or trade school = 0, college or some university = 1, university degree = 2)

outcome for population subgroups defined by place of work, time of survey, and smoking status were obtained by summing the sampling weights for all the respondents in that subgroup (Table 2). The first row of the table indicates that there were 76.9 respondents working in the city of Toronto in the pre-bylaw survey who had never been a regular smoker and who supported prohibition of smoking in the workplace. The corresponding percentage is a row percentage, indicating that 35% preferred that smoking be prohibited rather than restricted or unrestricted. One feature to be noted concerns the subgroups of former smokers: the data tend to be sparse, particularly for the third outcome category, and some subgroups are empty.

Table 2   Weighted Frequencies for Population Subgroups

Place of Work	Time of Survey	Smoking Status	Attitude toward Smoking in the Workplace					
			Prohibited		Restricted		Unrestricted	
			n	$\%$	n	$\%$	n	$\%$
City of Toronto	Pre	Never smoked	76.9	35	138.1	63	3.9	2
		Quit >12 months	24.4	39	37.0	59	1.0	2
		Quit 6–12 months	0	0	20.5	97	0.6	3
		Quit < = 6 months	6.7	24	20.0	70	1.8	6
		Current smoker	15.7	11	104.6	76	18.0	13
		Total (n = 469.3)	123.7	26	320.3	68	25.3	6
	Post	Never smoked	76.0	35	135.8	62	5.5	3
		Quit >12 months	27.0	37	45.7	63	0	0
		Quit 6–12 months	4.4	37	6.6	55	0.9	8
		Quit < = 6 months	4.4	26	10.0	59	2.6	15
		Current smoker	15.9	13	93.2	77	12.7	10
		Total (n = 440.6)	127.7	29	291.3	66	21.6	5
Outside the city of Toronto	Pre	Never smoked	75.4	29	179.3	68	7.9	3
		Quit >12 months	19.3	24	58.2	74	1.6	2
		Quit 6–12 months	3.2	10	30.0	90	0	0
		Quit < = 6 months	3.8	15	20.3	82	0.8	3
		Current smoker	22.1	12	138.6	72	31.6	16
		Total (n = 592.1)	123.8	21	426.4	72	41.9	7
	Post	Never smoked	82.0	32	167.6	66	3.7	2
		Quit >12 months	22.7	26	62.8	73	0.9	1
		Quit 6–12 months	4.2	61	1.8	27	0.8	12
		Quit < = 6 months	3.7	27	10.1	73	0	0
		Current smoker	15.3	9	129.4	76	25.1	15
		Total (n = 530.0)	127.8	24	371.7	70	30.5	6
Not outside the home	Pre	Never smoked	72.5	34	137.7	64	4.3	2
		Quit >12 months	31.1	35	53.0	59	5.3	6
		Quit 6–12 months	4.4	30	10.6	70	0	0
		Quit < = 6 months	6.6	37	11.3	63	0	0
		Current smoker	13.4	14	76.9	80	6.4	6
		Total (n = 433.5)	128.1	29	289.5	67	15.9	4
	Post	Never smoked	81.8	39	127.7	60	2.1	1
		Quit >12 months	23.9	24	70.1	71	4.8	5
		Quit 6–12 months	1.6	32	3.4	68	0	0
		Quit < = 6 months	3.0	43	3.9	57	0	0
		Current smoker	12.8	17	59.3	77	4.8	6
		Total (n = 399.2)	123.1	31	264.5	66	11.6	3

3   METHODS AND MODELS

3.1   Polychotomous Logistic Regression

The polychotomous logistic regression model, first described by Cox (1966) and by Mantel (1966), has been applied in a variety of contexts, including cohort and case–control studies (Dyer et al., 1980; Raynor et al., 1981; Dubin and Pasternack, 1986), in problems in differential diagnosis and prediction (Wijesinha et al., 1983; Marshall and Chisolm, 1985; Albert and Harris, 1987), and in the analysis of survey data (Bloom et al., 1978; Pederson et al., 1989; Rao et al., 1989). Important theoretical developments concerning application under different sampling models were provided by Anderson (1972), Prentice and Pyke (1979), Scott and Wild (1986), Roberts et al. (1987), and Morel (1989). Albert and Lesaffre (1986) have reviewed relevant work, and several recent textbooks also include discussion of the model (Albert and Harris, 1987, Section 5.5; Hosmer and Lemeshow, 1989, Chapter 8; McCullagh and Nelder, 1989, Sections 5.2, 6.4, 7.5; Agresti, 1990, Section 9.2).

Definition of the Model
Assume that the categorical outcome of interest, Y, is a multinomial variable with categories $j = 0, \ldots, J$, and that $\mathbf{x}$ is a $1 \times p$ vector of covariates. The polychotomous logistic model specifies a conditional probability of the outcome given $\mathbf{x}$ to be of the logistic form

$$p_j(\mathbf{x}) = \Pr(\text{outcome falls in } j\text{th category} \mid \mathbf{x})$$

$$= \frac{\exp(\beta_{j0} + \mathbf{x}\boldsymbol{\beta}_j)}{1 + \sum_{k=1}^{J} \exp(\beta_{k0} + \mathbf{x}\boldsymbol{\beta}_k)} \quad \text{for} \quad j = 1, \ldots, J,$$

and

$$p_0 = 1 - \sum_{k=1}^{J} p_k.$$

For each category j there is a regression function, and a corresponding $(p + 1) \times 1$ vector $(\beta_{j0}\boldsymbol{\beta}_j^{\mathrm{T}})$ of regression parameters that formulates the log odds of response in category j, relative to category 0, as a linear function of the parameters:

$$\ln \frac{p_j(\mathbf{x})}{p_0(\mathbf{x})} = \beta_{j0} + \mathbf{x}\boldsymbol{\beta}_j.$$

The outcome $j = 0$ is the baseline category to which the other categories are compared. This choice is arbitrary except on substantive grounds, for example, when there is a natural baseline category such as survival in a mortality study or case status in a case–control study with multiple control groups, or for ease of interpretation.

As in dichotomous logistic regression, the regression parameter β_{js} can be interpreted as a log odds ratio, and $\exp(\beta_{js})$ as an odds ratio. [See Hosmer and Lemeshow (1989, Chapter 3 and Section 8.1.2) for further discussion of the interpretation of logistic regression parameters.] The logistic regression model is a multiplicative model in the sense that the effect of changing a covariate value from $x_s = c$ to $x_s = d$ is to multiply the odds of response by $[\exp(\beta_{js})]^{d-c}$. Similarly, the odds ratio for an individual with $x_1 = 1$ and $x_2 = 1$ relative to an individual with $x_1 = 0$ and $x_2 = 0$ is $[\exp(\beta_{j1})] \cdot [\exp(\beta_{j2})]$. Incorporation of a cross-product term such as $x_1 \cdot x_2$ into the regression in order to model interaction is thus examining interaction on the multiplicative scale.

Estimation and Inference

Let $\mathbf{Y}_i = (Y_{i0}, \ldots, Y_{iJ})$ represent the multinomial outcome for individual i, where $Y_{ij} = 1$ if the jth category is chosen and 0 otherwise. The maximum likelihood estimates (MLEs), $\hat{\boldsymbol{\beta}}_j$ and $\hat{\beta}_{j0}$, of the slope and intercept parameters are obtained by maximizing the likelihood for the observations $(\mathbf{Y}_i, \mathbf{x}_i), i = 1, \ldots, n$, based on the probabilities $p_{ij} = p_j(\mathbf{x}_i) = \Pr(\mathbf{Y}_i = j | \mathbf{x}_i)$. The log-likelihood can be expressed as

$$
l(\boldsymbol{\beta}) = \sum_{i=1}^{n} \sum_{j=0}^{J} w_i Y_{ij} \ln(p_{ij})
$$

$$
= \sum_{j=1}^{J} \left[\left(\sum_{i=1}^{n} w_i Y_{ij} \right) \beta_{j0} + \left(\sum_{i=1}^{n} w_i Y_{ij} \mathbf{x}_i \right) \boldsymbol{\beta}_j \right]
$$

$$
- \sum_{i=1}^{n} w_i \ln \left[1 + \sum_{k=1}^{J} \exp(\beta_{k0} + \mathbf{x}_i \boldsymbol{\beta}_k) \right], \tag{1}
$$

where w_i is an individual observation weight. Weights are useful in the analysis of sample survey data in which observations have been selected with unequal probabilities or in the analysis of data sets in which identical observations have been aggregated and summarized with a frequency weight.

The MLEs are the solution to the simultaneous score equations, $\mathbf{S}_j(\boldsymbol{\beta}) = \mathbf{0}$, found by taking the first partial derivatives of the log-likelihood with respect to the regression parameter vectors:

$$\mathbf{S}_j(\boldsymbol{\beta}) = \sum_{i=1}^{n} w_i(Y_{ij} - p_{ij})(1, \mathbf{x}_i)^{\mathrm{T}}, \qquad j = 1, \ldots, J. \tag{2}$$

The matrix of second partial derivatives, $\mathbf{H}(\boldsymbol{\beta})$, of dimension $J(p+1)$, has matrix elements

$$\mathbf{H}_{jk}(\boldsymbol{\beta}) = -\sum_{i=1}^{n} w_i v_{ijk}(1, \mathbf{x}_i)^{\mathrm{T}}(1, \mathbf{x}_i), \qquad j, k = 1, \ldots, J, \tag{3}$$

where v_{ijk} is $p_{ij}(1 - p_{ij})$ when $j = k$ and $-p_{ij}p_{ik}$, otherwise. The Fisher information matrix $\mathbf{I}(\boldsymbol{\beta})$ is the expectation of $-\mathbf{H}(\boldsymbol{\beta})$. A quadratic approximation to the log-likelihood is therefore

$$l(\boldsymbol{\beta}) = l(\hat{\boldsymbol{\beta}}) + \frac{(\boldsymbol{\beta} - \hat{\boldsymbol{\beta}})^{\mathrm{T}}\mathbf{H}(\hat{\boldsymbol{\beta}})(\boldsymbol{\beta} - \hat{\boldsymbol{\beta}})}{2} \tag{4}$$

which ignores higher-order terms in the Taylor series expansion of the log-likelihood around the MLE vector $\hat{\boldsymbol{\beta}}$.

In the asymptotic case (i.e., as n goes to infinity), the quadratic approximation to the log-likelihood is exact. When the model is specified correctly, the MLEs are unbiased and have a multivariate normal distribution with covariance matrix given by the inverse of the Fisher information matrix. The estimated variance–covariance matrix $\mathrm{Var}(\hat{\boldsymbol{\beta}})$ is usually obtained by inverting the observed information matrix evaluated at the MLEs: that is, $\mathrm{Var}(\hat{\boldsymbol{\beta}}) = [-\mathbf{H}(\hat{\boldsymbol{\beta}})]^{-1}$.

In the finite sample case, however, the log-likelihood may be asymmetric, particularly when one or more of the MLEs is large in absolute value, and the quadratic approximation may be inadequate. Furthermore, the estimates tend to overestimate the magnitude of the parameters and are only approximately normally distributed, sometimes with a skewed distribution (Cox and Snell, 1968; Jennings, 1986). Consequently, asymptotic confidence intervals may be inaccurate. In certain situations (e.g., when no responses are observed in a category for certain subgroups defined by the covariates), the estimates may not exist; this will be exhibited in lack of convergence in the maximum likelihood iterative process or in one or more estimates going to infinity. This problem, also referred to as complete and partial separation of populations, has been considered by several authors (Albert and Anderson, 1984; Santner and Duffy, 1986; Lesaffre and Albert, 1989a).

Testing of hypotheses concerning the regression parameters can include tests of a single parameter, tests involving several parameters from the same regression, and joint tests involving parameters from different regressions. In polychotomous logistic regression, tests for the contribution of one or more parameters from the same regression are usually conducted with a large sample Wald test, with test statistic

$$Q_W = \hat{\boldsymbol{\beta}}_B^T [\text{Var}(\hat{\boldsymbol{\beta}}_B)]^{-1} \hat{\boldsymbol{\beta}}_B, \tag{5}$$

where $\text{Var}(\hat{\boldsymbol{\beta}}_B)$ is the estimated covariance submatrix for the relevant parameters. This statistic is approximately distributed as a χ^2 random variable with q degrees of freedom under the null hypothesis that the q-dimensional vector $\boldsymbol{\beta}_B = \mathbf{0}$. When there is a single parameter β_{js} of interest, $Q_W = [\hat{\beta}_{js}/se(\hat{\beta}_{js})]^2$. More generally, linear contrasts of parameters can be used to test null hypotheses of the form $\mathbf{C}\boldsymbol{\beta}_B = \mathbf{0}$, where $\mathbf{C}$ is a matrix of contrasts. The Wald test statistic is then

$$Q_W = (\mathbf{C}\hat{\boldsymbol{\beta}}_B)^T [\mathbf{C}\text{Var}(\hat{\boldsymbol{\beta}}_B)\mathbf{C}^T]^{-1} \mathbf{C}\hat{\boldsymbol{\beta}}_B. \tag{6}$$

Testing of parameters from different regressions can also be performed with Wald tests, but it is often desirable to use a likelihood ratio test to assess the effect of excluding one or more variables on the remaining parameter estimates and because it may have better distributional properties for small samples (Cox and Snell, 1989). This requires estimating parameters in models both with $(\hat{\boldsymbol{\beta}}_A, \hat{\boldsymbol{\beta}}_B)$ and without $(\hat{\boldsymbol{\beta}}_A^*)$ the parameters of interest. The likelihood ratio test statistic,

$$Q_R = -2[l(\hat{\boldsymbol{\beta}}_A^*, \boldsymbol{\beta}_B = \mathbf{0}) - l(\hat{\boldsymbol{\beta}}_A, \hat{\boldsymbol{\beta}}_B)], \tag{7}$$

is approximately distributed as a χ^2 random variable with q degrees of freedom under the null hypothesis that the q-dimensional vector $\boldsymbol{\beta}_B = \mathbf{0}$. Specific examples of Wald and likelihood ratio tests are described in Section 3.2.

Model Assessment
Several different approaches have been proposed to assess the goodness-of-fit of an estimated model, including residual analysis, influence and leverage statistics and other regression diagnostic techniques, and omnibus goodness-of-fit tests (Pregibon, 1981; Lesaffre and Albert, 1989b; Hosmer and Lemeshow, 1989, Section 8.1.4; Hosmer et al., 1991). The latter approach, proposed by Hosmer and Lemeshow (1980) for dichotomous logistic regression, provides a single summary statistic and is appropriate when it is not important to identify deviations from fit for a small number of individual observations. An extension for polychotomous regression can be obtained by calculating the Pearson chi-squared statistic Q_H from the $(J + 1) \times G$ table of observed (o_{jg}) and expected (e_{jg}) probabilities as follows:

$$Q_{\rm H} = \sum_{g=1}^{G} \sum_{j=0}^{J} \frac{(o_{jg} - e_{jg})^2}{e_{jg}}, \tag{8}$$

where

$$o_{jg} = \sum_{i=1}^{n_g} w_i Y_{ij} \quad \text{and} \quad e_{jg} = \sum_{i=1}^{n_g} w_i \hat{p}_{ij}$$

and n_g is the number of observations (unweighted) in group $g, g = 1, \ldots, G$. The estimated probabilities $\hat{p}_{ij}$ are calculated as

$$\hat{p}_{ij} = \frac{\exp(\hat{\beta}_{j0} + \mathbf{x}_i \hat{\boldsymbol{\beta}}_j)}{1 + \sum_{k=1}^{J} \exp(\hat{\beta}_{k0} + \mathbf{x}_i \hat{\boldsymbol{\beta}}_k)} \quad \text{for} \quad j = 1, \ldots, J \tag{9}$$

and

$$\hat{p}_{i0} = 1 - \sum_{k=1}^{J} \hat{p}_{ik}.$$

The groups of size n_g can be determined in several ways. Equally sized groups can be defined by percentiles of one of the $J + 1$ estimated probabilities, giving random cutpoints on the probability scale. The distributional properties of this extension, or of a statistic involving weights, have not been investigated, although results for the dichotomous case suggest that $Q_{\rm H}$ may be approximately chi-squared with $(JG - 2)$ degrees of freedom (Hosmer and Lemeshow, 1980; Korn et al., 1986; Hosmer et al., 1988). Another approach, suggested by the work of Shillington (1978) and Tsiatis (1980), is to define groups of random size by fixed levels of the covariates, for example, by 10-year age groups. The appropriate chi-squared distribution for $Q_{\rm H}$ in this case, however, is not clear. Omnibus goodness-of-fit measures do not appear to have been well evaluated for polychotomous regression, but in combination with comparisons of observed and expected proportions, they do serve as a general indicator for regions where the model is not performing well.

3.2 Application: Evaluation of Determinants of Attitudes toward Workplace Restrictions

Logistic regression has several features that were desirable in analysis of the categorical attitude data. It models the logit of the outcome probability, the log odds, which has an unrestricted range, rather than the probability itself, which can range from zero to 1; this was important in the application because the distribution of attitudes was such that the regression model was required to model probabilities over most of the range from zero to 1. The hypothesis concerning interaction could be assessed in a straightforward manner by examination of the regression coefficients for cross-product terms and both categorical and continuous determinants could be included in the regression model. The polychotomous extension of the usual dichotomous outcome model does not require any assumptions about ordering in the categories. This allowed for the possibility that implementation of the bylaw was associated with polarization of attitudes into the categories of *prohibited* and *unrestricted*, or with centralization into the *restricted areas* category.

Specification, Estimation, and Inference
The polychotomous model was specified with two regression equations. The *first* equation modeled the log odds of the probability of preference for *prohibition* of smoking in the workplace as a function of the determinants of interest, comparing respondents who expressed preference for *prohibition* of smoking to those who expressed preference for smoking in *restricted* areas only. The *second* equation modeled the log odds of the probability of preference for *unrestricted* smoking in the workplace, comparing respondents who preferred that smoking be *unrestricted* to those who expressed preference for *restricted* areas. In the primary analysis, the first model of interest included an indicator variable for time of survey (x_1), two indicators for place of work (x_2, x_3), and their interactions. A second model excluded the interactions. No adjustments were made for the smoking-related and sociodemographic characteristics of the respondents. The models were specified as

$$\text{U1:} \quad \ln\left(\frac{p_j}{p_0}\right) = \beta_{j0} + x_1\beta_{j1} + x_2\beta_{j2} + x_3\beta_{j3}$$
$$+ (x_1 \cdot x_2)\beta_{j4} + (x_1 \cdot x_3)\beta_{j5}$$

and

$$\text{U2:} \quad \ln\left(\frac{p_j}{p_0}\right) = \beta_{j0} + x_1\beta_{j1} + x_2\beta_{j2} + x_3\beta_{j3}$$

for $j = 1, 2$. The coding for the indicators defined in Table 1 is such that the intercept parameter β_{j0} is interpreted in both models as the log odds of response in pre-bylaw city workers. In model U1, the parameter β_{j1} is interpreted as the log odds ratio of response associated with the implementation of the bylaw among city workers only, because of the presence of the interaction terms. Similarly, the parameter β_{j2} is interpreted as the log odds ratio of response associated with working outside rather than inside the city among pre-bylaw respondents only. The interaction parameter β_{j4} is the increment in the log odds ratio associated with the implementation of the bylaw among the workers outside the city over the city workers. In model U2, however, β_{j1} is the log odds ratio associated with implementation for all respondents and β_{j2} is the log odds ratio associated with working outside the city for both pre- and post-bylaw respondents.

For each variable included in the model, maximum likelihood estimation produced a regression coefficient and estimated standard error for each of the two regression equations, so that there were two sets of regression coefficients and standard errors. The regression coefficients were interpreted as estimates of log odds ratios, and confidence intervals were calculated for the odds ratio estimates by taking the exponent of the upper and lower endpoints of the asymptotic confidence interval for the log odds ratio. For the place-of-work indicators, the signs of the coefficients were reversed in order to compare city workers to each of the other groups of workers. The a priori hypothesis that changes in attitudes associated with the bylaw would be greater in the city workers than in either of the other two groups was evaluated with a likelihood ratio test of the null hypothesis that $\beta_{14} = \beta_{24} = 0$ and $\beta_{15} = \beta_{25} = 0$ in model U1. This required fitting models with and without the variables of interest and examining the change in the log-likelihood using Q_R defined at (7).

To assess the associations between a single variable, such as time of survey (x_1), and the three-category outcome, overall Wald tests (2 d.f.) were conducted using the estimated covariance matrix. In this case, $\boldsymbol{\beta}_B = (\beta_{11}, \beta_{12})^T$, the null hypothesis is $\beta_{11} = \beta_{21} = 0$, and the Wald test statistic (5) reduces to

$$Q_W = \frac{(\hat{\beta}_{11}/\sigma_{11})^2 + (\hat{\beta}_{21}/\sigma_{21})^2 - 2\rho(\hat{\beta}_{11} \cdot \hat{\beta}_{21}/\sigma_{11} \cdot \sigma_{21})}{1 - \rho^2} \qquad (10)$$

where σ_{j1} is the estimated standard error of $\hat{\beta}_{j1}$, and ρ is the estimated correlation between $\hat{\beta}_{11}$ and $\hat{\beta}_{21}$. A large value of this statistic provided evidence that β_{11} or β_{21} or $(\beta_{11} - \beta_{21})$ is different from zero.

Likelihood ratio tests were used to assess the overall contribution of multiple variables, such as the place of work indicators (x_2, x_3) in model U2, by fitting models with and without the variables of interest and examining the change in the log-likelihood. Wald tests of the single parameters corresponding to x_2 and x_3 compared the attitudes of workers outside the city and nonworkers, respectively, to those of workers in the city. To compare workers outside the city to nonworkers, that is, to test the null hypothesis $(\beta_{j2} - \beta_{j3}) = 0$, linear contrasts of the parameters: $\mathbf{c}(\beta_{j2}, \beta_{j3})^T$ with $\mathbf{c} = (1, -1)$ were required. In this case, the Wald statistic (5) is

$$Q_W = \frac{(\hat{\beta}_{j2} - \hat{\beta}_{j3})^2}{\sigma_{j2}^2 + \sigma_{j3}^2 - 2\rho\sigma_{j2} \cdot \sigma_{j3}}, \qquad (11)$$

where ρ is the estimated correlation between $\hat{\beta}_{j2}$ and $\hat{\beta}_{j3}$.

Model-Fitting Strategy

The analysis was conducted by fitting a series of regression models that included various combinations of the variables of interest (as defined in Table 1). For models in this series, including the unadjusted models introduced above, Table 3 summarizes the variables used, the number of parameters estimated, and the value of the log-likelihood, expressed as $-2l(\hat{\boldsymbol{\beta}})$. The adjusted models were of

Table 3   Summary of Fitted Models

Model	Variables Included	Number of Parameters	-2 Log-Likelihood
U1	Time, work, time × work	12	4342.28
U2	Time, work	8	4342.73
U3	Time	4	4365.98
A1	Time, residence, work, time × work, smoking, knowledge, time × smoking sex, age, age^2, education, education^2	42	3980.83
A2	Time, residence, work, smoking, knowledge, time × smoking sex, age, age^2, education, education^2	38	3981.36
A3	Time, residence, smoking, knowledge, time × smoking sex, age, age^2, education, education^2	34	3987.62
A4	Time, work smoking, knowledge, time × smoking sex, age, age^2, education, education^2	36	3983.87
A5	Time, residence, work, smoking, knowledge, sex, age, age^2, education, education^2	30	3998.76
A6	Time, residence, work, knowledge, sex, age, age^2, education, education^2	22	4129.24
A7	Time, residence, work, smoking, time × smoking sex, age, age^2, education, education^2	36	4067.45
A8	Time, residence, work smoking, knowledge, time × smoking age, age^2, education, education^2	36	3989.03
A9	Time, residence, work, smoking, knowledge, time × smoking sex, education, education^2	34	4006.93
A10	Time, residence, work, smoking, knowledge, time × smoking sex, age, age^2	34	4003.30
A11	Time, residence, work, smoking, knowledge, time × smoking	28	4038.54

the form

$$\ln\left(\frac{p_j}{p_0}\right) = \beta_{j0} + \mathbf{x}\boldsymbol{\beta}_j + \mathbf{z}\boldsymbol{\Gamma}_j \quad \text{for } j = 1, 2,$$

where $\mathbf{x}$ and $\mathbf{z}$ represent vectors of covariates, including interactions. Models A1 to A3 added variables for place of residence (z_1), smoking status (z_2, z_3, z_4, z_5), interaction between time and smoking status ($x_1 \cdot z_2$, etc.), knowledge score (z_6), sex (z_7), and linear and quadratic terms in age (z_8, z_8^2) and in level of education (z_9, z_9^2) (see Table 1). The interaction between time and smoking status allowed for the impact of the bylaw to depend on smoking status.

The time × place of work interaction in adjusted model A1 and other overall tests of the association between single or multiple variables and attitude were conducted using the likelihood ratio test statistic Q_R (7), which required fitting models with and without the variables of interest (models A2 to A11). Model A6, for example, did not include any main effects or interactions for smoking status. Comparison to model A2, which was otherwise the same, indicated the overall contribution of smoking status. Several other models were fitted to explore interactions for smoking status and place of work, smoking status and sex, and age and sex, but none of these contributed significantly and therefore are not presented. Table 4 summarizes the overall likelihood ratio test statistics (Q_R) used to assess each of the effects of interest. The values of Q_R were derived from the values of the log-likelihood given in Table 3, using (7). For

Table 4   Summary of Overall Likelihood Ratio Test Statistics (Q_R) in Unadjusted and Adjusted Models

Effect	Models	Q_R	d.f.	p-Value
Time × place of work	U1, U2	0.45	4	0.99
	A1, A2	0.53	4	0.97
Place of work	U2, U3	23.25	4	0.0001
	A2, A3	6.26	4	0.18
Residence	A2, A4	2.51	2	0.28
Time × smoking and smoking	A2, A6	147.88	16	0.0001
Time × smoking	A2, A5	17.40	8	0.03
Knowledge	A2, A7	86.09	2	0.0001
Sociodemographic (sex, age, education)	A2, A11	57.18	10	0.0001
Sex	A2, A8	7.67	2	0.02
Age	A2, A9	25.57	4	0.0001
Level of education	A2, A10	21.94	4	0.0002

example, in the first line of Table 4, Q_R = 4342.73 − 4342.28 = 0.45 with d.f. of 12 − 8 = 4.

For the final model A2, Wald test statistics (Q_W) were also used to assess the variables of interest. These were calculated from the estimated variance matrix using (5). The triplet of estimated probabilities for each respondent was calculated from the MLEs and the regression functions (9). The respondents were ranked according to the estimated probability of preference for smoking in restricted areas and 20 subgroups were formed using cutpoints at five percentile intervals in the cumulative weighted frequency distribution. Expected proportions for each subgroup were calculated by summing the estimated probabilities for respondents in the subgroup and were compared to the observed proportions using the Hosmer–Lemeshow goodness-of-fit statistic Q_H (8). Other comparisons were made between observed and expected proportions using subgroups defined by values of the covariates. For knowledge of the health effects of smoke, six subgroups were defined by the score levels: (0–2, 3–4, 5–6, 7–8, 9–10, 11–12). For age, there were six subgroups: (18–24 years, 25–34, 35–44, 45–54, 55–64, over 64 years). The subgroups for education were defined by the original levels of the covariate.

4 RESULTS

The overall likelihood ratio test of the interaction between time of survey and place of work in model U1 did not provide evidence to reject the null hypothesis that the impact of the bylaw was the same regardless of place of work (first line of Table 4). In model U1 (Table 5a), the overall Wald test provided no evidence of changes in city workers between the pre and postimplementation surveys (Q_W = 0.82 in the first line of the table). The estimated values of the coefficients given in the second and third lines of Table 5a indicated that at the time of the pre-bylaw survey, city workers tended to be more likely than those working outside the city to prefer prohibition rather than restriction: the odds ratio was 1.33 with a 95% confidence interval of (1.00, 1.79). The confidence intervals for the odds ratios for the interaction terms, given in the last two lines of Table 5a, indicated that odds ratios larger than 3.1 (in either direction) would have been excluded.

In model U2 (Table 5b), the changes associated with the bylaw implementation were small: the odds ratios for prohibited versus restricted smoking and for unrestricted versus restricted were 1.12 and 0.86, respectively, with 95% confidence intervals of (0.95, 1.33) and (0.61, 1.20). The overall Wald test value was Q_W = 3.02. Based on a likelihood ratio test (Q_R = 23.25 in the third line of Table 4), there was evidence for an overall association between attitude and place of work. Both before and after bylaw implementation, city workers were more likely than those working outside the city to prefer complete prohibition rather than restricted areas (Q_W = 7.94): the odds ratio for prohibited versus restricted was 1.30 with a 95% confidence interval that excluded 1.00 (second

Table 5 Estimates and Confidence Intervals for Models U1 and U2

Comparison	Overall Wald Test (2 d.f.)		Prohibited vs. Restricted		Unrestricted vs. Restricted	
	Q_W	p-Value	Odds Ratio	95% CI	Odds Ratio	95% CI
(a) Model U1						
Post vs. pre (city workers only)	0.82	0.66	1.14	0.85, 1.52	0.94	0.52, 1.70
Place of work (for pre only)						
City vs. work outside	5.01	0.08	1.33	1.00, 1.77	0.80	0.48, 1.34
City vs. not work	2.31	0.31	0.87	0.65, 1.17	1.43	0.75, 2.74
Time × place of work						
City vs. work outside	0.15	0.93	0.96	0.64, 1.44	1.13	0.52, 2.43
City vs. not work	0.21	0.90	1.08	0.72, 1.64	1.18	0.44, 3.12
(b) Model U2						
Post vs. pre (all respondents)	3.02	0.22	1.12	0.95, 1.33	0.86	0.61, 1.20
Place of work						
City vs. work outside	7.94	0.02	1.30	1.06, 1.60	0.85	0.58, 1.24
City vs. not work	4.43	0.11	0.91	0.74, 1.12	1.54	0.95, 2.50

line of Table 5b). Comparison of nonworkers to outside-city workers, using linear contrasts (11), also indicated that nonworkers were more likely to prefer prohibition and less likely to prefer unrestricted smoking.

Adjusting for the other determinants (models A1 and A2) produced the same conclusion about the interaction hypothesis, that is, no differential changes ($Q_R = 0.53$ in the second line of Table 4). It did change, however, the conclusion about the association between attitude and place of work: Q_R was reduced from 23.25 to 6.26 (lines 3 and 4 in Table 4). The magnitude of the coefficients for city versus outside city workers was reduced and the confidence intervals were wider (compare Table 6 to Table 5b). Examination of the regression coefficients in models with and without the smoking and the sociodemographic variables (not presented) suggested that adjustment for sociodemographic characteristics reduced differences between city and outside city workers.

The individual predicted probabilities calculated from the final model A2 ranged from 0.05 to 0.66 for prohibited, from 0.33 to 0.93 for restricted, and from 0.001 to 0.50 for unrestricted. The goodness-of-fit procedures found good agreement between the observed and expected proportions for the most part (Figure 1). The Hosmer–Lemeshow statistic was 49.66 for the percentile-based test, which does not exceed the conventional 5% critical value of 53.38 for

Table 6   Estimates and Confidence Intervals for the Final Model (Model A2)

Comparison	Overall Wald Test (2 d.f.)		Prohibited vs. Restricted		Unrestricted vs. Restricted	
	Q_W	p-Value	Odds Ratio	95% CI	Odds Ratio	95% CI
Bylaw related						
Post vs. pre (for never smokers only)	2.29	0.32	1.14	0.91, 1.43	0.69	0.32, 1.51
City vs. work outside	2.98	0.23	1.20	0.97, 1.52	0.97	0.64, 1.49
City vs. not work	2.82	0.24	1.11	0.86, 1.43	1.56	0.88, 2.78
City reside vs. other	2.52	0.28	1.18	0.96, 1.45	1.10	0.71, 1.68
Smoking related						
Smoking (for pre only)						
Current vs. never	49.82	0.0001	0.38	0.27, 0.53	3.14	1.74, 5.68
Recent quitter vs. never	1.39	0.50	0.72	0.40, 1.28	1.16	0.29, 4.54
Quitter vs. never	1.21	0.55	0.98	0.70, 1.36	1.64	0.66, 4.04
Short vs. long quitter	12.40	0.002	0.26	0.12, 0.59	0.13	0.10, 1.82
Knowledge score	81.82	0.0001	1.11	1.07, 1.15	0.78	0.73, 0.84
Post vs. pre × smoking						
Current vs. never	0.69	0.71	0.85	0.52, 1.39	1.24	0.50, 3.04
Recent quitter vs. never	0.94	0.63	1.38	0.54, 3.51	2.19	0.30, 16.04
Quitter vs. never	1.57	0.46	0.75	0.48, 1.18	0.87	0.22, 3.42
Short vs. long quitter	14.85	0.001	8.48	2.54, 28.34	28.36	1.09, 740.9
Sociodemographic						
Male vs. female	7.46	0.02	0.99	0.82, 1.19	1.68	1.15, 2.44
Linear age	13.32	0.001	1.10	1.03, 1.17	0.85	0.73, 0.99
Quadratic age	7.46	0.02	1.04	1.01, 1.07	1.06	0.99, 1.14
Linear education	16.41	0.0003	0.91	0.84, 0.98	0.75	0.63, 0.88
Quadratic education	7.48	0.02	1.08	1.02, 1.14	0.98	0.86, 1.11

a chi-squared distribution with 38 degrees of freedom (p-value = 0.10). Relatively larger discrepancies occurred in subgroups with larger proportions for prohibition (Figure 1a) and in the high knowledge score group (Figure 1b). It may be that the same group of respondents are contributing in both cases, because of the strong association of knowledge with support for prohibition, but residual analysis and other regression diagnostic techniques would be required to identify the individual cases.

As expected, smoking status was a highly significant determinant of attitudes. The overall likelihood ratio test statistic for the association between attitude and smoking status, including interactions with time of survey, was quite large (Q_R = 147.88, line 6 of Table 4). In specific comparisons of smoking status categories for the pre-bylaw survey, current smokers were more likely

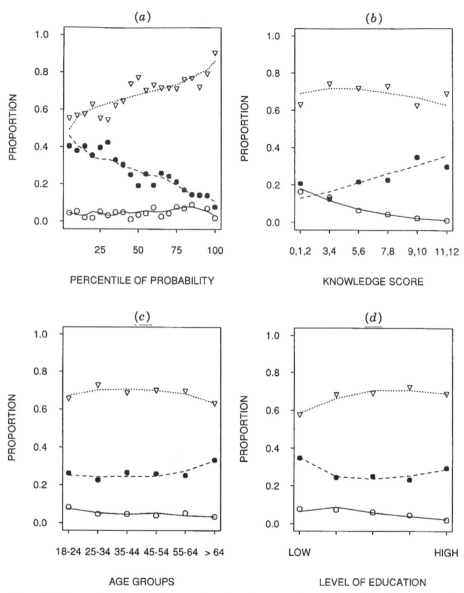

Figure 1. Observed and expected proportions for subgroups of respondents: (*a*) subgroups based on the estimated probability of preference for restricted smoking; (*b*) subgroups based on levels of the knowledge score; (*c*) subgroups based on 10-year age groups; (*d*) subgroups based on level of education. The symbols indicate the observed proportions and the lines indicate expected proportions from the fitted model: observed proportion for restricted (∇), expected proportion for restricted (·····), observed proportion for prohibited (•), expected proportion for prohibited (- - - - -), observed proportion for unrestricted (○), expected proportion for unrestricted (———).

than nonsmokers to prefer no restrictions rather than restricted areas, and less likely to prefer prohibition (Q_W = 49.82, second section of Table 6). The odds ratios (95% confidence intervals) were 0.38 (0.27, 0.53) for prohibited versus restricted and 3.14 (1.74, 5.68) for unrestricted versus restricted for this comparison.

A somewhat unexpected interaction was found for former smokers and time of survey, indicating that the association between attitudes and smoking status depended on time of survey (Q_R = 17.40, line 7 of Table 4; and Q_W = 14.85, second section of Table 6). Before bylaw implementation, former smokers of duration 6 to 12 months (short-term quitters) were less likely than longer-term quitters to prefer prohibition or unrestricted smoking; that is, the odds ratios were less than 1.00. After implementation, short-term quitters, that is, those who quit around the time of bylaw implementation, were more likely to prefer prohibition or unrestricted smoking, (i.e., odds ratios greater than 1.00), indicating a polarization of attitudes. This is evident in Table 7, which summarizes the observed percentage preference for smoking restriction in short- and long-term quitters from all places of work. It is also important to note from Table 2 that much of this change appears to have occurred in those who work outside the home, either inside or outside the city, and not in those not working outside the home. However, because of some empty cells (see Table 2), it was not possible to estimate the relevant parameters for the time × smoking × work interaction. The wide confidence intervals for some of the time × smoking parameters in Table 6 also reflect the sparseness of the data for former smokers.

Other findings included the following (see Table 6). Knowledge of the health effects of environmental tobacco smoke was strongly related to attitude: those with higher scores were more likely to prefer prohibition and less likely to prefer no restrictions. The relationship between attitude and knowledge is depicted in Figure 1b. At all knowledge levels, preference for restricted areas was usually in the majority. However, preference for prohibition increased with the knowledge score. Men were somewhat more likely than women to prefer unrestricted smoking. Preference for prohibition increased with age, particularly in the older age groups, with a concurrent decrease in preference for no restrictions (Figure 1c). Level of education was also related to attitude in a nonlinear fashion, with preference for prohibition higher for the extremes than for the intermediate levels and preference for unrestricted smoking higher in those with lower levels of education (Figure 1d).

5 CONCLUSIONS

In summary, there was little evidence to support the hypothesis that the impact of the bylaw on attitudes depended on place of work, either with or without adjustment for place of residence, smoking status, knowledge score of the

Table 7   Percentage Distribution for Unexpected Interaction among Former Smokers

Group of Former Smokers	Number of Observations, n	Attitude toward Smoking in the Workplace (%)		
		Prohibited	Restricted	Unrestricted
Short-term (6–12 months)				
Pre	69.3	11	88	1
Post	23.7	43	50	7
Long-term (>12 months)				
Pre	231.0	32	64	4
Post	257.9	29	69	2

health effects of environmental tobacco smoke, age, sex, and level of education, and there was little evidence to indicate large changes in attitudes in the eight-month period used to assess the impact of the bylaw. Before bylaw implementation, however, workers in city of Toronto workplaces were already more likely than noncity workers to prefer prohibition rather than restriction, so that larger changes in city workers may have been more difficult to achieve. These differences were partially explained by differences in sociodemographic characteristics that were related to attitudes. Smoking status had a strong association with attitudes: current smokers were more likely than nonsmokers to prefer no restriction rather than restricted areas, and less likely to prefer prohibition. Nevertheless, there was little indication that smokers were less supportive of restrictive measures after implementation of the bylaw than smokers had been before implementation. Knowledge of the health effects of environmental tobacco smoke was also strongly related to attitudes; those with higher scores were more likely to prefer prohibition and less likely to prefer no restrictions. Level of education was related to attitudes, with those more educated tending to be more likely to prefer restricted smoking compared to those with lower levels of education.

Several factors need to be kept in mind when interpreting the results. First, since the pre- and postsurveys were independent, inferences can be made about changes in population groups but not about changes in attitudes within individuals. Second, the residents of metropolitan Toronto were not randomly assigned to workplaces covered by the bylaw intervention, so that the effect of place of work may have been confounded by other factors related to attitudes. Third, cross-sectional data can only indicate associations, not cause and effect, so that although knowledge of the health effects of environmental tobacco smoke exhibited a strong association with attitudes, for example, this does not imply that an increase in knowledge would be followed by a change in attitudes. Furthermore, some of the so-called determinants of attitude may also have been affected by the bylaw implementation. For example, some respondents in the postimplementation survey indicated that they had quit smoking or tried to quit smoking because of the new law. Finally, the two control groups of noncity workers may have been influenced by secular changes or spillover effects, due to the bylaw being widely publicized, and this would have reduced the interaction effect hypothesized.

Given the sparse data for former smokers, and the considerations just discussed, the interaction observed between quitting and time of survey must be interpreted with caution. One possible explanation is that complete prohibition is useful for the maintenance of smoking cessation. However, this specific effect was not hypothesized in advance and may have arisen from sampling variability, nonresponse bias, or because of the number of hypothesis tests conducted.

Although it is natural to interpret the logistic regression equations in terms of log odds ratios and to use the odds ratio as a measure of association, this does not preclude presentation and interpretation of the fitted models in terms of proportions, as has been done in Table 2 and Figure 1. This is frequently desirable in the context of public health and public policy, in which interest is more often in the proportions or numbers of individuals affected rather than in the relative risks of an outcome.

In allowing for the effects of the survey design on the analysis, it was sufficient in these surveys to weight the estimates, because the households were selected with equal probabilities, that is, with simple random sampling. The adjustments for selection within the household and for poststratification were incorporated to make the results more closely represent the metropolitan Toronto population. Aside from the weighting, no adjustments were made to the estimate of the covariance matrix, as might be necessary had the data been collected using a complex multistage design with stratification and cluster sampling (see Bull and Pederson, 1988; Morel, 1989; Korn and Graubard, 1991).

With the mounting scientific evidence that adverse health outcomes are associated with exposure to environmental tobacco smoke, there have been marked changes in attitudes toward and acceptance of this exposure (U.S. Department of Health and Human Services, 1989a). These changes have been accompanied by the implementation of both voluntary and legislated restrictions on smoking in public places and in workplaces. While the primary objective of legislative measures to restrict smoking in the workplace is to reduce exposure to environmental tobacco smoke, positive attitudes toward such measures may be a co-requisite to effective implementation, compliance, and enforcement. Information about the impact of restrictions and determinants of attitudes toward restrictions is useful to investigators in understanding the role of legislation in changing social norms (Pederson et al., 1991) and to health policy analysts in developing, implementing, and evaluating public policy. Statistical models such as polychotomous logistic regression are useful in modeling established and hypothesized relationships, in identifying population subgroups with positive and negative attitudes toward restrictions in order to target relevant programs, and in evaluating policy changes.

ACKNOWLEDGMENTS

The author thanks L. L. Pederson (Department of Epidemiology and Biostatistics, University of Western Ontario) and M. J. Ashley (Department of Preventive Medicine and Biostatistics, University of Toronto) for many discussions and for their careful reading of the manuscript. Kathy Sykora and Janice Smith provided assistance with data analysis, and Min Gao prepared the figures. The telephone interviews were conducted by the Institute for Social Research at York University, Ontario, Canada. This research was supported by the National Health Research and Development Program, Health and Welfare Canada, through Project Grant 6606-3346-46 and through a National Health Research Scholar Award to the author.

QUESTIONS AND PROBLEMS

1. Using the estimates, variances, and covariances for β_{j2} and $\beta_{j3}, j = 1, 2$, given in Table 8, verify that the Wald test (2 d.f.) of the null hypothesis $\beta_{12} = \beta_{22} = 0$ is $Q_W = 7.94$ [using equations (5) or (10)], and verify that the Wald test (1 d.f.) of the linear contrast $\beta_{12} - \beta_{13} = 0$ is $Q_W = 11.94$ [using equation (5) or (11)].

Table 8   Maximum Likelihood Estimates and Variance Matrix for Selected Parameters in Model U2

Comparison	Parameter	MLE	Variance–Covariance ($\times 10^2$)			
			β_{12}	β_{13}	β_{22}	β_{23}
Prohibited vs. restricted						
Work outside vs. city (x_2)	β_{12}	−0.2643	1.08	0.56	0.28	0.16
Not work vs. city (x_3)	β_{13}	0.0984	0.56	1.14	0.16	0.34
Unrestricted vs. restricted						
Work outside vs. city (x_2)	β_{22}	0.1662	0.28	0.16	3.80	2.30
Not work vs. city (x_3)	β_{23}	−0.4335	0.16	0.34	2.30	6.09

2. Suppose that the time of survey variable was coded as 1 and −1 instead of 1 and 0. What would be the interpretation of the regression parameter estimates in a model that included variables for time, place of work, and their interaction? What are the advantages and disadvantages of this alternative coding scheme?

3. Show how the odds ratio estimates for model U1 given in Table 5a are related to the odds ratios that can be calculated directly from the data in the total rows of Table 2. Why is it not possible to do this for model U2? [*Hint:* Solve the score equations (2) for model U1.]

4. Other statistical models might also be appropriate to meet the objectives of this investigation. An ordinal model, for example, in which the degree of restriction (none, some, complete) was built into the model formulation would be attractive from the point of view of parsimony because there would be only one regression function instead of two. [See Anderson (1984) and McCullagh and Nelder (1989) for a review of various ordinal models.] However, some of these models force certain constraints that require the odds of response in one category relative to the adjacent category to be similar for all categories. Does this appear to be appropriate for all the covariates in the final model reported in Table 6? How would you compare the goodness of fit of an ordinal model to that of the polychotomous model?

5. Using a logistic regression package, fit model A2 and calculate the triplet of predicted probabilities for each observation in the data set. [*Note:* If you have a binary logistic regression program but not a polychotomous logistic regression program, an approximate solution can be obtained by fitting two separate binary regressions (see Hosmer and Lemeshow, 1989, Chapter 8). The first should exclude all respondents in the unrestricted category, and the second should exclude all respondents in the prohibited category.] Using the regression diagnostic techniques described by Lesaffre and Albert (1989b) and Hosmer et al. (1991), attempt to identify the individual observations that contribute to the discrepancies between the observed and expected proportions in Figure 1 noted in Section 4.

PART V

Clinical Trials

CHAPTER 14

Interpretation of a Leukemia Trial Stopped Early

Scott S. Emerson and Phillip L. C. Banks

1 MOTIVATION AND BACKGROUND

In this chapter we report the outcome of a phase III clinical trial designed to confirm the benefit of a new drug indicated for the treatment of acute myelogenous leukemia (Berman et al., 1991). The analysis presented here focuses mainly on the way in which the results of this clinical trial were used as evidence in support of approval of a new drug application to the U.S. Food and Drug Administration (FDA). Attention is directed more toward the analysis of the data following termination of a study rather than the issues involved in deciding to stop the study.

1.1 Acute Myelogenous Leukemia

Leukemias are cancers in which blood-forming cells undergo changes resulting in uncontrolled, malignant growth. Patients with leukemia exhibit excessive numbers of abnormal white blood cells in their circulation. Normally, white blood cells play a major role in the body's defense against infection. The white blood cells that predominate in leukemias, however, are generally quite immature and limited in their ability to fight infections. Furthermore, the cancerous cells replace the normal blood-forming cells in the bone marrow, and thus a patient with leukemia will often have anemia, low numbers of platelets in the circulating blood, and other hematologic abnormalities.

The causes of leukemias have not been fully identified, although there is some evidence linking leukemia with environmental exposures such as ionizing

Case Studies in Biometry, Edited by Nicholas Lange, Louise Ryan, Lynne Billard, David Brillinger, Loveday Conquest, and Joel Greenhouse.
ISBN 0-471-58885-7 © 1994 John Wiley & Sons, Inc.

radiation, chemicals such as benzene, or certain viral infections. There is also some evidence that genetic factors may play a role.

There are several types of leukemia. They are classified by the type of blood-forming cell that has become malignant (lymphocytic versus myelogenous) as well as by the aggressiveness of the disease (acute versus chronic). Medical treatment of leukemia varies with the exact classification of the disease. The main treatment for acute myelogenous leukemia is administration of anticancer drugs which target rapidly dividing cells. Because these drugs are not perfectly selective for cancer cells, there are generally high levels of toxicity associated with cancer chemotherapy. In the process of killing the cancer cells, some nondiseased cells are also affected, especially those with a naturally high rate of growth (e.g., in hair follicles, the blood-forming cells in the bone marrow, and the cells in the lining of the gastrointestinal tract). The doses of anticancer drugs that can be administered are limited by the extent of this toxicity. Thus, leukemia chemotherapy usually proceeds through several phases. In the first phase (termed *remission induction*), an intensive course of chemotherapy is administered in an attempt to eliminate the leukemic clones. If this treatment is successful, microscopic examination of the circulating blood and bone marrow cells will reveal few or no cancer cells, and the patient is then said to have had a remission induced. In some cases, multiple courses of remission induction chemotherapy must be administered before a remission is achieved. Sometimes, no remission will be achieved, and some patients die during early courses of chemotherapy.

After the patient enters remission, further courses of intensive chemotherapy (consolidation treatments) are often administered in an effort to kill any remaining leukemic cells. Following consolidation, patients generally continue to receive periodic, less intense courses of chemotherapy called *maintenance therapy*. These maintenance treatments can continue for years after initial diagnosis, and often include treatments which target areas of the body that are known to be poorly treated during the induction phase (e.g., the brain, spinal cord, and testes).

Despite the consolidation and maintenance therapies, leukemia often reappears in patients who have had a successful induction of remission. In such cases, the patient will often undergo additional remission induction treatments, sometimes with different drugs. With each succeeding relapse, however, the success rate of remission induction decreases. In recent years, bone marrow transplantation has been used to treat patients who have had one or more relapses. There has also been some investigation of the use of bone marrow transplantation prior to leukemic relapse while the patient is still in remission. In a bone marrow transplant, all blood-forming cells in the patient are destroyed by chemotherapy, radiation, or both. Nondiseased bone marrow is then transplanted into the patient in the hopes that the transplanted marrow will be able to provide the blood-forming cells needed to ensure adequate response to infections.

1.2 Clinical Trials

Drugs that demonstrate effectiveness after extensive laboratory and animal testing can be evaluated in clinical trials involving human volunteers. The highly toxic nature of the drugs demands that such testing proceed cautiously. There is much literature about the proper conduct of clinical trials (see, e.g., Pocock, 1983). Briefly, the clinical trials of new anticancer drugs proceed through three phases. In phase I testing, the new treatment is given to small numbers of human volunteers in order to find appropriate doses. Often phase I trials are conducted in patients for whom standard treatments have failed. Phase II trials investigate preliminary measures of treatment efficacy along with further assessment of treatment safety in slightly larger numbers of patients. Traditionally, phase II trials do not attempt to compare the new treatment to an existing treatment; instead they focus on demonstrating any anticancer activity of the drug.

Treatments which show promising anticancer activity at tolerable doses are then tested in a larger phase III trial, with the goal of comparing its performance with existing standard treatment or, if no standard therapy exists, to a placebo. Whenever possible, these trials are conducted double blind so that neither the patient nor the study investigators know which treatment is being administered. This helps to prevent patient or investigator bias affecting the outcome of the experiment.

Each patient in a clinical trial is followed for treatment outcome. Typically, there are multiple ways to measure treatment success (e.g., length of patient survival, percent of patients surviving for two years, or percent of patients experiencing tumor regression). Important secondary measures of treatment success might include percent of patients experiencing toxicities and the severity of those toxicities. At the conclusion of the study, these and other endpoints are analyzed, and the results are used to establish the net benefit of the new treatment.

1.3 Clinical Trial of Idarubicin in Acute Myelogenous Leukemia

In 1984, a comparative clinical trial was initiated to test the difference in therapeutic effect between two chemotherapies indicated for the treatment of adult acute myelogenous leukemia. Patients from the Memorial Sloan Kettering Cancer Center were randomized with equal assignment probability to two treatment arms. Since it was not possible to make the two treatments identical in appearance, the investigators and the patients were not blinded as to which treatment the patients received. However, the pathology data used to determine remission status were reviewed without knowledge of treatment assignments.

The two treatments being compared were each of the class of chemicals called anthracyclines. One of the treated groups was given the newly synthesized anthracycline idarubicin, while the other treatment group (or treatment arm) received the standard anthracycline agent, daunorubicin. As is common in many cancer chemotherapy regimens, the usual induction treatment of acute myelogenous leukemia involves multiple drugs. Thus, both treatment arms were dosed with cytosine arabinoside (ARA-C) in addition to the anthracyclines.

The trial permitted both induction and consolidation phases of treatment. Induction therapy consisted of an intravenous bolus of 25 mg/m^2 of ARA-C, followed immediately by 200 mg/m^2 of continuously infused ARA-C for five days. The anthracyclines were given by slow intravenous injection for the first three days of the ARA-C dosing period. The idarubicin and daunorubicin doses were 12 and 50 mg/m^2, respectively.

Patients failing to achieve complete remission status following this initial induction course received a second induction course identical in schedule to the first. Patients not responding to the second course were considered treatment failures and were subsequently withdrawn from the study.

Complete responders (i.e., patients achieving complete remission) proceeded to the consolidation phase of the study following a three- to four-week rest period. The treatment plan for the consolidation phase was the same as that used for the induction period, except that the ARA-C was given for 4 days with the anthracycline administration coinciding with the first two days of ARA-C infusion. A maximum of four consolidation courses could be given to each patient.

The study protocol was amended early during the trial to omit a maintenance treatment period and to modify criteria for identifying patients to receive bone marrow transplantation. The maintenance course, offered to only a few patients, consisted of randomizing patients who remained in complete remission one month after their first consolidation course to receive either no treatment or a regimen of subcutaneous ARA-C.

Originally, patients 40 years of age or less with a suitable donor were eligible for bone marrow transplantation after achieving a complete response. No consolidation therapy was to be given. Under the revised design, all potentially eligible patients in complete remission received one course of consolidation therapy. Then patients 50 years of age or less proceeded to bone marrow transplantation if a suitable donor were available, or, if not, were eligible for bone marrow harvest and autologous bone marrow transplantation (i.e., re-infusion of their own bone marrow cells). A patient declining autologous transplantation could undergo bone marrow harvest, with the opportunity for autologous bone marrow transplantation should relapse occur and a second complete remission be achieved.

As indicated by the study protocol described above, great care was exercised in the conduct of the clinical trial to promote comparability of the treatment arms. The primary study objective was to demonstrate a difference between the treatment arms with respect to the rates of patients achieving a complete remission. Secondary objectives included the assessment of differences between the treatment arms with respect to patient toxicity rates and patient survival. It is not uncommon that survival be relegated to secondary status, due to the larger sample size and longer study duration required to achieve adequate statistical power to detect clinically important differences.

During the early portion of the trial, the data were reviewed for patient safety and compliance. The data were also informally monitored for treatment efficacy. Periodic monitoring of the data in a clinical trial is usually indicated to satisfy the ethical considerations involved in human experimentation. It is important that a trial be terminated if there is reliable evidence that patients are being harmed by continuing the study.

In the case of this study, however, the protocol, though well specified in most other respects, initially failed to specify adequately the methods by which the data would be monitored. As discussed in Section 3, if decisions to terminate a clinical trial are based on repeated analyses of the accruing data, the type I statistical error of hypothesis tests may be inflated over the desired level, confidence intervals may not have the correct coverage probabilities, and bias may be introduced into the estimates of treatment effects. Although the researchers retroactively imposed a formal stopping rule on the study, the FDA was reluctant to trust that the final reported study results were not unduly affected by the early unplanned analyses, which showed a favorable trend for the idarubicin arm. The remainder of this chapter focuses on the statistical problems introduced by unplanned interim analyses of clinical trials.

2 DATA

2.1 Study Design and Stopping Rules

The original study protocol called for a single formal analysis of the data following the accrual of the entire planned sample size. However, after early, unplanned analyses of the data suggested some advantage of idarubicin over daunorubicin in inducing complete remission, a level 0.05 O'Brien–Fleming (1979) group sequential design with a maximum of $m = 4$ analyses was adopted at the time that 69 patients had been accrued. Although only three formal analyses were planned for the study, the O'Brien–Fleming design based on $m = 4$ was chosen to account for the unplanned early looks at the data that had already taken place. For the case of equal group sizes accrued between analyses, $\alpha = 0.05$, and $m = 4$, the critical value specifying the stopping boundaries (see Section 3) is $c^* = 2.0243$.

Additional analyses were then planned after groups of approximately 40 response-evaluable patients had been randomized and assessed for their remission status. The maximum sample size was adjusted upward so that the resultant test would still have 80% power to detect absolute differences in complete response rates ≥ 0.20. The new estimate called for 160 response evaluable patients. A slight excess of patients was to be enrolled to ensure that sufficient numbers of evaluable patients were accrued, bringing the maximum sample size to be accrued to 90 patients per treatment arm.

The first formal analysis was performed after a total of 90 patients had been accrued, and the second (and last) such interim analysis was performed after 130 patients had been accrued in June 1989. At the second analysis, 10 of the patients were judged nonevaluable for determination of complete response (due primarily to improper diagnosis at study entry). However, this case study will report on the entire randomized study population, to avoid any possibility of selection bias.

2.2 Description of Variables

Data collected on the patients at the time they entered the study included a complete medical history, physical examination, and an evaluation of ambulatory status. In the analysis of the clinical trial results, these data are used to assess the comparability of treatment groups prior to receiving the treatment, that is, to assess the adequacy of the randomization. Such baseline measurements can also be used to evaluate treatment effects within subsets. Baseline data of greatest interest in this trial include demographic data (patient sex and age), classification of disease into subtypes, objective measurements of disease severity (white blood cell count, platelet count, and hemoglobin level), and a subjective measurement of patient condition (Karnofsky scale of performance status).

Measurements were also made while each patient was on the trial to determine whether a remission had been induced. These measurements included a bone marrow aspiration and biopsy with histochemical stains, a complete blood count, a lumbar puncture and a routine biochemical profile of the blood. Other data were collected at specified intervals to assess patient safety and compliance. Surviving patients were followed routinely after their last course of chemotherapy to ascertain their continued survival and continued remission. This included patients failing both induction courses as well as those completing all or a portion of the consolidation period.

Determination of the primary endpoint of induction of complete remission was conditioned on the results of the bone marrow and peripheral blood counts, and the presence or absence of continued leukemic disease outside the bone marrow. A complete response was defined as a bone marrow of normal cellularity or at least not hypocellular with some evidence of normal maturation. Moreover, there had to be ≤5% blasts (immature blood-forming cells) in two consecutive specimens over a four-week period. Finally, the peripheral counts had to recover and there could be no evidence of extramedullary disease. Secondary measures of treatment effect included the number of courses of chemotherapy required to induce remission and patient survival. Also included in the data are measurements of the time at which a patient was judged to be in complete remission, and indicators of whether the patient received a bone marrow transplant. Since bone marrow transplantation might affect survival, adjustment for this last variable may be desirable in assessing the secondary endpoint of patient survival. As the study progressed, some patients were identified as having some form of leukemia other than acute myelogenous leukemia, and thus they had been entered into the study by error. For this and other reasons, some patients were judged by the primary researchers to be nonevaluable for remission status. An indicator of this evaluability is included in the data.

Table 1 displays the data available for a sample of the patients in the clinical trial. It should be noted that the statistical problems posed by these data revolve around the interim analyses performed on the data as they accrued. To reproduce the results of those analyses, an indicator of those cases available for analysis at the first formal analysis is included. This analysis took place on June 30, 1988. The analysis at which the study was terminated used data available through December 31, 1989. The patient survival data available for an analysis must be computed from the date on study, the date of last follow-up, the status variable, and the date of analysis. For a survival analysis, the observation times and indicators of failure are needed. The observation time will be zero if the date

Table 1   Sample of the Data

Variable	Case Data[a]			
Patient ID	1	2	3	4
Date on study (MMDDYY)	072384	071984	082984	090184
Treatment arm (D, daunorubicin; I, idarubicin)	D	D	I	I
Sex (M, male; F, female)	M	M	M	M
Age (years)	27	43	36	54
FAB classification (1–6)	5	3	1	1
Karnofsky score (0–100)	80	90	90	70
Baseline white blood cells ($10^3/mm^3$)	179.0	0.9	1.8	31.9
Baseline platelets ($10^3/mm^3$)	51	14	71	46
Baseline hemoglobin (g/dL)	8.8	13.1	6.9	10.8
Evaluable (Y, yes; N, no)	Y	Y	Y	Y
Complete remission (CR) (Y, yes; N, no)	N	N	N	Y
Courses of chemotherapy to CR	NA	NA	NA	1
Date of CR (MMDDYY)	NA	NA	NA	100884
Date of last follow-up (MMDDYY)	072984	082184	082585	010286
Status at last follow-up (D, dead; A, alive)	D	D	D	D
Bone marrow transplant (Y, yes; N, no)	N	N	N	N
Date of bone marrow transplant (MMDDYY)	NA	NA	NA	NA
Inclusion in June 30, 1988 analysis (Y, yes; N, no)	Y	Y	Y	Y

[a]NA, not applicable or not available.

on study is after the date of analysis. Otherwise, the observation time will be the minimum of the difference between the date of last follow-up and the date on study and the difference between the date of analysis and the date on study. The indicator of failure should be 1 if the date of last follow-up is prior to the date of analysis and the status variable is 1, and it should be 0 otherwise.

3 METHODS AND MODELS

To facilitate discussion, the data analysis is first discussed in the fixed sample (no interim analysis) setting; then the methods appropriate for group sequential monitoring of a clinical study are described.

3.1 Fixed-Sample Methods

In the classical study design, a clinical trial protocol specifies the number of patients to be accrued to each treatment arm. After all patients have been entered on study and their treatment outcomes observed, the data are analyzed. Such an analysis typically involves calculating point estimates, confidence intervals, and p-values, and deciding to reject or not to reject a null hypothesis.

In this clinical trial of idarubicin versus daunorubicin, the primary measure of treatment outcome was the induction of complete remission, a binary outcome. Comparisons of drug effectiveness can be modeled by assuming a binomial distribution for the number of patients Y_I and Y_D achieving a complete remission in the idarubicin and daunorubicin arms, respectively. That is, if N_I and N_D patients are accrued to the idarubicin and daunorubicin treatment arms, respectively, it is assumed that $Y_I \sim \mathscr{B}(N_I, p_I)$ and $Y_D \sim \mathscr{B}(N_D, p_D)$. The parameters p_I and p_D can be interpreted as the probabilities that a randomly selected patient receiving idarubicin or daunorubicin would achieve a complete remission.

The objective of detecting a difference in complete response rates by treatment can then be addressed statistically by testing the null hypothesis H_0: $p_I = p_D$ of no treatment effect versus the alternative H_1: $p_I \neq p_D$ of one treatment being more likely to result in induction of a complete remission. Estimates of the effect of treatment response rates can be based on the difference $p_I - p_D$ in treatment response rates.

With sufficiently large sample sizes, tests of H_0 versus H_1 are traditionally based on looking at the standardized difference between the two estimated response probabilities $\hat{p}_I = Y_I/N_I$ and $\hat{p}_D = Y_D/N_D$. The test statistic is

$$Z = \frac{\hat{p}_I - \hat{p}_D}{[\hat{p}(1 - \hat{p})(1/N_I + 1/N_D)]^{1/2}}, \tag{1}$$

where $\hat{p} = (Y_I + Y_D)/(N_I + N_D)$ is the estimate of a common response rate for the two arms under H_0. For sufficiently large sample sizes, the test statistic Z has an approximately standard normal distribution under the null hypothesis. Thus, an approximate two-sided level α test rejects H_0 in favor of H_1 whenever $|Z| \geq z_{1-\alpha/2}$, the $1 - \alpha/2$ quantile of the standard normal distribution. The p-value associated with a particular observation $Z = z$ is $2[1 - \Phi(|z|)]$, where $\Phi(\cdot)$ is the cumulative distribution function for a standard normal random variable. An approximate $100(1 - \alpha)\%$ confidence interval for the difference in treatment response rates is

$$(\hat{p}_I - \hat{p}_D) \pm z_{1-\alpha/2} \left[\frac{\hat{p}_I(1 - \hat{p}_I)}{N_I} + \frac{\hat{p}_D(1 - \hat{p}_D)}{N_D} \right]^{1/2}.$$

3.2   Group Sequential Test Designs

Due to the need for satisfying both ethical demands and efficiency considerations, studies involving human subjects are increasingly being monitored on interim bases. The primary objective of these analyses is to decide whether the trial should be prematurely stopped, and, subsequently, to curtail patient exposure to an inferior therapy. However, the naive practice of repeatedly applying fixed sample methods to accumulating data has the undesirable effect of inflating the type I statistical error above the presumed level (Armitage et al., 1969). Therefore, methods specific to the sequential nature of the clinical trial must be used.

Since Wald's seminal work (Wald, 1947) on sequential hypothesis testing, there has been much progress in developing practical statistical methods to account for interim analyses of data as they accrue (e.g., Pocock, 1977; O'Brien and Fleming, 1979; DeMets and Ware, 1980; Lan and DeMets, 1983). These approaches all provide stopping rules which define the conditions under which a clinical trial should be terminated. Most often, this stopping rule is specified by identifying those test statistic values that are sufficiently extreme to warrant rejection of or failure to reject the null hypothesis, even though the planned maximal sample size has not been accrued.

In the present trial, for example, the stopping rule might be defined for a maximum of m interim analyses, where the kth analysis would be performed after a total of N_{Ik} and N_{Dk} subjects have been accrued in the idarubicin and daunorubicin treatment arms, respectively. At each analysis, a test statistic Z_k would be computed as in (1). A commonly used form of a stopping rule consists of defining values $c_k, k = 1, \ldots, m$, such that the trial should be terminated when $|Z_k| \geq c_k$ or at the mth analysis.

The choice of the limits c_k affects the operating characteristics of the hypothesis test. In the form of the stopping rule considered here, the usual strategy is to choose the c_k's so that the statistical decision is to reject the null hypothesis H_0 in favor of the alternative H_1 if the study is terminated early at the kth analysis with $|Z_k| \geq c_k$ or if $|Z_m| \geq c_m$ at the mth analysis, and to fail to reject

H_0 if $|Z_m| < c_m$ at the final analysis. Thus, to achieve the desired type I error, the c_k's must be chosen to guarantee that $\Pr(|Z_k| < c_k, k = 1, \ldots, m) = 1 - \alpha$. This formulation of a stopping rule is a straightforward extension of the fixed sample setting, since in that case $m = 1$ and $c_1 = z_{1-\alpha/2}$ for a level α two-sided hypothesis test. However, as documented by Armitage et al. (1969), the naive choice of $c_k = z_{1-\alpha/2}$, the critical value for the fixed sample test, will not satisfy this constraint when $m > 1$.

It should be noted that more complicated stopping rules are easily fashioned. In general, a group sequential design is uniquely identified by specifying the maximum number of analyses m, and for $k = 1, \ldots, m$, the cumulative sample size N_k, the continuation set $\mathscr{C}_k$, and the stopping sets $\mathscr{S}_k^0$ and $\mathscr{S}_k^1$. At each analysis, a test statistic T_k is computed and compared to the corresponding continuation set $\mathscr{C}_k$. If $T_k \in \mathscr{C}_k$, the trial is continued to observe the $(k+1)$th group. Otherwise, the trial is stopped and the null hypothesis H_0 is accepted or rejected according to whether T_k is in $\mathscr{S}_k^0$ or $\mathscr{S}_k^1$, respectively. The continuation and stopping sets at each analysis are chosen such that the resulting hypothesis test has the desired operating characteristics (e.g., type I and II statistical errors). In the simple example given in the preceding paragraph for test statistic $T_k = |Z_k|$ with Z_k computed according to (1), the continuation sets and stopping sets are given by

$$
\begin{aligned}
\mathscr{C}_k &= [0, c_k), & k &= 1, \ldots, m-1, \\
\mathscr{C}_m &= \varnothing, \\
\mathscr{S}_k^0 &= \varnothing, & k &= 1, \ldots, m-1, \\
\mathscr{S}_m^0 &= [0, c_m), \\
\mathscr{S}_k^1 &= [c_k, \infty), & k &= 1, \ldots, m.
\end{aligned}
\tag{2}
$$

In this case study, only stopping rules of the form given by (2) are considered, although more general notation will be used at times for convenience. In the group sequential setting, the constraint imposed by fixing the type I error leaves some flexibility in the choice of the c_k's in (2). There are infinite ways to choose those limits and still have the desired type I error. Most often, there are still many choices available even if other operating characteristics (e.g., statistical power) are specified. To reduce the complexity of choosing suitable stopping rules, many designs proposed in the literature have parameterized the relationships among the c_k values, the boundaries of the continuation sets. That is, to reduce the complexity of choosing suitable stopping rules, many designs impose relationships between successive continuation sets. For instance, the Pocock (1977) designs are based on choices such that $c_k = c$, a constant, for all $k = 1, \ldots, m$. The O'Brien–Fleming (1979) designs choose the c_k values such that testing is extremely conservative at the earlier analyses and closer to the fixed sample test at the mth analysis. Specifically, if $N_{Ik} = N_{Dk} = N_k$ at each of the analyses, an O'Brien–Fleming design for the idarubicin trial would choose $c_k = c^*(N_m/N_k)^{1/2}$ where c^* is some constant. It should be noted that the constant c or c^* chosen for a particular stopping rule under either the Pocock or O'Brien–Fleming boundary relationships will depend on the desired overall type I error for the resulting group sequential test, as well as the choices for m and the N_k's.

An iterative, trial-and-error search is usually required to find a stopping rule that has the desired type I error. Such a search involves repeatedly guessing continuation and stopping sets, and then integrating the sampling density for the sequentially collected data over the stopping sets $\mathscr{S}_k^1, k = 1, \ldots, m$, under the assumption that the null hypothesis is true. When the continuation sets are parameterized by a single value, the search only involves refining estimates of that parameter to obtain the value corresponding to a test with the desired type I error, and thus the search for the appropriately sized test is greatly simplified.

Since the sample sizes used in this trial are sufficiently large for asymptotic results to be a good approximation, stopping rules appropriate for normally distributed data can be used. The approximate sampling distribution for the group sequential data can similarly be based on the normal distribution.

To find that sampling distribution, it is convenient to consider the individual observations of treatment outcome. Let Y_{Ij} be the indicator of complete remission for the jth subject on the idarubicin treatment arm as before, and let the Y_{Dj}'s be the similar measurements for the daunorubicin arm. Let

$$S_k = \sum_{j=1}^{N_{Ik}} Y_{Ij} - \sum_{j=1}^{N_{Dk}} Y_{Dj}.$$

If the accrual to the two treatment arms is balanced at each analysis, then $(S_k - S_{k-1})$, the data on the primary endpoint added between the $(k-1)$th and kth analyses, has an approximate $N(n_k\mu, n_k\sigma^2)$ distribution, where $\mu = p_I - p_D$, $\sigma^2 = p_I(1-p_I) + p_D(1-p_D)$, and n_k is defined by $N_k = N_{Ik} = N_{Dk} = \sum_{i=1}^k n_i$. Also, the independence among the individual patients guarantees the independent increment structure necessary for the usual group sequential test designs: $(S_k - S_{k-1})$ is independent of $S_{k-1}, k = 2, \ldots, m$. The problem of estimating the treatment effect thus reduces to estimating the mean of a normal distribution following a group sequential test of a fixed null hypothesis H_0: $\mu = 0$.

Since interest in the sampling distribution is directed toward the information the sample contains about the unknown parameter μ, the statistical problem can be reduced to finding the distribution of a statistic that is sufficient for μ (Bickel and Doksum, 1977, p. 63). For a clinical trial that terminates at analysis M, it can be shown that the bivariate statistic (N_M, Z_M) is a sufficient statistic for $\mu = p_I - p_D$. The distribution of (N_M, Z_M) can be derived from the density of (M, S_M), because $S_k = \sigma\sqrt{N_k} Z_k$. The density for the (M, S_M) can be computed using the method of Armitage et al. (1969) as

$$p(k, s; \mu) = \begin{cases} f(k, s; \mu), & \text{if } s \notin \mathscr{C}_k, \\ 0, & \text{otherwise,} \end{cases} \tag{3}$$

with $f(k, s; \mu)$ defined recursively by

$$f(1, s; \mu) = \frac{1}{\sqrt{n_1}\, \sigma} \phi\left(\frac{s - n_1 \mu}{\sqrt{n}\, \sigma}\right),$$

and

$$f(k, s; \mu) = \int_{\mathscr{C}_{k-1}} \frac{1}{\sqrt{n_k}\, \sigma} \phi\left(\frac{s - u - n_k \mu}{\sqrt{n_k}\, \sigma}\right) f(k - 1, u; \mu)\, du,$$

$$k = 2, \ldots, m,$$

where $\phi(\cdot)$ is the standard normal density. Although this form of the density appears complicated, computationally it is quite efficient. Heuristically, it can be seen that the density is reasonable. Since S_k is only defined if the clinical trial is not terminated prior to the kth analysis, the distribution of S_k for $k > 1$ is described by a subdensity, which does not integrate to 1. The function $f(1, s; \mu)$ is the density for S_1, and because $\Pr(S_k < s) = \Pr[(S_k - S_{k-1}) + S_{k-1} < s | S_{k-1} \in \mathscr{C}_{k-1}]$ with S_{k-1} and $(S_k - S_{k-1})$ independent, the subdensity for S_k is the convolution $f(k, s; \mu)$ of the density for $(S_k - S_{k-1})$ and the subdensity for S_{k-1}.

The density in (3) cannot be integrated in closed form, and computer programs are therefore needed to compute the type I error and other operating characteristics of a particular group sequential design. Furthermore, in that density, the unknown parameter μ is not a simple shift parameter. Thus, unlike the normal density, no standardized form of the density can be tabulated.

3.3 Estimation Following a Group Sequential Trial

The use of a group sequential stopping rule affects the sampling density for parameter estimates, thereby causing the usual fixed-sample point estimates to be biased toward the extremes and the fixed-sample confidence intervals to have incorrect coverage probabilities. More recently, exact methods for statistical inference about the estimation of treatment effects have received attention (e.g., Whitehead, 1983, 1986a,b; Tsiatis et al., 1984; Rosner and Tsiatis, 1988; Emerson and Fleming, 1990b).

When analyzing studies with fixed sample designs, it is common practice to provide a p-value as a quantification of the strength of evidence against the null hypothesis, and to provide point and interval estimates of the parameter measuring treatment effect to be able to judge the clinical importance of the trial results. A similar approach would be useful for studies designed with sequential stopping rules. A naive approach would be to use the results of the trial as if they arose in a fixed sample study, and to assume that the test statistics have the same approximate normal distributions as they would have under fixed-sample testing. In fact, however, the group sequential testing alters the sampling distribution of the test statistics in a complicated fashion. Figure 1 displays the distribution of that estimated difference in response rates, $\hat{p}_I - \hat{p}_D$, for selected values of $p_I - p_D$ when the group sequential nature of the sampling is taken into account. From this figure it can be seen that the group sequential distribution is markedly nonnormal and that the shape of the distribution varies as the difference in response rates changes. Because of this nonnormality, the usual fixed sample estimation techniques do not suffice. Instead, estimates based on the true sampling distribution for the test statistic must be found.

Using the density (3), estimates for the primary treatment effect which adjust for the stopping rule of the clinical trial can be found. Integration of the density over those outcomes more extreme than that observed allows p-values to be computed. Confidence intervals can be calculated by a search for the values of

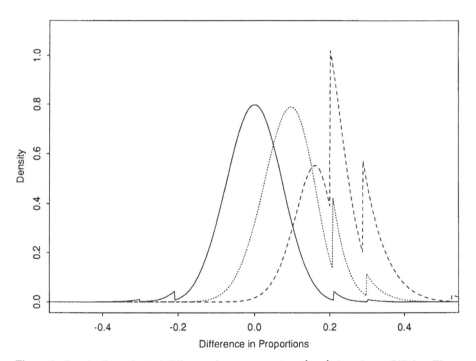

Figure 1. Density for estimated difference in response rates, $(\hat{p}_I - \hat{p}_D)$, under an O'Brien–Fleming (1979) group sequential design with analyses after accruing 25, 45, 65, and 90 patients per arm, and when the true difference in proportions is 0 (solid line), 0.1 (dotted line), and 0.2 (dashed line).

μ for which the observed outcome is not extreme. Point estimates can be derived using methods similar to those used in fixed-sample settings as follows:

1. The maximum likelihood estimate (MLE) is the sample mean S_M/N_M, just as in the fixed-sample case.
2. The uniform minimum variance estimate (UMVUE) can be found by conditioning any unbiased estimator on the complete sufficient statistic (Bickel and Doksum, 1977, p. 120). Emerson (1993) has described an algorithm for the computation of this estimate in the group sequential setting.
3. The bias adjusted mean (Whitehead, 1986a) assumes that the observed outcome is the expected value of the MLE under the true distribution of the group sequential test statistic. Thus, the bias adjusted mean is that value of μ for which the expectation of S_M/N_M (as computed using the above density) is equal to the observed sample mean.
4. A median unbiased estimate (MUE) assumes that the observed outcome is the median of the distribution of the group sequential test statistic.

In the fixed-sample, normal theory case, the four estimates listed above coincide. In the group sequential setting, however, the MLE is generally biased toward the extremes, and these four estimates tend to differ. The MLE, UMVUE, and bias-adjusted mean can be computed directly using the density. Calculation of p-values, confidence intervals, and the median unbiased point estimate, however, require the definition of an ordering of the two dimensional sample space. Because of the lack of monotone likelihood ratio in the unknown mean parameter, there is no universally optimal choice for that ordering.

Several orderings of the sample space have been proposed and compared by a number of authors for the problem of estimating the mean from normally distributed observations (Tsiatis et al., 1984; Rosner and Tsiatis, 1988; Chang, 1989; Emerson and Fleming, 1990b; Whitehead and Facey, 1992). We shall focus here on the estimates and p-values based on the sample mean ordering, which Emerson and Fleming (1990b) found to be well behaved with respect to a variety of criteria. In this case, the ordering of possible outcomes observed at different stopping times is dictated by the magnitude of the maximum likelihood estimate for the parameter measuring treatment effect. The ordering investigated by Tsiatis et al. (1984) is not as universally applicable and tends to average slightly wider confidence intervals, but because that ordering places more emphasis on the time at which the trial is stopped, it provides a useful comparison to the sample mean ordering. The estimates from the two orderings most often agree closely. When they disagree, it is usually a sign that the later accrued data were more extreme than the earliest data. For this reason we will also present estimates based on this "Tsiatis ordering."

3.4 Methods for Imprecisely Specified Stopping Rules

The methods for group sequential tests described above provide significant improvements in the conduct of clinical trials. However, application of these methods still entails as much art as science due to the complexity of clinical trial testing and the limitations of the methods developed to date.

Some of the ways in which the conduct of clinical trials departs from the methods described above do not present particularly difficult problems. For instance, in the earliest group sequential designs, the maximum number of analyses, m, and the cumulative sample sizes, the N_k's, were fixed in advance of the trial (Pocock, 1977; O'Brien and Fleming, 1979). The continuation and stopping sets were derived based on the sampling distribution of the prespecified test statistics, Z_k. Later designs did not completely specify the exact group sequential test prior to the study, thereby allowing the value of m and/or the value of some or all of the N_k's to be random (Slud and Wei, 1982; Lan and DeMets, 1983). Generally, these variations in the specification of the stopping rules have been addressed for the estimation techniques described above (Emerson and Fleming, 1990b).

There are other features of the typical clinical trial that pose problems for which statistical methods are not yet well defined. For example, before a trial is prematurely stopped, a data monitoring committee usually considers not only whether the group sequential boundary for the primary endpoint has been crossed, but also whether the data are sufficiently accurate and complete for all endpoints of interest, whether the magnitude of the observed effect is clinically relevant, whether the results for the primary endpoint are consistent with secondary measures of treatment effect and within meaningful subgroups, and whether the results are in line with concurrent studies. Statistical techniques cannot fully address all of these concerns. Therefore, the group sequential stopping rule does not generally function as a strict "rule" but rather as an important guideline to aid in the overall monitoring process (DeMets, 1984). Thus, at the end of a group sequential trial, the exact stopping rule may not be precisely known or may deviate from the stopping rule believed to have been used.

The situation is worsened when the decision to terminate the study early is driven by early, unplanned analyses of the data. In such cases, those early analyses should be considered as part of the stopping rule. The problem is that these unplanned analyses are often informal and poorly documented. This then raises the question of the extent to which inappropriate repeated significance testing early in a trial has caused the true type I error to be inflated above the nominal level. This problem is also present when unplanned analyses have been used to impose retrospectively a group sequential design, such as occurred in the idarubicin trial. In cases such as this, a p-value is more useful than the simple dichotomous decision of a hypothesis test. The situation in which group sequential methods have been improperly applied is similar to the problem of reporting only the conclusion of a hypothesis test. In fixed-sample hypothesis testing, if only the decision to reject or accept the null hypothesis is reported, all observers must agree on the level used to judge statistical significance. A decision to reject a null hypothesis using a 0.10 level of significance is noninformative to someone having a more stringent criterion for statistical significance. When a p-value is available, observers with more stringent criteria for rejecting a null hypothesis can evaluate the results of the study with respect to their own criteria.

Suppose that unplanned, informal analyses early in a study mean that the true stopping rule applied to the data corresponds to a group sequential test having a higher type I error than that originally planned. If the result of the hypothesis test is considered to be linked inextricably to the original stopping sets defined in the group sequential design, the decision to reject the null hypothesis is kept constant and the level of the test is altered. If the test had been performed properly, the conclusion of the study might be to reject H_0 using a 0.05 level of significance, but due to the errors in the conduct of the test, the early termination now corresponds to a decision to reject H_0 using a 0.10 level of significance. Again, reporting a p-value will allow other observers to evaluate the hypothesis test with respect to other standards.

In effect, the strategy proposed here dissociates the stopping rule from the hypothesis test. The stopping rule can be regarded as merely a sampling scheme which determines how many subjects are accrued to the study. Since the stopping rule is based on a measurement of the primary outcome estimated from the data accumulated prior to each analysis, the sampling density of the test statistic is clearly affected by the stopping rule (as shown in Figure 1). Thus, the stopping rule must be used to describe the distribution of the test statistic. Given the true stopping rule and some ordering of the outcome space, however, the probability, under H_0, of observing data more extreme than the results of the clinical trial can be computed, and that p-value used to make the decision regarding rejection of the null hypothesis. Thus, when the p-value is sufficiently small, the fact that the stopping rule might have corresponded to, say, a level 0.25 test need not affect our ability to reject the null at a much lower level of significance.

Such dissociation of the stopping rule and the hypothesis test is possible because the density of the test statistic is dependent only on the continuation sets, and is unaffected by the way in which the stopping sets are partitioned into $\mathscr{S}_k^0$ and $\mathscr{S}_k^1$ at the kth analysis. Thus, different observers can use different stopping sets to decide whether the null hypothesis is rejected, as long as they use the same continuation sets. Using the p-value based on some ordering of the outcome space as the criterion for rejecting H_0 simply redefines the stopping sets in such a way as to ensure the desired type I error. In this redefinition, it is possible that the study is terminated early due to the observation of a relatively high value of the test statistic (i.e., smaller values of the test statistic would have caused the study to continue), but the p-value associated with that early outcome is too large to allow rejection of the null hypothesis of a small or no-treatment effect. This may result in markedly inefficient statistical tests but does not affect the size of the test.

In this manner, the sensitivity of the analysis to misspecification of the stopping rule can be explored by considering a class of plausible stopping rules. To do this, some restricted set of designs must be chosen which covers the spectrum of likely stopping rules. Consideration is restricted here to a class of designs similar to those of Wang and Tsiatis (1987), but expanded to include testing after unequal group sizes in the manner used by Emerson and Fleming (1989) for the symmetric group sequential designs.

The Wang and Tsiatis designs are all of the form specified by (2). For a given level of significance α and analysis times specified by $\mathbf{N} = (N_1, N_2, \ldots, N_m)$, the c_k values are defined by $c_k = c(\alpha, \mathbf{N}, p)/(N_k/N_m)^{0.5-p}$, where the critical value $c(\alpha, \mathbf{N}, p)$ can be found by integrating the density for the group sequential test statistic in an iterative search to find the test which has the appropriate size.

By using this family of group sequential test designs, a spectrum of reasonable estimates for the unknown stopping rule can be considered by varying the following parameters:

1. *The Boundary Relationship Parameter p.* This parameter measures the degree of conservatism applied at earlier analyses relative to the later analyses. When $p = 0$, this corresponds to an O'Brien and Fleming (1979) type of boundary relationship; when $p = 0.5$, the test is similar to a Pocock (1977) design. These two values for p tend to lie at the extremes of boundary relationships commonly used in applications of group sequential test designs.

2. *The Sample Sizes at Each of the Analyses* $\mathbf{N}$. For the idarubicin trial, the putative stopping rule is based on $N_m = 180$ and roughly equally spaced analyses, but the possibility that the true sample size would have been different from what was planned must also be considered, as well as the effect of more frequent monitoring prior to stopping.

3. *The Level of Significance of the Group Sequential Test Which Corresponds to the Stopping Rule* α. As stated above, there is no real interest in using the stopping rule to define the critical region for a hypothesis test. However, for specified values of p and the N_k's, the size of the resulting test is a convenient measure of the location of the critical value at each analysis. For the idarubicin trial, bounds can be placed on the size of the test by considering the results of the analysis when the accrued sample size was 45 per arm and the study was continued, and the results when the accrued sample size was 65 per arm and the study was stopped. Thus, it is reasonable to consider only those test designs which are consistent with those two decisions.

Several test designs are identified which tend to include the worst cases among the plausible stopping rules. Obviously, the choices are somewhat arbitrary, but they can nevertheless serve to quantify the degree to which the uncertainty regarding the true stopping rule affects our inference about the benefit of idarubicin versus daunorubicin. For each such design, the bias adjusted mean, sample mean–based 95% confidence interval, and sample mean–based p-value are computed. Of the various stopping rule parameters open to question in this clinical trial, the most uncertainty was expressed about the number of interim analyses which had been performed and which might have influenced the decision to terminate the trial. A secondary issue was the possible effect that varying maximum sample size might have had on the operating characteristics of the test. There was relatively little concern about the boundary relationships or the nominal size of the test since the level 0.05 O'Brien–Fleming boundaries had been specified prior to the first formal analyses. Thus, exploration of the effect of varying the latter parameters is primarily for illustrative purposes, but it should be noted that the earliest informal looks at the data could have influenced the choice of stopping rules.

4   RESULTS

4.1   Results of the Hypothesis Test

Discussion of the results of the clinical trial shall be limited to those analyses based on comparison of the two treatment arms without adjustment for other variables. Because the treatment groups accrued to the study were comparable with respect to baseline characteristics, such a restriction should not unduly bias the results. Table 2 presents the results of analyses of the primary remission endpoint, as well as the secondary survival endpoint analyzed using the logrank test, at each of the analyses. Also included is the stopping boundary dictated by the O'Brien–Fleming group sequential test design adopted for use in this study. The first analysis of response rates did not exhibit sufficiently strong evidence of a difference between treatment arms to warrant termination of the study. Based primarily on the results of the second analysis, however, patient accrual to the daunorubicin arm was stopped in June 1989. At that time, 78% of patients on the idarubicin arm had achieved a complete remission compared to 58% on the daunorubicin arm. The test statistic $Z_2 = 2.454$ exceeded the O'Brien–Fleming stopping boundary of 2.382. The final results of other selected secondary endpoints are also included in Table 2, and these results also influenced the decision to terminate the study, although not through a formal stopping rule. Patients on the idarubicin arm who achieved complete remission tended to be less likely to require two induction courses (31% for idarubicin versus 50% for daunorubicin), and there was also a trend toward more treatment failures due to resistant disease on the daunorubicin arm than on the idarubicin arm. Follow-up survival data were collected for all patients up to December 31, 1989, and the Kaplan–Meier survival curves are displayed in Figure 2.

Table 2 Summary of Efficacy Analyses

	Treatment Arm[a]		Test Statistic[b]	Group Sequential Critical Value
	IDR	DNR		
	First Analysis			
Number of patients	45	45		
Number of complete remissions (%)	35 (78%)	25 (56%)	2.236	2.863
Number of CR[c] after one course (% of CR)	24 (69%)	12 (48%)		
	Second Analysis			
Number of patients	65	65		
Number of CR (%)	51 (78%)	38 (58%)	2.454	2.382
Number of CR after one course (% of CR)	35 (69%)	19 (50%)		
Number of resistant disease (% of failed CR)	8 (57%)	20 (74%)		

[a]IDR, idarubicin; DNR, daunorubicin.
[b]Value of test statistic for test of binomial proportions Under the null hypothesis of no treatment effect, the statistic has a standard normal distribution.
[c]CR, complete remission.

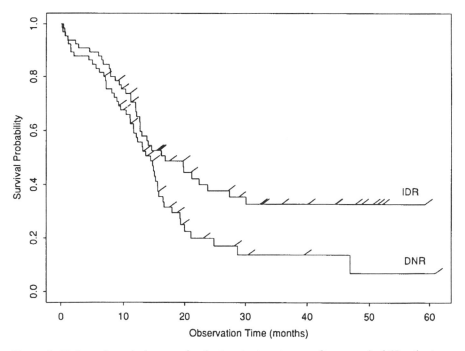

Figure 2. Estimated survival curves for the two treatment arms after accrual of 65 patients per arm. (IDR = idarubicin, DNR = daunorubicin).

4.2　Estimates Adjusting for the Putative Stopping Rule

The clinical trial investigators, guided by the early stopping under the O'Brien–Fleming design, concluded from these data that idarubicin represented a potential improvement in the chemotherapy of acute myelogenous leukemia (Berman et al., 1991). The results of this study and three other controlled comparative clinical trials (Mandelli et al., 1991; Wiernik et al., 1992; Vogler et al., 1992) were used in part to support a New Drug Application filed in August 1989 with the FDA to gain approval for the marketing of idarubicin for the treatment of acute myelogenous leukemia. During such a process, it becomes important to derive estimates for the magnitude of the treatment effect, in addition to reporting the outcome of the hypothesis tests. During their review of the application, the FDA raised two major questions regarding the interpretation of the final results of this study. First, since the interim analyses were not planned in advance, can it be trusted that the probability of type I error had not been inflated above the nominal 0.05 level? Second, since it is presumed that induction of a complete remission influences the chances of long-term survival for these patients, is it not likely that the reported estimate of treatment effect on survival is biased by the group sequential test of complete response rates? The first of these questions is addressed in detail here. Space limitations preclude discussion of the question related to survival.

A naive approach to these more detailed analyses is to use the results presented in Table 2 as if they arose in a fixed-sample study. Such an approach would suggest that the best estimate of the difference between response rates was 0.2 (95% confidence interval 0.04 to 0.36, p-value 0.014). These estimates are based on the assumption that the test statistic is approximately normally distributed, as it would be under fixed-sample testing. It is interesting to note that in their report of this trial, Berman et al. (1991) reported only these naive estimates and p-values.

More appropriate estimates will be obtained by using methods that adjust for the interim analyses. Under the supposition that the retroactively imposed O'Brien–Fleming stopping rule accurately reflects the true sampling scheme, Table 3 presents the adjusted estimates of treatment effect on the primary endpoint of the difference between proportions of patients attaining a complete remission. For comparison, the naive estimates based on the usual fixed-sample methods are also included. It should be noted again that the fixed sample point estimate is also the MLE for the group sequential setting, although it is biased by the use of an early stopping rule. Emerson and Fleming (1990b) observed that the bias-adjusted mean had less bias than the MLE or the median unbiased estimate based on either the sample mean or Tsiatis ordering, and tended to have lower mean-squared error than the UMVUE, and recommended the use of the bias-adjusted mean for those reasons. In this trial, the bias adjusted mean is approximately 10% less than the MLE. There is also relatively less of a difference among the adjusted estimates (bias adjusted mean, median unbiased estimate, UMVUE) compared to the difference between any adjusted estimate and the MLE.

Table 3 Estimates of Treatment Effect Adjusted for Interim
Analyses

	Induction of CR[a] $(p_I - p_D)$
Fixed-sample analysis	
p-Value	0.014
Maximum likelihood estimate	0.2000
95% confidence interval	0.044, 0.356
Estimates adjusted for interim analyses	
Bias-adjusted mean	0.1837
UMVUE	0.1931
Sample mean ordering	
p-Value	0.017
Median unbiased estimate	0.1858
95% confidence interval	0.034, 0.334
Tsiatis ordering	
p-Value	0.016
Median unbiased estimate	0.1995
95% confidence interval	0.038, 0.361

[a]CR, complete remission.

With respect to 95% confidence intervals, there is relatively little difference between the intervals derived from the two orderings. The sample mean ordering produces a slightly narrower confidence interval, which is in keeping with the trend in the results observed by Emerson and Fleming (1990b). Both of these adjusted confidence intervals are wider and closer to the null value than is the fixed-sample interval. These adjusted confidence intervals are guaranteed to agree with the results of the group sequential test in that they will not contain the null value if and only if the group sequential test rejects the null hypothesis. This property is not always satisfied by the fixed-sample confidence intervals, nor by some adjusted confidence intervals based on other orderings of the sample space (Emerson and Fleming, 1990b).

The adjusted p-values are quite similar to those based on the fixed-sample p-value. This is primarily a reflection of the O'Brien–Fleming boundary relationships which test extremely conservatively at earlier analyses. From these results it can be concluded that idarubicin represents a statistically significant and clinically important improvement over daunorubicin with respect to induction of complete remission in acute myelogenous leukemia.

4.3 Sensitivity Analysis of Misspecified Stopping Rules

Table 4 presents the adjusted estimates for representative designs. The focus is on designs that vary in the number of early analyses which are performed.

Table 4   Sensitivity of Analyses of Remission Rates to Variation in Stopping Rules

Timing of Interim Analyses (N_k's)[a]	O'Brien–Fleming (1979) Boundaries ($p = 0$)		Pocock (1977) Boundaries ($p = 0.5$)	
	Best Case[b]	Worst Case[b]	Best Case	Worst Case
45 65 90				
Size[c]	0.043	0.187	0.030	0.084
p-Value	0.017	0.046	0.024	0.046
95% Confidence interval	0.035, 0.327	0.003, 0.348	0.025, 0.325	0.003, 0.343
Bias-adjusted mean	0.1854	0.1816	0.1823	0.1807
UMVUE	0.1950	0.1569	0.1795	0.1567
25 45 65 90				
Size	0.043	0.188	0.039	0.107
p-Value	0.017	0.048	0.033	0.073
95% Confidence interval	0.035, 0.327	0.001, 0.348	0.016, 0.324	−0.018, 0.339
Bias-adjusted mean	0.1845	0.1728	0.1710	0.1643
UMVUE	0.1949	0.1535	0.1662	0.1358
12 25 45 65 90				
Size	0.043	0.188	0.049	0.133
p-Value	0.017	0.048	0.043	0.100
95% Confidence interval	0.035, 0.327	0.001, 0.348	0.006, 0.323	−0.038, 0.337
Bias-adjusted mean	0.1845	0.1725	0.1614	0.1489
UMVUE	0.1949	0.1534	0.1553	0.1181
12 25 35 45 65 90				
Size	0.043	0.191	0.053	0.141
p-Value	0.017	0.054	0.047	0.110
95% Confidence interval	0.034, 0.327	−0.003, 0.347	0.003, 0.322	−0.044, 0.335
Bias-adjusted mean	0.1825	0.1684	0.1594	0.1471
UMVUE	0.1940	0.1487	0.1514	0.1133

[a] Sample size per treatment arm at the $k = 1, \ldots, m$ analyses.
[b] Best case assumes that the stopping rule was barely exceeded at the second formal analysis (sample size $N_2 = 65$ per arm). Worst case assumes a stopping boundary nearly as low as the results at the first formal analysis (sample size $N_1 = 45$ per arm).
[c] Size of group sequential test corresponding to stopping boundaries.

Although not presented here, there was very little difference in the estimates as the maximal sample size, N_m, was varied by ±17%. Such variation affected the sample mean ordering based p-values by ±0.0001 and the bias adjusted mean by ±0.004. This is in keeping with the findings of Emerson and Fleming (1990b) that the estimation techniques that are based on the sample mean ordering are relatively robust to misspecification of future analysis times. The Tsiatis ordering-based estimates, as well as the UMVUE, are unaffected by the choice of future analysis times.

In Table 4, the "best case" O'Brien–Fleming designs are closest to the putative stopping rule for the clinical trial. Varying the number of early analyses has little effect on the p-values or estimates of treatment effect. When the possibility is considered that less stringent O'Brien–Fleming stopping boundaries might have been used (i.e., corresponding to group sequential tests with larger type I errors), there is more variation in the estimates. However, the p-values generally suggest that using a 0.05 level of significance would still result in a conclusion that there is a statistically significant improvement in response rates associated with idarubicin therapy. Even if it is assumed that the true stopping rule corresponded to a 0.191-level O'Brien–Fleming test with a maximum of $m = 6$ analyses, the p-value for the observed results is 0.054.

The estimates based on Pocock stopping boundaries are also included in Table 4. There is more variability in the estimates for these designs, even for the best case designs, which correspond to the assumption that the results at the second formal analysis were just barely extreme enough to justify stopping the trial. Even so, for all of the best case designs presented, the decision would be in favor of a beneficial effect due to idarubicin therapy. For the worst case designs, on the other hand, it might have been decided that the study was inconclusive, because the observed results were not more extreme than those observed by random chance under the null hypothesis of no treatment effect. That is, when adjustment was made for an interim analysis occurring before the first formal analysis, the computed sequential p-value exceeded the 0.05 level of significance. This situation is an important case to consider when no formal stopping rule was specified because the naive practice of repeatedly applying fixed-sample hypothesis tests corresponds to monitoring with a Pocock boundary relationship. For this trial the worst case boundary would correspond to repeatedly performing level 0.04 hypothesis tests. Thus, repeatedly applying roughly level 0.05 hypothesis tests would provide less evidence against the null hypothesis, and would probably raise concerns on the appropriateness of stopping at $N_2 = 130$ patients.

Inference has been made primarily on the estimates based on the sample mean ordering and the bias adjusted mean. For all stopping rules explored with these data, the p-value based on the Tsiatis ordering varied by less than 0.013 from the sample mean ordering based p-value. For comparison purposes, the UMVUE estimates have been included in Table 4. These estimates are more affected by which stopping rule is assumed. This is in keeping with this estimator's tendency toward greater mean-squared error relative to the bias adjusted mean, which was observed by Emerson and Fleming (1990b).

5 CONCLUSIONS

Other approaches are available to address the problem of unplanned interim analyses or poorly quantified stopping rules, most notably repeated confidence intervals (RCIs) (Jennison and Turnbull, 1984, 1989) and Bayesian methods. The RCIs entail the same sort of sensitivity analyses as presented here, since they are in essence based on stopping rules. To make an inference using RCIs, they should ideally correspond to the sampling scheme used, so efforts must still be made to identify the stopping rule in effect. Furthermore, since they are generally more conservative than the estimates presented in this analysis, the use of RCIs will lead to less efficient analyses.

Bayesian methods are extremely attractive in sequential analysis primarily because they are unaffected by the number and timing of interim analyses performed. The major disadvantage of a Bayesian analysis, and the reason Bayesian approaches are not widely used in clinical trials, is the extreme sensitivity of the analysis to the choice of prior distribution for the unknown parameter. To circumvent this problem, a class of prior distributions can be considered, examining the consistency of results across choices of priors within that class. Such an approach is similar to the sensitivity analysis presented here and is preferred by some statisticians because they have greater interest in the Bayes posterior probability than in the frequentist p-value.

In this case study, attention has been restricted to the frequentist approach. In doing so, only certain estimators have been selected for presentation. There is not yet wide agreement on the best estimates to use following a group sequential test, and lacking theory to provide optimal choices, it is likely that multiple methods will continue to be used.

The common feature shared by almost all of the estimates that adjust for interim analyses is the requirement for relatively intricate computer software to compute the estimates. Conceptually, calculation of each of the estimates is based on integration of the density for the statistic (N_M, S_M). A relatively small number of routines suffice for computation of all the estimates considered here (Emerson, 1993). In practice, however, the required calculations involve extensive recursive numerical integration, and the necessary routines have not been incorporated into the more common statistical analysis packages. Specialized programs are available which are capable of handling specific group sequential designs and which can compute selected estimates (Whitehead and Marek, 1985; Emerson, 1992), and as sequential analysis of clinical trials becomes more widespread, the availability of software should likewise increase.

The problem of an unknown stopping rule is one that can be minimized by planning interim analyses in advance. If the stopping rule is specified completely and reliably, the analyses of Section 3.2 may suffice. However, there will almost always be some component of the stopping rule that is poorly quantified. Although there has been much progress in the development of methods that allow flexibility in the timing of interim analyses, statistical techniques are not well developed for analysis of multiple endpoints or for incorporating the results of concurrent trials into the decision to terminate a group sequential trial. Data monitoring committees usually must consider many factors beyond the putative primary endpoint, and thus the stopping rule is approximate at best.

For the clinical trial presented here, analyses along the lines presented in Section 4 were used successfully in support of the new drug application for idarubicin. In those analyses, the hypothesis test was not decided solely on the stopping sets of the group sequential test. Instead, the stopping rule was used to estimate the sampling density for a statistic estimating treatment effect, and a typical frequentist analysis based on that sampling density generated p-values, point estimates, and confidence intervals. To the extent that the stopping rule was unknown, a class of sampling densities was explored, and the consistency of the statistical inference across those candidate densities was examined.

The ultimate goal of the sensitivity analyses is to place bounds on the precision of estimates of treatment effect and level of significance when the stopping rule is poorly quantified. The variability in the adjusted estimates and sequential p-values as different stopping rules were considered also attests to the importance of presenting study results in a manner which accounts for any interim analyses performed on the accruing data. In particular, reporting p-values computed under standard fixed samples can be quite misleading and should be avoided.

ACKNOWLEDGMENTS

This research was supported in part by a grant from the National Cancer Institute. The authors thank Ellen Berman and Glenn Heller for permission to use the data from this clinical trial for our illustration.

QUESTIONS AND PROBLEMS

1. What are the relative advantages and disadvantages of the various estimators used to adjust for the effect of interim analyses?

2. In the sensitivity analyses presented here, little attention was paid to the number and timing of analyses which might have followed that at which the study was terminated. Why is this reasonable?

3. The analyses of the primary endpoint that were considered here did not adjust for baseline risk factors. What is the justification for that approach? How would group sequential methods be applied to analyses adjusted for covariates such as age, sex, and baseline hematologic measurements?

4. There are several subtypes of acute myelogenous leukemia as classified by the FAB (French, American, British) classification scheme. Is there any evidence that the difference between idarubicin and daunorubicin treatment effects was dependent upon the FAB classification of the patients' disease? How would an analysis of this question adjust for the interim analyses?

CHAPTER 15

Early Lung Cancer Detection Studies

Betty J. Flehinger and Marek Kimmel

1 MOTIVATION AND BACKGROUND

The Cooperative Early Lung Cancer Detection Program was a set of three parallel clinical trials sponsored in the early 1970s by the National Cancer Institute. The trials were conducted at the Johns Hopkins Medical Institutions in Baltimore, Maryland; the Memorial Sloan-Kettering Cancer Center in New York, New York; and the Mayo Clinic in Rochester, Minnesota. In each of these trials, approximately 10,000 men at high risk of lung cancer were recruited and randomly assigned to two groups with contrasting levels of screening. Screening continued through 1982, with two additional years of follow-up. Numerous papers have been written presenting and analyzing various aspects of the data that were carefully collected by the three institutions (Berlin et al., 1984; Flehinger et al., 1984; Fontana et al., 1984, 1986; Frost et al., 1984; Melamed et al., 1977, 1981, 1984, 1990). This case study is intended to summarize the design of the trials, the methods of analysis used, and the results obtained.

According to recent estimates (Boring et al., 1992), lung cancer is responsible for more than 135,000 deaths in the United States, more than double the mortality attributable to cancer of any other site. In the 50 years from 1940 to 1990 the lung cancer death rate for men increased from 10 to 75 per 100,000; in women this increase has been from 3 to 30 per 100,000. This dramatic change is caused primarily by cigarette smoking, and the success of smoking cessation programs has been limited to restricted segments of the American population.

Survival of lung cancer patients in the general U.S. population is currently limited to 13% at five years after detection. The treatment of choice is surgical resection, but the possibility of cure rests primarily on detection of the cancer in

Case Studies in Biometry, Edited by Nicholas Lange, Louise Ryan, Lynne Billard,
David Brillinger, Loveday Conquest, and Joel Greenhouse.
ISBN 0-471-58885-7 © 1994 John Wiley & Sons, Inc.

an asymptomatic, localized stage. Therefore, much attention has been focused on methods of detecting lung cancer before it becomes symptomatic.

In the years before 1970, there were three studies of chest roentgenography as a tool for early detection (Brett 1969; Nash et al., 1986; Weiss et al., 1982). None of them demonstrated any significant reduction in mortality attributable to x-ray screening. In 1971, there were two available methods for detection of early lung cancer, the chest x-ray and sputum cytology. Sputum cytology had been successful in identifying cases of squamous cell lung cancer while it was still radiologically occult. However, before 1968, cases so identified were difficult to localize prior to surgery and sputum cytology did not appear to be a promising method of early detection. In 1968 (Ikeda et al., 1968), with the introduction of the fiber-optic bronchoscope, it appeared that very small radiographically occult tumors that were shedding cancer cells could be accurately localized and surgically resected, preferably by lobectomy.

At that point it appeared possible that lung cancer mortality might be substantially reduced by screening with sputum cytology in addition to periodic chest x-rays, coupled with a systematic procedure for diagnosis and treatment. Therefore, clinical trials were initiated simultaneously at the Johns Hopkins Medical Institutions (Hopkins), the Mayo Clinic (Mayo), and the Memorial Sloan-Kettering Cancer Center (MSKCC). The trials were designed to determine "(1) whether detection of lung cancer can be improved by adding modern sputum cytologic screening techniques to the examination at regular intervals by chest radiography, and (2) whether the mortality from lung cancer can be reduced significantly by this type of screening program followed by newer localizing methods and appropriate treatment" (Berlin et al., 1984, p. 545).

Each of the three institutions enrolled approximately 10,000 men over the age of 45 who smoked at least a pack of cigarettes daily. These participants were randomly assigned, half to study groups to be screened intensively and half to control groups which received less intensive screening. Enrollment was complete by 1978; all participants were screened for at least five years and followed for at least one extra year.

Study Design

The Hopkins and MSKCC studies had identical designs (Flehinger et al., 1988) (Figure 1), intended to compare the efficacy of adding periodic sputum examinations to the annual chest x-ray with the efficacy of the annual chest x-ray alone. The control group was offered posterior–anterior and lateral chest x-rays at enrollment and annually thereafter; the study group was asked to submit sputum specimens every four months in addition to the annual radiographic examinations. Active screening was continued until all participants had been enrolled for at least five years. Any positive or suspicious findings were carefully investigated, and surgery was offered whenever resection of lung cancer seemed feasible. Follow-up staffs in both centers urged all participants to follow their assigned screening schedules, and all enrollees were followed through

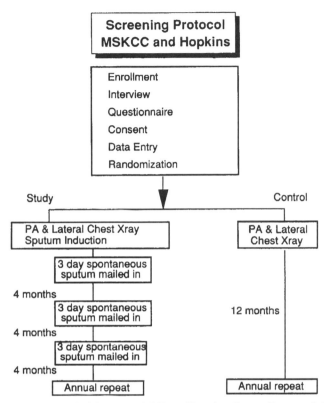

Figure 1. Screening protocol of the Memorial Sloan-Kettering Cancer Center and the Johns Hopkins Medical Institutions.

1984 to determine their survival and cancer status even if they failed to comply with the screening schedules. Approximately 0.5% were lost to follow-up at the end of 10 years. All deaths in the study population were individually reviewed by a mortality review committee, consisting of pulmonary physicians, pathologists, and biostatisticians from the cooperating institutions to determine whether death was due to lung cancer (Flehinger et al., 1988, p. 388). The only reason for exclusion was a reported history of lung cancer prior to enrollment.

The Mayo Lung Program (MLP) was designed to compare a program of four-monthly dual-modality screening to simple Mayo Clinic advice about annual screening (Figure 2). According to Fontana et al. (1984):

The MLP used Mayo Clinic outpatients as study and control groups. The design of the MLP is as follows: 10,993 Mayo outpatients who were men over 45 years old without known lung cancer and who were smokers of at least one package of cigarettes daily received 36 cm × 43 cm chest roentgenograms and three-day "pooled" sputum cytology tests. If either test proved positive for lung cancer on this

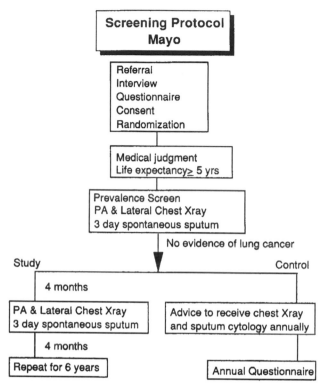

Figure 2. Screening protocol of the Mayo Clinic.

initial screening the patient became a "prevalence" case. There were 91 such cases, a prevalence rate of 8.3 per thousand offered the screening. The rate increased rapidly with age, from one per thousand among men 45 to 49 years old to 17 per thousand among men age 65 and older.

There were 9,211 men who completed the initial screen with results that were reported as satisfactory and negative and who also met certain other criteria for continued screening (life expectancy at least five years, mentally competent, pulmonary resection—at least lobectomy—possible). These men were subsequently studied in two randomized groups.

In the screened group, there were 4,618 patients who were asked, and reminded, to have chest roentgenograms and three-day "pooled" sputum cytology tests at 4-monthly intervals for a period of six years. Intensive efforts were made to secure compliance. Non-compliant patients and those who had completed six years of screening were contacted yearly by letter.

The control group of 4,593 patients received only the standard 1970 Mayo recommendation concerning yearly chest x-ray films and sputum tests. No reminders or questions about tests were sent, but contact was maintained by annual follow-up letter.

Thus, the Mayo study focused on evaluating intensive screening with both sputum cytology and chest x-ray compared to little or no screening, while Hopkins and MSKCC tried to determine the additional value of sputum cytology with the chest x-ray used identically in both study and control groups. Another major difference is that Mayo screened study and control participants with both chest x-ray and sputum cytology at enrollment and excluded all detected "prevalence" cases from their comparison study. At MSKCC and Hopkins, only the study group received cytologic screening initially and detected "prevalence" cases were included in comparison statistics.

The following statistical considerations applied to each of the three studies: In the enrolled populations, the annual death rate from lung cancer was estimated to be 3 per 1000 person-years. Assuming that the screening procedure might reduce the death rate by one-half, it was estimated that approximately 20,000 person-years of observation would be required in each arm of each study to achieve 90% probability of demonstrating a mortality difference significant at the 5% level. It was recognized that imperfect compliance and contamination of the control group would increase the required person-years of observation.

2 DATA

The basic results of the three parallel studies are summarized in this section and in Table 1. In addition, Section 2.1 describes an assessment of the effect of surgery on survival from stage I non-small cell lung cancer. In Table 1, total lung cancers and non-small cell lung cancers are listed separately, because

Table 1   Cooperative Early Lung Cancer Group Major Statistics[a]

	MSKCC		Hopkins		Mayo	
	Study	Control	Study	Control	Study	Control
Population	5226	5161	4968	5072	4618	4593
Total lung cancers[b]	147	146	226	241	151	121
Non-small cell[b]	126	124	186	200	115	87
Stage I non-small cell[b]	55	52	90	78	55	21
Lung cancer deaths[c]	94	95	139	165	80	72
Non-small cell deaths[c]	74	74	102	128	50	43

[a]The MSKCC data were abstracted from files maintained by the investigators; the Hopkins and Mayo data were abstracted from a tape obtained from the National Cancer Institute.

[b]The cancer counts refer to cancers detected by screening or diagnosed as interval cases during the years when active screening was offered.

[c]The cancer death counts refer to deaths from cancer of the patients described above. In MSKCC, deaths before the end of 1986, in Hopkins those who died by the end of 1983, and in Mayo those who died within seven years of enrollment were included.

small-cell lung cancer progresses too rapidly to be amenable to early detection and treatment. If screening is to have any value, it must lie in the detection of stage I non-small cell lung cancer, since all other cases have extremely small five-year survival probability. Hence, a separate line indicates the number of stage I cancers. It is to be noted that the Mayo comparison demonstrated a substantial excess of stage I cancers found in the study group. However, this did not seem to affect mortality since the number of lung cancer deaths was actually somewhat greater in the study group than among the controls. The MSKCC study resulted in closely matched results for study and control groups although 14 cases of squamous cell cancer were detected by sputum cytology while still radiographically occult. In Hopkins, where the total number of lung cancers was very large, more were found among controls than in the study group, although 22 radiologically occult cases were detected cytologically. Correspondingly, there were slightly more cancer deaths among controls. None of these comparisons were statistically significant. The conclusion was that these studies failed to prove that the addition of four-monthly sputum cytology to a program of periodic x-ray examinations would decrease lung cancer mortality. Table 2 shows a sample of the data available on each of the 1,032 cancers diagnosed during the period of active screening.

Effect of Surgical Treatment on Survival

The results of the Hopkins and MSKCC studies indicated that sputum cytology provides no significant mortality benefit over annual chest x-ray examinations. However, since both study and control groups were offered the same program of annual chest x-rays, a comparison of deaths in the two groups provides no information about the value of radiographic screening. In the Mayo study, where four-monthly sputum and x-ray examinations were contrasted with Mayo Clinic advice, no mortality benefit was demonstrated. In a recent article (Eddy, 1989), this result was explained with an analysis which concluded that "the data are consistent with the hypothesis that many of the lesions detected by screening and labeled as cancers were not clinically important in the sense that they would never have become clinically evident during the time of the clinical trial and follow-up (approximately twelve years)." If this explanation were correct, the survival of stage I patients would be the same whether they were treated surgically or not. Ethical considerations have always precluded randomized clinical trials comparing resection of stage I lung cancer to no treatment at all. However, a careful review of data gathered by all three institutions revealed that a sizable number of stage I cancers failed to be resected either because patients refused surgery or because the surgeons believed that there were medical contraindications to surgery. Since these were all stage I cancers, the decisions not to operate were in no case related to the resectability of the tumor. Therefore, a comparison of times to lung cancer death in surgical versus nonsurgical cases sheds light on the efficacy of surgical treatment of early lung cancer (Flehinger et al., 1992).

Table 2   Sample of Data Collected on 1032 Men Diagnosed with Lung Cancer during the Period of Active Screening in the Cooperative Early Lung Cancer Group[a]

id	inst	gr	det	ct	st	T	N	M	op	surv	stat
1	0	0	3	1	1	1	0	0	1	2672	0
2	0	0	1	1	2	2	1	0	1	819	1
3	0	1	2	0	3	2	2	0	0	518	1
4	0	1	0	0	1	1	0	0	1	2590	0
5	0	1	1	1	1	1	0	0	1	3862	0
6	0	0	1	3	1	1	0	0	1	561	1

[a]Data elements and their codes:

Patient ID (id): Integer
Institution (inst): 0   Memorial Sloan-Kettering
                   1   Mayo Clinic
                   2   Johns Hopkins
Group (gr): 0   Control
            1   Study
Means of detection (det): 0   Routine cytology
                          1   Routine x-ray
                          2   Both x-ray and cytology
                          3   Interval
Cell type (ct): 0   Epidermoid
                1   Adenocarcinoma
                2   Large cell
                3   Small cell
                4   Other
Stage: four digits   1st digit (st) $(1, 2, 3)$ Overall stage
                      2nd digit (T) $(1, 2, 3)$ Tumor
                      3rd digit (N) $(0, 1, 2)$ Lymph nodes
                      4th digit (M) $(0, 1)$ Distant metastases
Operated (op) : 0   No
                1   Yes
Survival (surv): Integer   Days from detection to last date alive
Status (stat): 0   Alive
               1   Dead of lung cancer
               2   Dead of other causes
Missing values: '–'

All cases of early stage non-small cell lung cancer diagnosed in the years 1974 to 1984 in the populations enrolled in the studies were identified. For each case identified, it was determined whether the patient was surgically explored and the tumor resected. The survival probability after detection for the surgical group was compared to that of the nonsurgical group (Kaplan and Meier, 1958). Endpoints for this analysis were death due to lung cancer, including postoperative deaths. Deaths from other causes were treated as censored observations. Survival estimates for surgical patients were almost identical for all three institutions (Flehinger et al., 1992). Every death of a man enrolled in this program had been reviewed by a committee of chest physicians and pathologists from all three institutions who met every four months to examine all records and to determine whether death was due to lung cancer. The statistical significance of all survival comparisons was computed by both the log-rank test and the modified Wilcoxon test (Elandt-Johnson and Johnson 1980, Chapter 8).

The estimated survival distributions are plotted in Figure 3. The five-year survival probability after surgery was 70% and the five-year survival probability of the nonsurgical patients was 10%. This difference is significant at $p = 0.02$ by the log-rank test and at $p < 0.001$ by the modified Wilcoxon test. There were only two five-year survivors in the nonsurgical group. Additional analysis was used to investigate possible effects of circumstances of detection and institutions of treatment. The basic results were unaffected.

The decision not to operate on stage I lung cancers was based on the patient's refusal or the surgeon's evaluation of the patient's ability to survive surgery. The extent of the cancer played no role in the decision. If it were true that a sub-

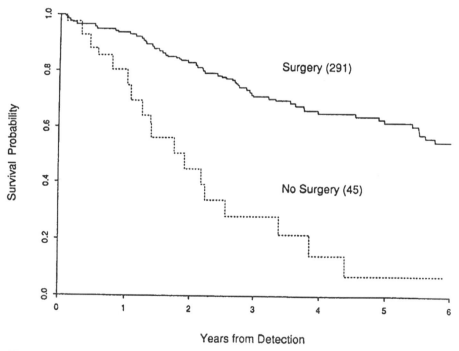

Years from Detection

Figure 3. Kaplan–Meier estimates of survival from stage I lung cancer in surgical and nonsurgical patients in Cooperative Early Lung Cancer Detection Program. Deaths are due to lung cancer; deaths from other causes are treated as withdrawals. Significance levels: log-rank test $p = 0.02$, modified Wilcoxon test $p < 0.001$.

stantial number of x-ray film-detectable lung cancers would remain dormant for many years without treatment, then a substantial proportion of the 45 untreated stage I patients would have survived lung cancer for more than five years.

3 METHODS AND MODELS

The results of the Cooperative Early Lung Cancer Detection Program involve a perplexing contradiction. On the one hand, more than one-third of all lung cancers were detected in stage I through periodic radiographic screening. Moreover, most of the early cancers were resectable and approximately 70% survived five years after detection, contrasted with 13% survival in the general population. Nevertheless, in the Mayo study, the only one that focused on a comparison of periodic x-rays with no systematic screening, no mortality advantage was demonstrated. This might be interpreted as implying that screening was finding some tumors that would not have led to death for many years if undetected and untreated.

In other words, it appears likely that lead-time bias and length-biased sampling were present. Lead-time bias occurs because the time from early detection to the time when the cancer would have become symptomatic is added to the survival time of each stage I case. Length biased sampling occurs because cancers grow at random rates and the sample of cases detected by screening contains an excess of slow-growing cancers compared to the sample found because of symptoms. The definitions of these and other biases associated with screening are discussed thoroughly in the book by Morrison (1985, p. 14). Analysis of the effect of surgical treatment on survival indicates that the influence of these biases is not too strong.

In an attempt to resolve this contradiction and as a means for drawing inferences about x-ray screening from the studies, a mathematical model of the progression kinetics of lung cancer in a screening program was developed (Flehinger and Kimmel, 1987; Flehinger et al., 1988, 1993; Kimmel and Flehinger 1991). This modeling effort was strongly influenced by the pioneer work of Zelen and Feinleib (1969) and other contributors to the theory of screening for chronic diseases (Prorok, 1976a,b; Walter and Day, 1983; Day and Walter, 1984). Briefly, there is a population of individuals born free of disease. At some unobservable time, an individual develops lung cancer, initially stage I. If he is enrolled in a screening program, he undergoes an examination shortly after the onset of disease; this examination and each subsequent examination may or may not detect the disease. If detection occurs, treatment is initiated. If treatment is successful, the patient's health is as good as if he had never contracted the cancer; if unsuccessful, he dies as quickly as if he had never been treated. Some cancers progress to advanced symptomatic stage without detection; these cause death very quickly.

The precise assumptions of the model are the following:

1. In a high-risk population selected for screening, a subgroup of the participants is susceptible to carcinoma of the lung. The probability that an individual belongs to this subgroup is ρ.

2. In the absence of screening and treatment, lung cancer, after its onset, progresses through two stages: early and advanced, followed by cancer death.

3. For an individual in the susceptible subgroup, the age of onset of the early stage τ_0 is a random variable with a trapezoidal distribution (i.e., the density is linear on an interval and zero elsewhere).

4. The durations τ_1 and τ_2 of the early and advanced stages are independent exponential random variables with means μ_1 and μ_2, respectively.

5. The screening program consists of examinations at fixed intervals intended to detect the cancer.

6. Given the presence of early cancer, the first examination detects it with probability p. Subsequent examinations lead to detection with probability λp, where the detectability factor $\lambda \leq 1$.

7. Advanced cancers are detected immediately after the stage transition.

8. When a cancer is detected, screening is aborted and the patient is treated. The probability of "cure" for early stage is equal to c, there is no possibility of cure in an advanced stage. Cure is defined pragmatically in terms of the patient's survival after detection: If the patient is cured, his survival distribution is the same as if he had never had cancer; if he is not cured, his survival distribution is the same as if his cancer had not been detected through screening.

9. Screened individuals are subject to the competing risks of death from lung cancer and death from other causes. Ages at enrollment and death from other causes are random variables with distributions characteristic of the screened population.

These assumptions were selected because of their relative simplicity, and some discussion of their implications and robustness is appropriate. Assumption 2 permits the natural history of an individual who contracts lung cancer to be treated as a semi-Markov process with only three states, the last one, death, an absorbing state. Lung cancer is characterized by clinicians in four stages, of which only stage I corresponds to a localized lesion that can be removed surgically with a high probability for long disease-free survival. Furthermore, stage I lung cancer is almost invariably asymptomatic, while disease that comes to clinical attention because of symptoms usually has spread to lymph nodes or other parts of the body and usually leads rapidly to death. Hence, the three-state model is well justified.

In assumption 3 the trapezoidal distribution of age of onset was selected for computational simplicity. It has two parameters and is always associated with increasing hazard rate. Since lung cancer incidence increases sharply with age, the increasing hazard and two parameters are a minimum requirement. Exploratory analysis satisfied the investigators that the major results of the modeling effort were insensitive to the specific parametric structure of the distribution of age of onset.

Assumption 4, regarding the exponentiality of the duration of the early and advanced stages, is a strong assumption introduced to minimize the required number of parameters. It implies that the probability of transition from early to advanced cancer does not depend on the time since disease onset; similarly, the probability of death does not depend on the time since transition to advanced cancer. Furthermore, the assumption of independence of τ_1 and τ_2 is at variance with the concept that some cancers are slow growing while those that grow quickly in early stages pass rapidly through the advanced stage and lead to early death. To investigate the robustness of this assumption, comparative modeling was carried out using, first, fixed times in early and advanced stages, and second, an advanced-stage duration exactly proportional to the exponentially distributed duration of the early stage. It was found that these modifications did not make any substantial difference in the results of the modeling. The choice of the exponential distribution for disease progression is not related to a biological model of tumor growth in any obvious way. The problem of finding such a connection is of importance but beyond the scope of this study. Papers by Atkinson et al. (1983) and Kimmel and Flehinger (1991) discuss different approaches to this problem.

Assumption 6, regarding the detection probability of early-stage cancer was introduced to incorporate the concept that a lesion that is missed on first examination is more likely to be missed on subsequent examinations, often because of its location in the chest cavity. A more comprehensive model would represent the dependence of detection probability on the size of the cancer, but that refinement is also beyond the scope of this study.

The definition of "cure" in assumption 8 is somewhat at variance with other models and with the point of view of the clinician. In essence, it requires that the patient's survival time after detection be switched from one distribution to another. Under this definition, if lengthy survival after cancer onset without treatment has high probability, it is very difficult to distinguish between cure and long survival without cure.

In order to project the results of the clinical trials to an understanding of the possible benefits associated with screening it was necessary first to estimate the key parameters of the model. Based on these estimates, bounds on the mortality improvement that might result from annual x-ray screening over many years using currently available technology were calculated. In addition, assumptions about the parameter changes that would come from improved technology were considered and were used to project the long-term effect on mortality. Finally, designs for clinical trials that would demonstrate the mortality benefit from the improved technology were analyzed. Both fixed-duration and sequential trials were examined.

The key parameters in the model are the susceptibility ρ, the mean duration of the early stage μ_1, the detectability of the early stage p, and the cure probability of the early stage c. None of these quantities can be estimated directly. It is impossible to determine whether an individual is susceptible to lung cancer if he or she does not develop the disease. Furthermore, even for a patient who is diagnosed with lung cancer, there is no direct way of knowing the length of time between onset and date of detection. If early-stage disease is not detected by chest x-ray or sputum cytology, there is generally no method of ascertaining its presence. Therefore, p cannot be estimated as the number of detected cases divided by the total number of early-stage cases. Finally, if a patient survives many years after treatment for lung cancer, it is impossible to know how long he or she would have survived in the absence of treatment, so that c cannot be estimated directly as the proportion of patients surviving treatment. Several instructive examples of different scenarios of disease progression and detection can be found in Morrison (1985, Chapter 2).

Since direct estimation is usually not feasible, parameter estimation must consist primarily of determining those values of susceptibility, mean duration of early stage, early-stage detectability, and early-stage cure probability that are consistent with data observed in the context of the model. All the key parameters of the model depend strongly on the population being screened, on the techniques of carrying out the chest x-ray examinations, and on the methods of treatment, in addition to the natural history of the disease.

Two major methods of parameter estimation were used in this study, a likelihood-based approach (Flehinger and Kimmel, 1987) and computer simulation. In both approaches, an extensive multidimensional region of parameter values was explored. Outputs of the model were calculated using parameter sets selected from this region. The estimates were then those parameter sets for which the outputs agreed with data collected during the screening study.

In the analytic approach, the outputs that were matched to data were the survival probability of early and advanced lung cancer, the numbers of early and advanced cases, and age-dependent cancer mortality rates. Maximum likelihood estimates of the mean time in advanced stage μ_2 and the distribution of age at death from other causes were calculated directly from data. Then the survival distribution of early lung cancer cases was used to establish a functional relationship between estimates of cure probability c and the mean time in the early stage μ_1. The estimate $c(\mu_1)$ is a decreasing function of μ_1, since the same survival distribution can result from zero cure probability coupled with long early-stage durations or from high cure probability coupled with short sojourns in the early stage. A confidence interval around this function was based on normal approximations. A joint confidence interval for the detection probability p and the mean time in early stage μ_1 was bounded by curves obtained from likelihood expressions for the proportion of early cases and for age-specific cancer mortality rates. Estimates of all the important parameters ρ, μ_1, c, and p

were highly correlated. In particular, there exists a strong negative correlation between the estimates of μ_1 and p. This reflects the fact that the number of early cases detected in the study is crudely proportional to the product of these two quantities.

The second approach to parameter estimation was based on computer simulation of the screening program. Each simulation run started with the selection of a set of parameter values $\rho, \mu_1, \mu_2, p, \lambda$, and c. Then a sequence of simulated participants equal in number to the screened population was generated. These participants were characterized by numbers selected from distributions with the appropriate parameters to represent their natural history of onset of cancer, progression through cancer stages, and competing risk of death from other causes. Each simulated study participant was "screened" periodically; early stage cancers were detected with probability p and cured with probability c, while advanced cancers and uncured early cancers proceeded to death. Cancer incidence by stage and cancer deaths were counted. One hundred runs (of 10,000 participants each) were carried out for each parameter set, so that expected values and standard deviations of cancer incidence and survival were calculated, in simulated "study" groups screened periodically, compared to simulated "control" groups, which received no scheduled screening. A review of relevant simulation methods and techniques can be found in the book by Lewis and Orav (1989).

The confidence region estimates of the mean duration of stage I μ_1, the susceptibility ρ, the early-stage detectability p, the detectability factor λ, and the early-stage curability c were remarkably consistent in all three arms of the program and based on the two different approaches to estimation. For simplicity only the results of the Mayo analysis based on simulation are presented. In Table 3, three typical sets of parameter values are labeled cases A, B, and C. The susceptibility ρ is acceptable in a very narrow range around 0.18; and the mean duration μ_1 ranges from four to eight years. Smaller values correspond to too many cancers in the control group, while larger values correspond to too few cancer deaths. A good-fitting value of λ is 0.5 (i.e. the second examination is half as likely to detect an early cancer as the first). The estimated values of both detection probability p and cure probability c are decreasing functions of the duration μ_1, with p ranging from 0.25 down to 0.13 and c ranging from 0.35 down to zero as μ_1 ranges from four to eight years.

4   RESULTS

4.1   Effect of Long-Term Annual Screening

To assess the possible benefit of long-term screening for lung cancer, a program of annual examination of a population of 5000 participants from age 45 to age 80 or death was simulated, using the parameters presented in Table 3. The results are displayed in Table 4. "Lung Cancers Found" refers to all cases

Table 3   Fitted Parameters from Simulation of Mayo Clinic Data ($\lambda = 0.5$)

Case	μ_1	ρ	p	c
A	4	0.174	0.245	0.35
B	6	0.177	0.165	0.16
C	8	0.182	0.130	0.00

that came to medical attention for any reason, because of screening ("screening detections") or symptoms. "No screen" refers to the group that received no x-ray examinations in the absence of symptoms, while "Annual x-rays" denotes the screened group. Noting first the numbers of lung cancer deaths in the population screened annually compared to the group not screened at all, we observe that there may be a modest reduction in lung cancer mortality due to screening ranging from zero to 13%. Next, in the screened population, 9 to 16% of the cancers found would never be discovered or diagnosed before the patients died of other causes or reached age 80 if they did not receive chest x-rays. Finally, only 40% of the cancers found are in stage I and detected by screening examinations.

It is obvious that the limited estimated benefit associated with screening arises from the low estimated values of the probabilities of early stage detection and early stage cure in this data set. Table 5 presents some estimates of the mortality benefit that might accrue from improved detection or treatment or both. It is noted that if detection were perfect and cure probability remained unchanged, mortality would be reduced by at most 32%. Conversely, if detection remained unchanged and treatment of early stage disease were always successful, mortality would be reduced by at most 37%. Even if detection and cure were both perfect ($p = c = 1$), the reduction in mortality would still be less than 100%; this is due to the presence of some patients who pass through the early stage in the

Table 4   Results of Simulation of 35 Years (Age 45–80) of Lung Cancer Incidence and Mortality of 5000 Men with No Routine Screening and with Annual Chest X-rays

	Lung Cancers Found		Stage I Screening Detections	Lung Cancer Deaths		
Case	No Screen	Annual X-rays	Annual X-rays	No Screen	Annual X-rays	Mortality Reduction (%)
A	426	469	200	368	319	13.3
B	389	444	179	335	317	5.4
C	362	429	172	312	310	0.6

Table 5   Results of Simulation of 35 Years of Lung Cancer Mortality in 5000 Participants with Improved Detection and Cure[a]

μ_1	ρ	p	c	Lung Cancers Found	Stage I Screening	Lung Cancer Deaths	Mortality Reduction
4	0.174	0	0	426	0	368	
		0.25	0.35	469	200	319	13
		1	0.35	516	456	250	32
		0.25	1	469	200	231	37
		0.5	0.5	491	322	255	31
		1	0.5	516	456	207	44
		0.5	1	491	322	147	60
		1	1	516	456	53	86

[a]Based on case A, annual chest x-rays, compared to no screening.

time interval between two successive screens. Thus, detectability and curability must both be increased to achieve mastery of lung cancer. One detection mode currently under consideration is the use of limited computed tomography (CT) scans for screening asymptomatic high-risk individuals. It is thought that this approach might increase both detection and cure probabilities, because smaller nodules would be visible.

4.2   Design of Clinical Trials

Current methods of detection and treatment of lung cancer offer little hope of stemming the mortality from the disease. While widespread smoking cessation might change the picture in the future, it appears that the lung cancer incidence rate will continue to rise in the next few years. Therefore, the major hope must rest on improved imaging techniques or other methods of early detection and on improved methods of treatment. When such techniques are discovered, there will be a demand for new clinical trials to demonstrate the benefit associated with their implementation. The insight about the natural history of lung cancer that has been gleaned through these 20 years of data gathering and statistical analysis can be used in the design of these trials.

As examples of this point consider two simple designs of clinical trials for significant mortality improvement associated with improved detection and treatment. The first design is fixed length, while the second is sequential. In the fixed-length design, 5000 study participants are screened simultaneously at the outset of the trial and annually thereafter for a fixed number of years (2, 4, 6, 8, or 10 years) while 5000 controls are contacted annually. All detected cancers are treated. At the end of the designated trial duration, the ratio D_1/D_2 of the number of control deaths to the number of study deaths is computed. If this ratio exceeds a prespecified cutoff value, which varies with the duration of the trial, the hypothesis that the methodology results in mortality benefit is accepted.

In the sequential design, once again 5000 study participants are screened simultaneously at the outset and annually thereafter, with all detected cancers treated for cure. Again, the controls are contacted annually. The trial is terminated when an appropriate likelihood ratio (based on a Poisson approximation) crosses one of the two boundaries, corresponding to acceptance of the null hypothesis that no mortality benefit is present or the alternative that the death rate can be reduced by a specified factor.

Planning the fixed-length design required an assumption about the parameters characterizing the natural history of lung cancer, primarily the mean time in stage I μ_1, the susceptibility ρ, and the detectability factor λ. Given that assumption, cutoff values for significance at the 0.05 level were calculated by simulation. First, lung cancer development, detection, treatment, and death of 5000 participants were simulated for periods of time ranging from 2 to 20 years. One thousand repetitions were carried out. The expected numbers of cancer deaths for the no-screening case, in which the detectability p and the curability c are both equal to zero were estimated. By using these estimates as parameters in Poisson distributions, cutoff values for 0.05 significance were calculated (i.e., values of the ratio D_1/D_2 of control deaths to study deaths that were exceeded in 5% of the simulations). Cutoff values as functions of trial duration are displayed in Figure 4.

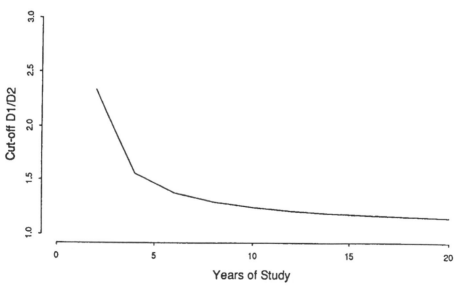

Figure 4. Cutoff value of D_1/D_2 for significant difference (at level 0.05) in mortality between study and control group ($\mu_1 = 4, \rho = 0.174, p = 0, c = 0$) (5000 study, 5000 control).

Table 6 Power of Fixed-Length Clinical Trials[a]

p	c	Mortality Reduction[b] (%)	Probability of Significant D_1/D_2				
			2 yr	4 yr	6 yr	8 yr	10 yr
0.25	0.35	13	0.09	0.12	0.16	0.19	0.23
0.5	0.5	31	0.17	0.29	0.41	0.51	0.61
1	0.5	44	0.35	0.59	0.75	0.84	0.90
0.5	1	60	0.35	0.65	0.83	0.92	0.96
1	1	86	0.92	1.00	1.00	1.00	1.00

[a]Statistic = D_1/D_2; μ_1 = 4, ρ = 0.174, sample size = 5000 study, 5000 control; significance level = 0.05.
[b]The mortality reduction figures are taken from Table 5 and refer to the benefit possible through annual screening starting at age 45.

Thus, the design of a trial involves selecting an appropriate duration and using Figure 4 to find the corresponding cutoff value of D_1/D_2. Now consider the power associated with a specified design and various values of the detectability p and the curability c. For each p, c pair, simulation was used to estimate the expected numbers of lung cancer deaths in the study group for durations ranging from 2 to 10 years, and again the Poisson approximation was used to estimate the probability of exceeding the 0.05 cutoff of D_1/D_2. The results are displayed in Table 6. The first row of the table is related to the most favorable estimate of the mortality benefit possible with the technology in use today. With detectability p = 0.25 and curability c = 0.35, the probability of demonstrating a significant mortality reduction after 10 years of screening is only 0.23. If both detectability and curability could be increased to 0.5, 10 years of screening would produce a significant outcome with probability 0.61. If either detectability or curability were perfect and the other were equal to 0.5, a 10-year trial would have power greater than 90%.

This design is based on an idealized situation with complete recruitment on the first day of the trial, perfect compliance of the study participants, and no contamination of the controls. Any practical situation would require correction in the design for the imperfections in the conduct of the trial.

The plan for a sequential trial based on the Wald (1947) sequential probability ratio test (SPRT) involves a design in which the deaths of study and control patients are monitored until specified boundaries in the $D_1 - D_2$ plane are crossed or until 20 years has elapsed. It is assumed that the sequence of events in the model results in a cancer death rate that may be approximated by a constant, λ_1 for controls and λ_2 for study participants. Testing involves the null hypothesis $\lambda_1 = \lambda_2$ (no mortality reduction) against the alternative $\lambda_1 = k\lambda_2, k > 1$, (mortality reduction of $1 - k^{-1}$). The appropriate likelihood ratio may then be expressed as follows:

$$R = \frac{\sup_{\lambda_2}\{[(k\lambda_2 T_1)^{D_1}/D_1!]e^{-k\lambda_2 T_1}[(\lambda_2 T_2)^{D_2}/D_2!]e^{-\lambda_2 T_2}\}}{\sup_{\lambda_2}\{[(\lambda_2 T_1)^{D_1}/D_1!]e^{-\lambda_2 T_1}[(\lambda_2 T_2)^{D_2}/D_2!]e^{-\lambda_2 T_2}\}}$$

$$= \left[\frac{k(T_1 + T_2)}{kT_1 + T_2}\right]^{D_1}\left[\frac{T_1 + T_2}{kT_1 + T_2}\right]^{D_2},$$

where T_1 and T_2 are the person-years of exposure in control and study arms. Since there are equal sample sizes in the two arms, $T_1 \approx T_2$, so that

$$R = \left(\frac{2k}{k+1}\right)^{D_1}\left(\frac{2}{k+1}\right)^{D_2}.$$

If the trial is to have significance α and power $1 - \beta$, then in the usual style of an SPRT, the trial is terminated as follows:

If $R \geq (1 - \beta)/\alpha$, accept the alternative hypothesis, $\lambda_1 = k\lambda_2$.

If $R \leq \beta/(1 - \alpha)$, accept the null hypothesis, $\lambda_1 = \lambda_2$.

Since $\ln R = D_1 \ln[2k/(k + 1)] - D_2 \ln[(k + 1)/2]$, there are linear boundaries in the D_1–D_2 plane, as illustrated in Figure 5.

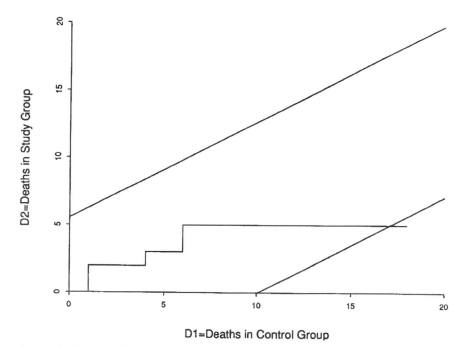

Figure 5. Example of sequential trial (sequential probability test: $k = 2, \alpha = 0.05, \beta = 0.10$).

In fact, the sequence of deaths in the model and in a clinical trial is not well approximated by a homogeneous Poisson process; the death rate tends to increase with time of study. Therefore, it is necessary to run the model through simulations to estimate the true significance and power associated with various values of k and the model parameters discussed in previous sections. The average duration of the trials must also be estimated.

5 CONCLUSIONS

In 1992, the American Cancer Society reported in *CA: A Cancer Journal for Clinicians* (Boring et al., 1992) that in 1988 the mortality from lung cancer in the United States was 133,284, more than double the number of deaths from any other cancer site. In the same issue (p. 45) there is a "Summary of American Cancer Society Recommendations for the Early Detection of Cancer in Asymptomatic People." Not one mention of lung cancer appears in that table. Thus, there exists a huge gap between the need for early detection of lung cancer and the availability of an accepted screening mode.

The design and results of the most recent American clinical trials to evaluate the effectiveness of screening with sputum cytology as an adjunct to periodic chest x-rays were summarized in this chapter. These trials required seven years of effort and many millions of dollars of investment. None resulted in rejection of the null hypothesis that screening conveys no mortality benefit. However, a great deal was learned about the natural history of lung cancer and it was determined that non-small cell lung cancers detected in stage I lead to 70% five-year survival if surgically resected. Those stage I cancers that fail to be resected because of patient refusal or medical contraindications lead quickly to death from lung cancer.

The outcome of the Cooperative Early Lung Cancer Detection Program is typical of many large-scale clinical trials which are systematically designed and carefully executed but result in equivocal answers. This often happens because the investigators are initially overoptimistic about the size of the effect they might observe. As a consequence, the trial design does not provide sufficient power to recognize valuable effects of smaller magnitudes than originally expected. From another point of view, trials of adequate power might require more time and more investment than anyone is willing to provide.

The information gathered from these clinical trials was used to develop a mathematical model of the natural history of lung cancer in the presence of a program of periodic screening chest x-rays. Parameters were estimated to fit major statistics collected during the progress of the trials. By using this model the possible mortality benefit that would accrue from annual x-ray screening of high-risk populations starting at age 45 has been projected. It was found that mortality reduction would be at most 13%. This benefit is limited both by the sensitivity of currently used detection methods for early lung cancer and by the cure probability associated with surgical treatment. Improved detection and treatment are required before the lung cancer epidemic can be brought under control through an early detection program.

When new techniques for early detection or treatment are proposed, a new round of clinical trials will probably be designed to evaluate their benefits. It is important that the information gathered by the Cooperative Early Lung Cancer Detection Program be utilized to design trials that will produce unequivocal results. Two simple study designs, one a fixed-length trial and the other a sequential trial, have been presented as examples of how this philosophy may be applied. Both designs require as input the estimates of parameters of disease progression as well as the estimates of sensitivity of detection and probability of cure. The parameters of disease progression can be assumed to belong to the confidence regions estimated from the Early Lung Cancer Detection Program data. The detectabilities for new screening modalities and cure probabilities for new treatment methods may be partly determined in a separate preliminary study but probably will have to be varied over a wide region of simulations. In this way, planners of new clinical trials will be well informed in advance about the extent of uncertainty in their outcome.

ACKNOWLEDGMENTS

The authors thank Myron R. Melamed, the principal investigator of the MSKCC program; Tatyana Polyak, who carried out the computations for this paper; and Margaret Cargiulo, who prepared the original manuscript.

QUESTIONS AND PROBLEMS

1. Assuming that deaths from lung cancer are a stationary Poisson process with an annual death rate of 3 per 1000 person-years, calculate the required person-years of observation to demonstrate a significant difference in mortality between study and control groups. It is required that significance level α be 0.05 and power $(1-\beta)$ be 0.90 to demonstrate a 33% difference between study and control groups.

2. In the mathematical model of the natural history of lung cancer in a screening program, discuss modifications in the assumptions that would represent the growth of a cancer in early stage and dependence of detection and cure probabilities on the size of the cancer.

3. Discuss modifications in fixed-length and sequential trial designs that allow for gradual accrual of participants, imperfect compliance of study group, and contamination of the control group.

4. Suppose that a new detection method is thought to be substantially more

sensitive than the chest x-ray. Describe the initial studies that should be carried out before a large-scale clinical trial to evaluate mortality reduction is initiated.

5. Suppose that cancers grow monotonically in early stage and make transition into advanced stage (metastasize) at random sizes X. Let $\phi(x)$ be the distribution function of these sizes at transition. The probability of detecting a cancer may depend on its size and stage. Let $F(x)$ be the probability that a cancer is in advanced stage if detected at size $X = x$. Discuss the relation between $F(x)$ and $\phi(x)$ and conditions under which they are identical (Kimmel and Flehinger 1991).

CHAPTER 16

Modeling Interrater Agreement for Pathologic Features of Choroidal Melanoma

B. Michele Melia and Marie Diener-West

1 MOTIVATION AND BACKGROUND

Many factors of biomedical interest cannot be measured objectively according to a definitive standard. Methods for classifying certain diagnoses, conditions, or characteristics of a disease are often based on the subjective evaluation of a clinician or technician using an ordered categorical scale. The reliability of such methods is usually assessed by examining the agreement of two or more independent raters of the same subjects. An $r \times r$ contingency table can be constructed for the comparison of two raters making classifications onto an ordered categorical scale of r categories.

For nominal data, agreement between two raters beyond that due to chance commonly has been evaluated using a kappa statistic κ as developed by Cohen (1960) of the form

$$\kappa = \frac{P_o - P_e}{1 - P_e},$$

where P_o is the observed proportion of agreement and P_e is the proportion of agreement expected if the two ratings are independent. A value of κ equal to 0 indicates no agreement beyond that due to chance, while a value of 1 indicates perfect agreement. A weighted *kappa* statistic (Cohen, 1968) can be used to describe agreement between two raters for ordered categorical data and is formed by multiplying the observed and expected proportions of disagreement by a weight that reflects the relative severity of disagreement. For two raters,

Case Studies in Biometry, Edited by Nicholas Lange, Louise Ryan, Lynne Billard, David Brillinger, Loveday Conquest, and Joel Greenhouse.
ISBN 0-471-58885-7 © 1994 John Wiley & Sons, Inc.

the weighted κ is easy to compute and can be used to summarize the overall agreement between observed cell counts and the expected cell counts on the main diagonal of each table. However, the choice of weights to account for the severity of differences in ratings is not always clear (Maclure and Willett, 1987). Other limitations of κ are that it depends on the number of categories specified (Maclure and Willett, 1987), is insensitive to differences between observed and expected patterns of agreement (Light, 1971), and may be negative for chance-generated multiple-rater data (Conger, 1980).

For multiple raters, κ-like statistics which measure agreement have been developed for nominal data (Davies and Fleiss, 1982) and for nominal or ordinal categories (O'Connell and Dobson, 1984). However, these statistics suffer from many of the same problems as does κ. In addition, the interpretation of the relative magnitude of both κ and κ-like statistics is problematic (Posner et al., 1990).

Within the past decade, parametric methods of modeling agreement have been suggested which describe the structure of the agreement and provide information on distinguishability of categories, characteristics not derivable from a single summary statistic such as κ. These methods include loglinear models, considered by Haberman (1974) and Goodman (1979, 1985), for the analysis of association in two-way tables where the row and column categories are ordered. Goodman proposed a class of models for analyzing association in a contingency table where the odds ratio is the measure of association for each of the 2×2 subtables formed from the full table. For these models, the chi-squared statistic is partitioned into separate components representing the general overall level of association, the row, column and other effects. The simplest model is the usual model of statistical independence. Tanner and Young (1985) noted that κ is based essentially on discrepancies between observed and expected cell counts under the loglinear model of independence. Goodman's model of uniform association adds a parameter to this model to describe linear-by-linear association between ratings. Tanner and Young (1985) later modified the independence model to examine agreement on nominal categorical scales by including a parameter for the main diagonal cells which is sensitive to discrepancies between observed and expected counts or to patterns of agreement on the main diagonal. Agresti (1988) generalized Goodman's uniform association model and Tanner and Young's agreement model to a single loglinear model for ordered categorical scales, which includes both the former models as special cases. This loglinear model of agreement plus linear-by-linear association analyzes the structure of the agreement by partitioning agreement into components, for example, due to chance, due to baseline association between the ratings, or due to exact agreement (beyond that due to the other two components), similar to the way in which an analysis-of-variance partitions variance. In this model, fixed scores, commonly assumed to be equally spaced, are arbitrarily assigned to each response category to account for ordering.

Becker (1989a, 1990) proposed a different log-nonlinear association model. This model partitions agreement similarly to the loglinear model but also includes an assessment of the degree to which raters can distinguish between categories. Particular attention is paid to distinguishability between adjacent categories. Scores for the categories are estimated from the data. Becker noted that fixing the scores as a linear function of the category numbers implies that all pairs of adjacent categories are equally distinguishable.

2 DATA

The histopathology data used in these analyses are from the Collaborative Ocular Melanoma Study (COMS) (1989), a set of multicenter clinical trials investigating treatment of choroidal melanoma, a rare cancer of the eye. Although rare, this condition is of special concern within the field of ophthalmology because of its life-threatening potential. The most widely used treatment has been enucleation (removal of the eye). However, over the past 10 to 20 years, various forms of radiation therapy have been employed as alternative treatments with the goal of saving the eye and, possibly, some vision in the eye. The COMS is sponsored by the National Eye Institute of the National Institutes of Health to evaluate the role of specific radiation modalities in prolonging survival of patients with choroidal melanoma. In the COMS, histopathology of tumors of enucleated eyes is evaluated independently by a review committee of three ophthalmic pathologists using grading schemes developed specifically for the study. Each pathologist reviews seven slides prepared from each enucleated eye and completes a standardized review form. Many of the tumor histopathologic features are graded onto an ordered categorical scale. These include tumor cell type, degree of tumor necrosis (tissue death), and extent of scleral extension (the extent to which the tumor has invaded the sclera or "white of the eye"). Scleral extension was coded by two raters for each of 885 eyes as one of five possible categories: (1) None or innermost layers; (2) Within sclera, but does not extend to scleral surface; (3) Extends to scleral surface; (4) Extrascleral extension without transection; and (5) Extrascleral extension with presumed residual tumor in orbit. Degree of necrosis was coded by three raters for each of 612 eyes and analyzed as one of three possible categories: (1) None; (2) Less than 10% of cells; and (3) Greater than or equal to 10% of cells (Table 1).

Agreement among the three pathologists has implications for the reliability of the new grading schemes for these histopathologic features, some of which are believed to be important prognostic indicators for the disease. At the end of patient follow-up within the study, analyses will be performed to investigate the correlation of these graded histopathologic features with survival time. Unreliable measurement could result in bias and increased error in estimation of parameters describing the prognostic significance of histopathologic features or in reduced power to detect association between prognosis and histopathologic features. Given these implications, it is useful to identify the patterns of disagreement in order to improve the reliability through refinement of the grading schemes by either collapsing categories or expanding grading definitions.

Table 1 Sample Data Display of Histopathology Ratings

Patient ID	Degree of Scleral Extension as Classified by	
	Rater A	Rater B
1	2	1
2	2	2
3	2	2
4	2	2
⋮	⋮	⋮
884	1	1
885	1	2

Patient ID	Degree of Necrosis as Classified by		
	Rater A	Rater B	Rater C
1	1	1	1
2	1	1	2
3	1	1	2
4	1	1	2
⋮	⋮	⋮	⋮
611	2	1	1
612	3	3	3

3 METHODS AND MODELS

Suppose that two raters, A and B, classify each of n subjects into one of the categories of an r-category ordered scale. An $r \times r$ contingency table may be constructed to describe the classifications, in which each cell $(i,j), i = 1, \ldots, r, j = 1, \ldots, r$, contains the number of subjects assigned to category i by rater A and category j by rater B. It is of interest to model the way in which the rater affects the relative number of subjects falling into each response category. If the classifications by rater A were statistically independent of the classifications by rater B, a possible model for the expected number of subjects, m_{ij}, appearing in each cell (i,j) is given by the loglinear model of independence:

$$\text{M1:} \quad \ln m_{ij} = \mu + \lambda_i^A + \lambda_j^B,$$

$$\text{with} \quad \sum_i \lambda_i^A = 0 \quad \text{and} \quad \sum_j \lambda_j^B = 0, \tag{1}$$

where μ is an overall mean across all cells (i,j), λ_i^A the additional effect of rater A for the ith category, and λ_j^B the additional effect of rater B for the jth category. However, this model is usually inappropriate for agreement data since the ratings are not usually statistically independent. For agreement data, given that rater A has chosen category i, rater B is usually more likely also to have chosen category i rather than category $j \neq i$.

Tanner and Young (1985) suggested a modification of model M1 as more appropriate for agreement data in which the response is a nominal category:

$$\text{M2:} \quad \ln m_{ij} = \mu + \lambda_i^A + \lambda_j^B + \delta I(i = j), \quad (2)$$

where $I(\cdot)$ is the indicator function, which takes the value 1 when the indicated event, in this case $(i = j)$, holds, and is zero otherwise. The $\delta I(i = j)$ term will be referred to as the *exact agreement term*, and model M2 as the *exact agreement model*, since it describes the discrepancies on the main diagonal between the observed and expected counts under the independence model, which can be thought of as due to exact agreement beyond that expected by chance.

Although this model is often appropriate for describing nominal scale agreement, it is usually inadequate for describing agreement when the response variable is ordered. Model M2 accounts for the high proportion of counts on the main diagonal, but not for the tendency of disagreement to fall close to the main diagonal, a feature which is common to agreement data with an ordered categorical response.

A model which could account for disagreements falling close to the main diagonal as well as sparse or no counts in cells far from the main diagonal was proposed initially by Goodman (1979) for the analysis of two-way tables. In this model, the association in the 2×2 subtables formed from adjacent rows and columns of the full table is inspected:

$$\text{M3:} \quad \ln m_{ij} = \mu + \lambda_i^A + \lambda_j^B + \beta u_i u_j, \quad (3)$$

where $u_1 < \cdots < u_r$ are fixed scores which are assigned to the categories. Since, within a row, the $\beta u_i u_j$ term describes deviations of row counts from independence as linearly related to the column scores, and within a column, deviation of column counts from independence as linearly related to the row scores, Agresti (1990) referred to it as the *linear-by-linear association* term, and model M3 as the *linear-by-linear association model*. For equally-spaced scores (e.g., $u_i = i$), model M3 reduces to Goodman's uniform association model. An important result regarding this model, shown by Goodman (1985), is that it is the discrete analogue of the bivariate normal distribution. However, model M3 is often inappropriate for describing agreement data because it cannot account sufficiently for the high frequencies appearing on the main diagonal.

For agreement data with ordered categories, Agresti (1988) suggested a model which combines the features of models M2 and M3:

$$\text{M4:} \qquad \ln m_{ij} = \mu + \lambda_i^A + \lambda_j^B + \beta u_i u_j + \delta I(i = j), \qquad (4)$$

where $u_1 < \cdots < u_r$ are the scores, usually, but not necessarily, equally spaced, assigned to the r categories. Since this model accounts for both the linear-by-linear association and additional exact agreement, which are typical of agreement data on an ordered scale, it is a more appropriate model of overall agreement for such data than either models M2 or M3. If model M4 is inadequate, an alternative is to replace the $\delta I(i = j)$ term with individual $\delta_i I(i = j)$ terms; however, this model is saturated on the main diagonal. Hence, M4 should be used whenever possible.

The β and δ parameters in this model have natural interpretations. A value of β greater than zero is evidence for the presence of linear-by-linear association in the data, (i.e., it implies that counts tend to fall close to or on the main diagonal). A value of δ greater than zero implies that there is additional exact agreement, [i.e., that there are additional counts appearing on the main diagonal beyond those expected due to chance (and linear-by-linear association, if $\beta > 0$)]. Since model M4 is hierarchical, the likelihood ratios for the full model, which contains both β and δ, versus reduced models, in which β and/or δ has been deleted, may be used to decide if these terms contribute significantly to the model, and whether linear-by-linear association and/or exact agreement are present in the data. Models M1 to M4 are loglinear, and may be fitted using standard statistical software.

The parameters of the model also have interpretations in terms of odds ratios. Let θ_{ij} be the odds ratio in the 2×2 subtable formed by the intersection of rows i and j and columns i and j (i.e., the odds of rater B choosing category i rather than j when rater A chooses category i versus the odds of rater B choosing category i rather than j when rater A chooses category j). Then

$$\theta_{ij} = \frac{m_{ii} m_{jj}}{m_{ij} m_{ji}} \qquad \text{for all } i \text{ and } j, \quad i \neq j,$$

and

$$\ln \theta_{ij} = (u_i - u_j)^2 \beta + 2\delta. \qquad (5)$$

Darroch and McCloud (1986) defined two categories i and j as indistinguishable if $\theta_{ij} = 1$ and $\theta_{ik} = \theta_{jk}$ for all $k \neq i,j$, and defined an index of distinguishability which is based on the odds ratios:

$$\nu_{ij} = 1 - \theta_{ij}^{-1}. \qquad (6)$$

The value of the index ν_{ij} achieves a maximum of 1 when there is perfect agreement. For odds ratios greater than 1 but finite, ν_{ij} is between 0 and 1, and for odds ratios less than 1, which is uncommon for agreement data, ν_{ij} is negative. Two categories i and j are indistinguishable and ν_{ij} is zero when $\theta_{ij} = 1$ (i.e., when the odds of rater B choosing category i are the same whether rater A chooses category i or j). Note that $\beta = \delta = 0$ in model M4 implies that all categories are indistinguishable. Becker (1990) derived necessary and sufficient conditions under which categories i and j are indistinguishable:

(1) $\beta = 0$ or $u_i = u_j$, and $\delta = 0$;

or

(2) $u_i = \pm 1/\sqrt{2}$, $u_i = -u_j$, and $u_k = 0$ for $k \neq m, n$, and $\delta = -\beta$.

More recently, Becker (1989a, 1990) and Becker and Agresti (1992) have discussed estimating the scores $u_1 < \cdots < u_r$ in model M4 from the data. Fitting the scores rather than making (somewhat arbitrary) assignments has the advantage of allowing inference about "distinguishability" of the categories. A disadvantage is that the estimated scores version of model M4 is no longer loglinear, and standard software packages may not be used directly for model fitting. Parameter estimates for this log-nonlinear model can be obtained by the algorithm developed by Becker (1989b). This algorithm uses standard software to estimate the loglinear model parameters, $\mu, \lambda_i^A, \lambda_j^B, \beta$, and δ keeping the scores fixed, and then modifies the scores using Newton's algorithm while holding the other parameter estimates fixed. The procedure is iterated until convergence has been reached for every score.

Valid standard errors for the estimates are not computed by this algorithm but may be obtained using the jackknife (Efron, 1982). The jackknife is a numerical method which allows direct approximation of the standard error of an estimate when its probability distribution is not assumed to be known. The method essentially involves deleting a single observation from the observed data and recalculating the parameter estimates based on the remaining $n-1$ observations. This procedure is repeated n times; with each procedure the ith observation is deleted, for $i = 1, \ldots, n$. The n parameter estimates obtained from the procedure are then used to calculate the standard error of the estimate. The jackknife is also recommended to identify influential observations (i.e., observations whose deletion from the data results in large changes in parameter estimates); this is of particular importance when the table is sparse, with many cells with small or zero observations.

To estimate the scores u_i from the data, it is necessary to constrain two of the scores; Becker recommends fixing the scores for the first and last categories. This constraint does not result in loss of generality as long as the two scores are not fixed to the same value—which is reasonable for ordered scales in which the first and last category scores are fixed, since it is unlikely that these categories would have equal scores. It should also be noted that the likelihood ratio statistic comparing a fixed score model and an estimated score model will not generally assume a χ^2 distribution, since the former model is loglinear and the latter is not. The choice of an estimated versus fixed scores model may be based on assessment of the goodness of fit of the fixed versus estimated scores model, appropriateness of using evenly spaced fixed scores as indicated by the estimated scores, and whether there is interest in examining category distinguishability through scores estimation.

Sparse tables are common for agreement data and can pose some problems. For sparse tables, the Pearson and likelihood ratio statistics used to judge the appropriateness of a model may not be chi-squared in distribution; the same is true for the deviance. Like the Pearson and likelihood ratio statistics, the deviance may be used to assess the appropriateness of a model. It is a measure of the discrepancy between the fitted and observed values in a model that is based on the log of the ratio of the maximum achievable likelihood to the likelihood of the model under investigation. Even when the sample size is large, the chi-squared approximation for the deviance may be poor. Given these difficulties, McCullagh and Nelder (1989) have recommended using the deviance only as a screening tool to identify obviously important terms in the regression without assigning p-values. In the next section, deviances without p-values are reported for model selection. Wald's statistic (Wald, 1943), defined as the square of the ratio of the estimate to its standard error, is used to test the hypotheses that the parameters are equal to zero and to assign p-values to terms in the models, using the approximate chi-squared distribution of the statistic for large sample sizes. Jackknife estimates of the standard error were used to calculate the Wald's statistics, since the asymptotic standard errors tend to be underestimates for sparse tables.

Model M4 can be extended to analyze agreement for three raters using a modification of the method of Tanner and Young (1985) for multirater agreement in the nominal scale situation:

$$\text{M5:} \qquad \ln m_{ijk} = \mu + \lambda_i^A + \lambda_j^B + \lambda_k^C + \beta_1 u_i u_j + \beta_2 u_i u_k$$
$$+ \beta_3 u_j u_k + \beta_4 u_i u_j u_k + \delta(i,j,k), \qquad (7)$$

where

$$\delta(i,j,k) = \delta_1 I(i=j) + \delta_2 I(i=k) + \delta_3 I(j=k) + \delta_4 I(i=j=k).$$

In this model, δ_1, δ_2, and δ_3 describe exact agreement between pairs of raters beyond that due to chance and linear-by-linear association, and δ_4 describes additional exact agreement among all three raters above that expected due to pairwise exact agreement and linear-by-linear association alone. Models constrained by $\delta_1 = \delta_2 = \delta_3$ will be referred to as homogeneous in pairwise δ, otherwise as heterogeneous in pairwise δ. Unlike the two-rater case, the model heterogeneous in pairwise δ is not saturated on the main diagonal. In the absence of three-way interaction, β_1, β_2, and β_3 are interpretable as measures of linear-by-linear association for each pair of raters. In the presence of three-way interaction, the interpretation becomes more complex, with the linear-by-linear association between a pair of raters dependent on the classification made by the third rater. For example, the linear-by-linear association for raters B and C at each level i of rater A is given by $\beta_3 + u_i\beta_4$, $i = 1,\ldots,r$. Similarly, linear-by-linear association for raters A and B at each level k of C is given by $\beta_1 + u_k\beta_4$, and for raters A and C at each level j of rater B by $\beta_2 + u_j\beta_4$.

Becker and Agresti (1992) have suggested a different approach for evaluating multirater agreement which describes simultaneous agreement in the second-order marginal tables. This approach may be preferable when the number of raters is greater than three and the contingency tables are correspondingly large and/or the data are very sparse. However, for three raters, if the tables are not too sparse, model M5 appears to summarize agreement well for many situations, may be fitted using the loglinear modeling procedures in standard software packages, and does not assume independence of the second-order marginal tables as does the approach suggested by Becker and Agresti (1992). Models M1 through M5 were used to describe the agreement between two raters and, when data were available, between three raters in grading histopathologic features of tumors obtained and processed from enucleated eyes.

4 RESULTS

In this section we summarize the results of modeling agreement on an ordered categorical scale for (1) scleral extension of the tumor as graded by two raters, and (2) degree of necrosis of the tumor as graded by three raters. The COMS owns the copyright to this data set; these data are considered preliminary due to the ongoing nature of the COMS clinical trials.

4.1 Scleral Extension

Table 2 summarizes the results of the classification by two raters, A and B, of extent of scleral extension of the choroidal melanoma in 885 eyes. The categories for this feature are ordered anatomically with respect to the sclera. The estimated weighted kappa, $\hat{\kappa}_w$, which gives 0.75, 0.50, 0.25, and 0.00 weight to counts falling 1, 2, 3, and 4 cells from the main diagonal, respectively, is 0.436, which indicates fair agreement according to the characterization suggested by Landis and Koch (1977).

The deviance for each of the hierarchical loglinear models and corresponding degrees of freedom are reported in Table 3. The category scores were assigned as the index of the category (i.e., $u_i = i$). Only model M4, that of agreement plus linear-by-linear association provides an adequate fit to the data. Both the β and δ terms are highly significant by Wald's test statistic (Table 4).

Table 2   Scleral Extension in 885 Eyes: Cross-Classification by Two Raters[a,b]

Rater A	Rater B				
	1	2	3	4	5
1	291	74	1	1	1
2	186	256	7	7	3
3	2	4	0	2	0
4	3	10	1	14	2
5	1	7	1	8	3

[a]Grading scale: 1, none or innermost layers; 2, within sclera, but does not extend to scleral surface; 3, extends to scleral surface; 4, extrascleral extension without transection; 5, extrascleral extension with presumed residual tumor in orbit.
[b]$\hat{\kappa}_w = 0.436$.

Table 3   Scleral Extension Data: Comparison of Loglinear Models

Model		Deviance	d.f.
M1	Independence	283.04	16
M2	Exact agreement	107.64	15
M3	Linear-by-linear association	59.15	15
M4	Agreement + linear-by-linear assoc.	15.35	14

Table 4   Scleral Extension Data: Parameter Estimates for Model M4 with Fixed Scores[a]

Parameter	Estimate	se	χ_w^2	p-Value
β (linear-by-linear assoc.)	0.508	0.0646	61.8	<0.001
δ (exact agreement)	0.589	0.0900	42.8	<0.001

[a]χ_w^2 is Wald's test statistic for the parameter of interest.

This model suggests that there is agreement in the data beyond that expected by chance alone, and that both linear-by-linear association, which can be interpreted as a tendency for counts to fall close to or on the main diagonal, and additional exact agreement are present.

Table 5 contains the parameter estimates for the agreement plus linear-by-linear association model in which the scores have been estimated. The reported standard errors for this log-nonlinear model were obtained using the jackknife. The first and last category scores were fixed to 1 and 5, respectively. Although a direct comparison of goodness-of-fit statistics is not possible, this model appears to fit better than did the fixed-scores model. This is not surprising given that the estimated category scores deviate considerably from the fixed scores assigned in the previous model, suggesting that the choice of fixed scores was inappropriate. For the estimated-scores model, both the β and δ terms are highly significant. Based on the estimated parameters and scores in Table 5, the θ_{ij} calculated from (5) are $\theta_{12} = 5.31, \theta_{23} = 4.90, \theta_{34} = 4.81$, and $\theta_{45} = 2.38$. Thus, the odds ratio is approximately twice as high for all other pairs of adjacent categories as it is for categories 4 and 5.

The estimated scores of 5.01 and 5.00 for the fourth and fifth categories (*extrascleral extension without transection* and *extension with presumed residual tumor in orbit*, respectively) are virtually identical; however, since δ is not zero, we cannot conclude that these two categories are indistinguishable. They are less distinguishable than the other pairs of adjacent categories, both by inspection of the scores and by $\nu_{ij} = 1 - \theta_{ij}^{-1}$, the index of distinguishability. Specifically, the estimated distinguishabilities (6) for each adjacent pair of categories are: $\nu_{12} = 0.81, \nu_{23} = 0.80, \nu_{34} = 0.79$, and $\nu_{45} = 0.58$.

Since the scores for categories 4 and 5 are nearly equal, the indices of distinguishability for category 4 and categories 1, 2, and 3 are equal to the indices of distinguishability for category 5 and categories 1, 2, and 3. In other words, the pathologist does not separate category 5 (*extrascleral extension with presumed*

Table 5 Scleral Extension Data: Parameter Estimates for Model M4 with Estimated Scores[a]

Parameter	Estimate	se	χ_w^2	p-Value
β (linear-by-linear assoc.)	0.418	0.090	21.6	<0.001
δ (exact agreement)	0.433	0.160	7.32	0.007
u_1	1.00 (fixed)	—		
u_2	2.39	0.203		
u_3 category scores	3.71	0.502		
u_4	5.01	0.410		
u_5	5.00 (fixed)	—		

[a]Residual sum of squares = 5.51 d.f. = 11; χ_w^2 is Wald's test statistic for the parameter of interest.

residual tumor in orbit) from categories 1 to 3 (*no extrascleral extension*), any more reliably than he separates category 4 (*extrascleral extension without transection*) from categories 1 to 3 (*no extrascleral extension*). However, category 5 (*extrascleral extension with presumed residual tumor in the orbit*) and category 4 (*extrascleral extension without transection*) are not indistinguishable; the odds of rater B choosing category 4 rather than 5 given rater A chose category 4 are 2.38 times higher than the odds of rater B choosing category 4 rather than 5 given that rater A chose category 5. In terms of the pathologist's ability to determine the extent of scleral extension, this suggests that rather than a five-point ordered scale, the scale actually has four ordered responses in which the fourth category of "extrascleral extension" is divisible into two subcategories, "extrascleral extension without transection" and "extrascleral extension with presumed residual tumor in orbit."

4.2 Degree of Necrosis

The cross-classification of degree of necrosis in 612 tumors by three raters is reported in Table 6. As is typical for agreement data, although the sample size is not small, the table is relatively sparse since most of the counts fall into a small number of cells. The estimated multiple-rater κ of Davies and Fleiss (1982), $\hat{\kappa}_{DF}$, is 0.234, which indicates poor agreement according to the standard of Landis and Koch (1977).

The deviances for the log-linear models are reported in Table 7. Scores were assigned as $u_i = i - 2$. As noted previously, the deviances should be interpreted

Table 6   Degree of Necrosis of Tumor in 612 Eyes: Cross-Classification by Three Raters[a,b]

		Rater C		
Rater A	Rater B	1	2	3
1	1	315	105	13
	2	14	22	3
	3	3	0	1
2	1	33	16	2
	2	8	16	7
	3	0	2	4
3	1	5	6	1
	2	1	3	4
	3	0	4	24

[a]Grading scale: 1, none; 2, <10%; 3, ≥10%.
[b]$\hat{\kappa}_{DF} = 0.234$.

Table 7   Degree of Necrosis Data: Comparison of Loglinear Models

Model	Deviance	d.f.
M1 Independence	384	20
M2 Exact agreement	114	16
M3 Linear-by-linear association:		
without three-way interaction	28.4	17
with three-way interaction	23.0	16
M5 Agreement + linear-by-linear association:		
Reduced by β_4, δ_4	19.2	14
Reduced by δ_4, homogeneous pairwise δ	15.6	15
Reduced by δ_4	9.69	13
Full model	9.54	12

as goodness-of-fit statistics with some caution because the chi-squared approximation may not be adequate, due to the sparseness of the table. However, for sparse data the p-values tend to be underestimated, so model fits may be better than indicated by the deviance. Model M5 appears to provide an adequate fit to the data, deviance = 9.54 with 12 d.f. Reducing the model by eliminating the δ_4 term increases the deviance only marginally, by $9.69 - 9.54 = 0.15$, and adds 1 more degree of freedom, leading to a more parsimonious model that still adequately describes the data. Further reduction of the model results in larger increases in the deviance. The change in deviance for homogeneous δ is $15.6 - 9.54 = 5.91$ with 2 d.f. Although the fit is still adequate, the relatively large increase in deviance combined with inspection of the estimates for pairwise δ in the model reduced by β_4 suggests that the model with homogeneous δ is not appropriate. Change in deviance for β_4 is $19.2 - 9.69 = 9.51$ with 1 d.f.; again, the relatively large increase in deviance suggests that the fuller model is more appropriate. Note that models not accounting for linear-by-linear association in the data are completely inadequate.

Jackknife estimates of standard error were obtained along with the asymptotic standard errors, since the asymptotic standard errors tend to be underestimates for sparse tables. The jackknife standard errors were then used to compute Wald's statistics for the parameter estimates in each of the models (data not shown). This led to selection of the full model reduced by δ_4 as the final model, the same decision as that resulting from using the deviance to test the importance of each parameter in the model.

The final model suggests that there is agreement beyond that expected due to chance in the form of linear-by-linear association, and additional exact agreement between pairs of raters, but no additional exact agreement between all three raters above that expected due to linear-by-linear association and exact pairwise agreement. The parameter estimates for the final model are given in

Table 8   Degree of Necrosis Data: Parameter Estimates for Model M5 Reduced by δ_4

Parameter	Estimate	Asymptotic se	Jackknife se
β_1	0.569	0.231	0.243
β_2	0.938	0.229	0.252
β_3	1.00	0.233	0.241
β_4	0.500	0.170	0.178
δ_1	0.661	0.209	0.218
δ_2	−0.0837	0.189	0.194
δ_3	0.363	0.193	0.202

Table 8. Since there is significant three-way linear-by-linear association as indicated by β_4, estimates of linear-by-linear association for each pair of raters by level of the third rater are given in Table 9.

Strength of the linear-by-linear association between any pair of raters increases as degree of necrosis as classified by the third rater increases. This suggests that in general the raters tend to agree better about which cases have a large degree of necrosis than they do about which cases have little or no necrosis, but that the degree of agreement depends on the pair of raters being considered. Linear-by-linear association is weaker between raters A and B than between A and C or B and C; however, raters A and B have the strongest additional exact agreement ($\delta_1 = 0.661$), which may explain the weaker linear-by-linear association. There is also a significant amount of exact agreement between raters B and C ($\delta_3 = 0.363$). Raters A and C exhibit no additional exact agreement beyond that due to linear-by-linear association ($\delta_2 = -0.0837$). The finding that raters A and B have strongest exact agreement while raters A and C and raters B and C have strongest linear-by-linear association suggests that rater C's evaluations may be shifted with respect to those of raters A and B. In fact, examination of the marginal distributions of each rater confirms this; rater C is less likely to assign cases to "no necrosis" (62%) than are raters A

Table 9   Degree of Necrosis Data: Estimates of Linear-by-Linear Association, $\beta_p + u_q\beta_4$ Each Pair of Raters by Level of Third Rater

Rater Pair, p	Level of Third Rater, q		
	1	2	3
1. A, B	0.069	0.569	1.07
2. A, C	0.438	0.938	1.44
3. B, C	0.500	1.00	1.50

and B (78 and 81%, respectively), and correspondingly, more likely to assign a higher degree of necrosis.

5 CONCLUSIONS

Our results in Section 4 provide examples of how loglinear (or log-nonlinear) models may be useful in describing agreement in grading of ordered categorical features among two or more raters. Overall agreement is partitioned into components to allow examination of types and patterns of agreement and provide estimation of the magnitude and significance of the agreement structure beyond that explained by chance or the baseline association of ratings. Advantages of the loglinear models developed by Tanner and Young (1985) and Agresti (1988) are that they make use of the ordering of the categories and result in easily interpretable parameters. In addition, the assumption of fixed scores for the rating scales can be assessed and the fit of the model may be improved by employing log-nonlinear models and using estimated scores (Becker, 1989a). The estimated scores may also prove helpful in identifying areas where refinement of category definitions is needed. However, it is important to note that this modeling may require a relatively large sample size and that this requirement increases with an increasing number of categories and/or raters. Also, as the number of raters increases, the number of sparse or empty cells may become problematic. Increasing sample size does not necessarily result in improved ability to fit the models; observations in a sparse extreme cell may become more extreme with increased sample size and may prove influential in the model-fitting process. For example, in grading degree of tumor pigmentation in COMS enucleated eyes (results not shown), deletion of a single observation out of 614 observations resulted in the adequate fit of a model, which was inadequate given the total data set.

The reliability of the COMS histopathology grading schemes was assessed as a result of an initial analysis using this modeling approach. The COMS Pathology Review Committee expanded the criteria for several histopathologic features in order to improve the validity of the grading schemes and to increase agreement among raters. For example, the evaluation of degree of inflammation was modified to include assessment of inflammatory cells surrounding the tumor as well as within the tumor. Similarly, the grading of tumor necrosis was expanded to include both empty spaces with macrophages and presumed necrosis in addition to evaluation of frank necrosis. Although three members of the pathology review committee review each case, a single adjudicated composite review is submitted to the COMS data coordinating center for inclusion in the study database. A possible learning effect from the adjudication procedure in addition to feedback from this analysis has hopefully resulted in increased reliability over time.

Future plans include assessing the importance of histopathologic features in the analysis of survival time by treatment group. The estimated scores from the log-nonlinear models may provide guidelines for combining histopathologic categories in the analysis of the data. Developing grading schemes for future studies of this and other cancers may also be enhanced.

ACKNOWLEDGMENTS

This work was supported under cooperative agreements EY-06287 and EY-06260 from the National Eye Institute, National Institutes of Health, Bethesda, Maryland. The authors appreciate the contributions of the COMS Pathology Review Committee, Daniel M. Albert, W. Richard Green, and Morton E. Smith, in developing the grading scheme, and reviewing and grading all of the materials represented by the data analyzed in this manuscript. The authors also thank Nancy L. Robinson for coordinating the review of materials and transmission of data.

QUESTIONS AND PROBLEMS

1. What additional information can loglinear and log-nonlinear models provide over κ or κ-like statistics in the analysis of interrater agreement?

2. What difficulties may be encountered in fitting loglinear or log-nonlinear models?

3. Using Table 5, verify the estimated odds ratios quoted in the text and the estimated distinguishabilities for each adjacent pair of categories.

4. Fit the models specified in Table 3. Calculate the estimated odds ratios for discrepant ratings for each model. What similarities/differences do you observe?

5. For three raters, is it possible to interpret the parameters of the association model in terms of odds ratios?

CHAPTER 17

Quality Control for Bone Mineral Density Scans

Suzanna Wong and Nancy Lane

1 MOTIVATION AND BACKGROUND

Most applications of statistics to quality control and process improvement are in the manufacturing and engineering areas. In this chapter we describe an application of statistical quality control to a multicenter clinical trial.

Multicenter clinical trials are commonly used to evaluate drugs, biologics, medical procedures and equipment in development. In such trials, certain operations decentralized to the individual centers can potentially lead to measurements with higher variability and lesser quality than if such activities are carried out at a central location. The variety of procedures, machines, personnel, and other factors at the different sites may all be contributing factors. A good process control plan may help reduce some of the variability and provide quality medical information for the final evaluation.

Within a multicenter clinical trial, the option of a decentralized, convenient, and practical operation is often weighed against a centralized, homogeneous operation. In this chapter we analyze the reading of the bone mineral density (BMD) scans of the lumbar spine in such a context and examine how standards can be set for individual center performance evaluation in order to begin a monitoring program.

1.1 Context

This study was performed in the context of a larger clinical trial designed to evaluate the effects of nafarelin [a drug which is an agonistic analogue of gonadotropin-releasing hormone (GnRH)] therapy on women with endometriosis. The study had a multicenter, double-blind, randomized, parallel design with

Case Studies in Biometry, Edited by Nicholas Lange, Louise Ryan, Lynne Billard, David Brillinger, Loveday Conquest, and Joel Greenhouse.

339

approximately 180 patients between 18 and 46 years of age randomized to either a six-month regimen or a regimen with three months' therapy and three months' placebo. Following six months of treatment, all patients were observed for a possible return of symptoms of endometriosis during a one-year follow-up period.

Endometriosis is a condition in which functioning endometrial tissue (the mucous membrane lining the uterus) is found outside the uterus anywhere throughout the peritoneal cavity. The disease usually results in severe pain in the abdominal area and sometimes leads to infertility. The GnRH agonists are often used to improve symptoms of endometriosis through their ability to lower circulating estrogen levels. The lower estrogen levels that result from the use of GnRH agonists can lead to increased bone resorption and an overall decrease in BMD. This phenomenon is similar to that which occurs in postmenopausal women. Previous studies of GnRH agonists have shown small but significant loss of lumbar spine BMD. Studies by Whitehouse et al. (1990) and Tummon et al. (1988) have also demonstrated that most, but not all of the lost BMD is regained 6 to 12 months after the medication has been stopped.

In the present study, BMD of the lumbar spine was monitored at pretreatment, during treatment, and for one year following treatment, to assess the degree of bone loss during treatment and the recovery of BMD after treatment stopped. Quality control was an important consideration in this trial because of the relatively long duration of the longitudinal study, and the BMD changes under evaluation were expected to be small.

The BMD measurements in the trial were to be made at regional bone density centers with investigators in the same geographic region referring patients to the bone density center of that region. Each participating bone density center was equipped with a Hologic QDR1000 densitometer (a dual-energy x-ray absorptiometer) with a Hologic computer algorithm in a workstation to provide the BMD measurements. The machine also came with a Hologic X-Caliber model DPA/QDR-1 anthropomorphic spine phantom (made of calcium hydroxyappitite encased in plexiglass) of the first through fourth lumbar vertebrae. A technician at each bone density center was trained on the densitometer by the manufacturer prior to the start of the study and had access to the Hologic Users' Manual for information on the functioning of the machine and the standard application of techniques and procedures in using the machine. The spine phantom was used daily at each center for calibration to lessen the drift effect of the instrument. Each participating center also had regular quality control evaluations and continual support by the manufacturer's application specialists. A single pair of spine and block phantoms (intersite phantoms) was transported to each site four times a year for an additional level of assessment of instrument stability and for intersite comparisons.

For each patient visit to the bone density center, two BMD scans were obtained on lumbars 1 through 4 (L1 to L4) of the patient, with repositioning of the patient for the second scan. Careful positioning of the patient was required each time, with the positions on subsequent visits duplicating as much as possible those at the pretreatment visit. The scans were recorded in a tape to be played back on the workstation screen at the time of reading. A technician at the center would perform the reading of the BMD scan by identifying a global region of interest of the scan and by setting limits to the vertebral body (L2 to L4) to be evaluated by the computer algorithm. If possible, the responsibilities were to be carried out by the same technician throughout the trial.

Centralized readings are generally thought to be more accurate, precise, and homogeneous since the technicians at the individual centers may not be fully familiar with the anatomy of the spine to identify correctly the limits of interest, and there may be abnormalities in the lumbar vertebrae which makes it hard to define the limits correctly (e.g., an extra lumbar vertebra, scoliotic curve of the spine, vertebral compression fractures, spinal disc degeneration with osteophytes, and disc space narrowing). A centralized reading could allow a professional radiologist knowledgeable about the anatomical variations in the lumbar spine to dedicate the time to the reading without interruptions. The uniformity in the setting of the bone limits and the appropriate labeling of the vertebrae are hence expected to reduce the variation in the scan readings in a centralized setting. However, centralized reading of all scans takes time in the transport and reading of the scans and incur extra cost for the centralized reader.

With the fairly new technology involved in the measurement of BMD, there was uncertainty in deciding on the decentralized (versus centralized) option despite the convenience of the procedure. The current study was designed to find out what was achievable under centralized reading, to gain an insight into what might at best happen in a decentralized setting, and if appropriate, to use the centralized readings to set standards to evaluate individual center performance and to start a monitoring program.

1.2 Experimental Design

An experiment was designed to simulate the theoretically ideal setting of both a centralized and a decentralized operation, and to evaluate the individual center's performance. A sample of scans was selected at random from those available at each center at a suitable time early in the study. All scans selected were pooled across the centers and read by three qualified individuals. The sample scans from a given center were also read at the center for evaluation of the center's performance.

The main constraint in the design of the experiment was to be able to fit this study into the main clinical trial with respect to the protocol, timing, and the budget of the trial. The bone density centers were the units to be evaluated, and all eight bone density centers with Hologic densitometers were included in the study. With uncertainty in the enrollment of the trial, a random sample of 10 pretreatment scans was planned for each center primarily from practical considerations of the limited resources. The sample size would require each centralized reader to read all sample scans in two days at a rate of about three or four scans per hour. This number of scans would also be desirable to assess center performance based on the percentage of readings outside the quality control limits. Pretreatment scans were to be used so that an early assessment, and if necessary, corrective actions could be in place for a timely evaluation of the data for the clinical trial. One scan per patient was chosen to provide a more varied sample for assessment. Equal representation of the treatment groups was not necessary but was employed in case an extended assessment to posttreated scans became necessary. To allow timely evaluation of the clinical trial, the study was conducted before all eight centers could enroll at least 10 patients. Thus a total of 68 sample scans (5 to 10 per center) resulted in the study.

Several precautionary measures were taken in the centralized reading of the BMD scans. Three qualified readers participated in the centralized reading session, to prepare for the future monitoring if needed, and to allow for possible cross-validation of the monitoring procedure with flexibility in the choice of the future monitor. The centralized readers first participated in a teaching session given by a technician both experienced on the Hologic QDR1000 densitometer and familiar with the nafarelin study protocol. The three readers then read four training scans (not from the study sample) and reached a consensus within 2% of the BMD of these scans. The entire set of sample scans was then read individually by each centralized reader, in an order randomized for the reader. The scan identities were blinded to the readers, and the randomized ordering was to allow potentially systematic factors such as fatigue to show up as disagreements among the centralized readers.

2 DATA

Table 1 shows a sample of the data collected in this study. The bone area, bone mineral content, and BMD were read for each sample scan of each participating center by the three centralized readers and by the participating center. The quantity BMD is the key variable for analysis in this study. The other measurements are for auxiliary information.

3 METHODS AND MODELS

3.1 Centralized Reading Analyses

The BMD measurements from the three centralized readers were analyzed with the following two objectives: (1) to ascertain that the three centralized readers were in agreement, thus depicting what might happen at best in the decentralized setting if each center had personnel, facilities, and maintenance of facilities as ideal as in the centralized setting, and to provide a background against which a monitoring procedure could be initiated and cross-validated; and (2) to evaluate the level of precision of the BMD measurements the centralized setting offered, and to provide information for the choice of the future monitor. Factor

Table 1 Representative Sample of Centralized and Individual Center Readings of BMD Scans[a]

#	C#	ID	BA1	BA2	BA3	BC1	BC2	BC3	BMD1	BMD2	BMD3	BA	BC	BMD
12	2	510	42.25	42.77	41.73	40.35	40.64	39.94	0.955	0.950	0.957	41.58	39.72	0.955
13	2	604	40.73	41.06	40.95	40.67	40.98	40.71	0.998	0.998	0.994	40.66	40.43	0.994
15	6	801	56.05	56.90	55.75	56.35	67.16	66.13	1.184	1.180	1.186	55.43	65.53	1.182
17	6	805	47.58	48.16	47.61	42.05	42.26	41.97	0.884	0.877	0.882	47.20	41.41	0.877
37	1	1301	50.50	50.54	50.84	55.08	55.13	55.11	1.091	1.091	1.084	50.60	55.15	1.090

[a]#, Observation number; C#, center number; ID, scan ID; BA, bone area (cm^2); BC, bone mineral content (g); BMD, bone mineral density (g/cm^2); postscript i, reading from centralized reader $i = 1, 2, 3$; no postscript. reading from participating center.

analysis was used to assess the agreement of the BMD measurements from the three centralized readers and to estimate the inherent precision of each centralized reader in the reading of the scans under this ideal setting.

Factor analysis is a statistical method originally developed in psychology; this method has since been applied to many other sciences. The method is usually applied to multidimensional data, which are accessible measures from different perspectives of some often unobservable yet common structures. The correlation induced from the common structures often exhibit patterns revealing the interrelationships of the different perspectives. The method is used to reduce the dimension of the data, condensing the data to a more manageable size with the underlying structural information preserved for examination. The method provides a framework to model the underlining structure either from preexisting theory or through the construct of an approximation based on the more accessible measurements. An expository description of the rationale and topics of factor analysis can be found in Bartholomew (1987, pp. 39–72).

In our discussion of the analyses, we assume the factor analysis framework using the orthogonal factor model in Press (1972, pp. 217, 283–319). Thus,

$$\mathbf{Y} = \mathbf{\Lambda F} + \mathbf{\Theta} + \mathbf{E}, \tag{1}$$

where $\mathbf{Y} = (Y_1, Y_2, Y_3)^T$ is the observable three-component measurement vector, with the Y_i component being the observed reading from the centralized reader i, $i = 1, 2, 3$, and $\mathbf{Y}$ is assumed to have a multivariate normal distribution with mean $\mathbf{\Theta}$ and covariance matrix $\mathbf{\Sigma}$, $\mathbf{F}$ is the m-component ($m \leq 3$) vector of unobservable underlying random factors with a multivariate normal distribution with mean $\mathbf{0}$ and covariance matrix $\mathbf{I}$ (the $m \times m$ identity matrix), $\mathbf{\Lambda}$ is the $3 \times m$ factor loading matrix, $\mathbf{\Theta} = (\theta_1, \theta_2, \theta_3)^T$ is a fixed unknown three-component vector, and $\mathbf{E} = (\epsilon_1, \epsilon_2, \epsilon_3)^T$ is the three-component random error vector with ϵ_i the random measurement error from centralized reader i. The random vector $\mathbf{E}$ is assumed independent of $\mathbf{F}$ and has a multivariate normal distribution with mean $\mathbf{0}$ and a diagonal covariance matrix $\mathbf{D}_e$.

The factor analytic framework is a good model for the current problem, as it involves a multidimensional observation ($\mathbf{Y}$, being readings from the three centralized readers) for each scan. The agreement of BMD readings from the three centralized readers is in part a question on the underlying correlation structure of the data, and in part a question on whether these specific readers have identical characteristics. A factor analysis would thus allow reduction of the three-dimensional data to a lower dimension, showing the common structure underlying the correlation pattern observed in the data. The other underlining structures modeled in the framework are the effects from the designated centralized readers. Different kinds of effects are modeled, and modeled separately for each centralized reader. Test results based on the data can therefore delineate clearly any characteristics that differ among the centralized readers. The three kinds of reader effects modeled are: location and scale shift characteristics, both modeled by different fixed-effect parameters and both of which can be tested for differences among readers, and precision characteristics, modeled by separate random error components which can be examined for each reader. The model is also more realistic in that tests for agreement among readers can be performed without restrictions on equal precisions from the three centralized readers.

The hypothesis to be tested is that if the three centralized readers are in agreement, the vector of underlying factors $\mathbf{F}$ is one-dimensional (there is only one underlying factor determined by the true value of the scan), common to the centralized readings explaining the correlation observed in the data. The underlying factor is transformed further by a systematic scale shift through the factor loading matrix $\mathbf{\Lambda}$ and by a systematic location shift through the fixed, unknown vector $\mathbf{\Theta}$. Agreement among the three readers implies that their effects on the location and scale shifts (and hence the underlying readings) are the same. Thus, the observed reading y_i from reader i is generated by the process

$$ y_i = y + \epsilon_i = \left(\frac{1}{\sqrt{3}} \right) \frac{(\sqrt{3}\sigma)(y - \theta)}{\sigma} + \theta + \epsilon_i, \tag{2} $$

where ϵ_i is the random error of reader $i, i = 1, 2, 3$. The one-dimensional unobservable underlying factor $\mathbf{F}$ is interpreted as the normalized value of the scan $(y - \theta)/\sigma$, with y being the unobservable "true" BMD value of a randomly selected scan, having a normal distribution with mean θ and variance σ^2. Thus, the readings from the centralized readers can be thought of as combinations of the true value of the scan with random errors.

The concordance between two readers has been examined using the notion of a concordance line in two dimensions as discussed in Miller et al. (1980) and Lin (1989). If two readers can read the scans perfectly without error, a plot of the readings of one reader against those of the other should be a straight line with intercept zero and slope 1. Since random error is expected, the analysis is to test whether the data are compatible with the diagonal concordance line.

The factor analytic approach here is actually an extension of the two-dimensional concordance line to higher dimensions. The analysis for the three-reader case is therefore done by testing the compatibility of the data with a diagonal concordance line in a three-dimensional plot. The following hypotheses were tested:

1. One factor (the true scan value) is fundamental to the data generation process (i.e., $m = 1$).
2. $\mathbf{\Gamma} = \mathbf{\alpha}_{10}$, where $\mathbf{\Lambda} = \mathbf{\Gamma D}_l^{1/2}$, $\mathbf{\Gamma}$ is the first normalized 3×1 eigenvector of $\mathbf{\Sigma}$, $\mathbf{D}_l$ is the first 1×1 eigenvalue of $\mathbf{\Sigma}$, and $\mathbf{\alpha}_{10}^{\mathrm{T}} = (1/\sqrt{3}, 1/\sqrt{3}, 1/\sqrt{3})$.
3. $\theta_1 = \theta_2 = \theta_3$; that is,

$$\mathbf{C\Theta} = \begin{pmatrix} 0 \\ 0 \end{pmatrix}, \qquad \text{where} \quad \mathbf{C} = \begin{pmatrix} 1 & -1 & 0 \\ 1 & 0 & -1 \end{pmatrix}. \qquad (3)$$

An approximate solution to the factor analysis was obtained using the principal component. The principal component was used to represent the concordance line. The diagonality of the concordance line was tested through hypotheses 2 and 3. Hypothesis 2 is analogous to testing for a unit slope for the two-reader case. Hypothesis 3 is analogous to testing for a zero intercept in the two-dimensional case. Tests on the one-factor hypothesis and on the concordance line were performed at the 0.05 significance level. Hypotheses 1 and 2 were tested using asymptotic methods given by Press (1972) and Morrison (1967). Hypothesis 3 was tested using the likelihood ratio test given by Anderson (1958).

Other analyses included tests of normal distribution for readings from each centralized reader, and a three-dimensional plot of the centralized readings. Profiles of the sample scans were summarized using the average of the three centralized readings to represent a scan. The coefficient of variation of random error was obtained for each centralized reader using the Winsorized residual standard deviation estimate from a prinicpal factor analysis with one factor and the mean Winsorized centralized readings for each reader. Details of the Winsorization and the estimation of the residual standard deviation are described in the results section below.

3.2 Cross-Validation and Individual Center Performance

An approach similar to quality control was taken here. [See, e.g., Duncan (1974) for a general introduction to quality control.] A monitoring procedure could be set up to determine if the individual centers were in control. The monitoring procedure would use the readings from two centralized readers who were in agreement (i.e., in control) to construct the quality control limits to evaluate whether the individual centers conform to their standard. One of the readers of the pair would be designated as the "future monitor" and the other as the "concording reader." If the individual centers were not in control, further monitoring may be necessary and the future monitor would carry the responsibility of reading new sample scans for such a monitoring program.

The quality control limits for evaluation of the individual center performance were set using the least-squares regression line to estimate the concordance line between readings of the future monitor (independent variable) and those of the concording reader (dependent variable) obtained at the centralized reading session. Simultaneous tolerance intervals for the linear regression model were then constructed via the product set procedure given by Limam and Thomas (1988), at the 95% confidence and 90% tolerance levels. The tolerance band was to contain with 95% confidence, simultaneously for all independent variable values, at least 90% of the dependent variable values centered at the regression line. Measurements of a reader or a center comparable to the concording reader (i.e., in control) were expected to fall within the tolerance band at least 90% of the time. Otherwise, an excessive percentage of the readings would fall outside the tolerance band.

Six monitoring procedures using different combinations of choices of the roles of the centralized readers were possible. Depending on the results of the analyses of the centralized readings, procedure(s) based on pair(s) of readers in agreement could be used to examine the individual center performance. If all three centralized readers were shown to be in agreement, all six procedures could be examined to investigate how sensitive the center performance results were to the choice of readers used in setting the limits. The extra centralized reader in each case could also be used to cross-validate the procedure. In each cross-validation, at least 90% of the 68 scan readings of the extra reader were expected to fall within the respective control limits. Due to the construction of the six tolerance bands by permutations of pairs of centralized readers, results of the six cross-validations and evaluations of center performances are expected to be somewhat related.

4   RESULTS

The individual centers that participated in the study and the number of sample scans from each center are shown in Table 2. Profiles of the sample scans ($N = 68$) are summarized in Table 3.

4.1   Centralized Reading Analyses

Figure 1 shows a three-dimensional plot for the centralized readings of BMD. The readings followed approximately the diagonal straight line in three dimen-

Table 2   Participating Centers and Number of Scans Analyzed

Center	Number of Sample Scans
1	10
2	10
3	5
4	9
5	10
6	9
7	8
8	7
	68

Table 3   Sample Scan Profiles (Based on 68 Average Centralized Readings)

	Bone Area (cm²)	Bone Mineral Content (g)	BMD (g/cm²)
Mean	49.39	53.23	1.075
SD	7.54	11.13	0.1315
Range	38.51–65.21	33.52–82.78	0.714–1.535

sions, suggesting agreement of the centralized readers in the reading of BMD in a centralized setting. The readings from each reader were compatible with an underlying normal distribution, tested using the Shapiro–Wilk statistic (Shapiro and Wilk, 1965). The p-values were 0.807, 0.852, and 0.573 for centralized readers 1, 2, and 3, respectively. The factor analysis model was judged to be a reasonable model to use.

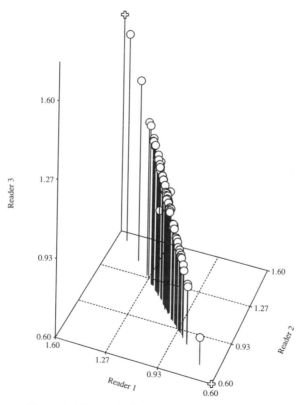

Figure 1. BMD (g/cm²) from three centralized readers.

Test of Hypothesis 1

The principal component solution of the factor analysis discussed in Press (1972) and Morrison (1967) was obtained. An unbiased estimate of Σ was given by

$$S = \begin{pmatrix} 0.01711 & 0.01726 & 0.01711 \\ 0.01726 & 0.01749 & 0.01727 \\ 0.01711 & 0.01727 & 0.01768 \end{pmatrix}, \tag{4}$$

with trace $S = 0.05228$. An estimate of the population eigenvalue vector was

$$(\hat{l}_1, \hat{l}_2, \hat{l}_3)^T = (0.051855, 0.000385, 0.000036)^T. \tag{5}$$

The 95% asymptotic confidence intervals for l_1, l_2, and l_3 were: (0.038737, 0.078406), (0.000288, 0.000582), and (0.000027, 0.000054), respectively. Expressed as fractions of the total variance trace S, the intervals were (0.7410, 1.4999), (0.0055, 0.0111), and (0.0005, 0.0010). By using these intervals as constraints on the three fractions and by observing the additional constraints that each fraction should be between zero and 1 and that the three fractions should sum to 1, linear programming can be used (essentially by solving the inequalities) to narrow down further the intervals for the three fractions. The lower bound for the fraction of the total variance explained by the first principal component was 0.9878. With the first principal component explaining a large proportion of the total variance, we concluded that $m = 1$.

Test of Hypothesis 2

The hypothesis was tested using the asymptotic distribution of the principal component solution under the null hypothesis in Morrison (1967). The estimate of the matrix of orthonormal eigenvectors of S was

$$(\alpha_1, \alpha_2, \alpha_3) = \begin{pmatrix} 0.57317 & 0.36685 & 0.73273 \\ 0.57919 & 0.45119 & 0.67895 \\ 0.57967 & -0.81354 & -0.04613 \end{pmatrix}. \tag{6}$$

The test statistic is

$$(N - 1)(\hat{l}_1 \alpha_{10}^T S^{-1} \alpha_{10} + \hat{l}_1^{-1} \alpha_{10}^T S \alpha_{10} - 2) = 1.939.$$

Under the null hypothesis, the test statistic had a chi-squared distribution with 2 degrees of freedom. Hence, the data were compatible in direction with the diagonal line in three dimensions (p-value = 0.379).

Test of Hypothesis 3

Under the null hypothesis, $\mathbf{C\overline{Y}}$ has a multivariate normal distribution with mean $\mathbf{C\Theta}$, covariance matrix $(1/N)\,\mathbf{C\Sigma C}^T$. The likelihood ratio test statistic is

$$[N(N - 2)/2(N - 1)](\mathbf{C\overline{Y}})^T(\mathbf{CSC}^T)^{-1}(\mathbf{C\overline{Y}}) = 2.413,$$

corresponding to a p-value of 0.097 according to the F distribution with 2 and 66 degrees of freedom as given by Anderson (1958). Hence the data were compatible with hypothesis 3, completing the test for the diagonal line in three dimensions.

Thus, the tests of hypotheses 1, 2, and 3 confirmed that the three centralized readers were in agreement.

Coefficient of Variation of Random Error

To evaluate the level of precision of the BMD measurements that the centralized setting offered, the coefficient of variations were obtained for each centralized reader. The residual correlation matrix $\mathbf{C}_r$ was estimated in the principal factor analysis with one factor. The residual standard deviation of the random error of centralized reader i was the ith diagonal element of $\mathbf{D}_e$ estimated by $\mathbf{D}_0\mathbf{C}_r\mathbf{D}_0^T$, where $\mathbf{D}_0$ is the diagonal matrix with the standard deviation of readings from the three centralized readers on the diagonal.

Two scans (ID 2210 and 2204 of center 8) appeared to have certain centralized readers having relatively outlying readings (see cross-validation results in Section 4.2 and discussion in Section 5). An ad hoc procedure was tried to Winsorize these readings to provide additional precision estimates more inherent to the readers for the basic scans in the clinical trial. The centralized readings for scan 2210 were (1.155, 1.152, 0.968). The Winsorization was performed so that the Winsorized value of the outlier (0.968 of reader 3) was the same distance from (but on the other side of) the resulting Winsorized mean as the most distant reading (1.155). The outlier value of 0.968 was Winsorized to a value of 1.149 in this case. Similarly, scan 2204 had centralized readings (1.077, 1.132, 1.072) and the outlier value 1.132 (of reader 2) was Winsorized to a value of 1.082.

The standard deviation estimation procedure was applied to the whole data set, to the Winsorized data set, and to the data set with the two scans deleted. The standard deviation, mean, and coefficient of variation estimates from the three procedures are shown in Table 4.

The Winsorized procedure resulted in very similar estimates as those with the two scans deleted and quite different from those when all original data were included. Whereas the estimates from the original data reflect more of the precision levels of the readers at the centralized reading session of this study, the Winsorized estimates were more robust against the outliers and reflect more of the precision levels of the readers under more typical conditions. The coefficient of variation of random errors in the BMD reading from the three readers

Table 4   Coefficient of Variation (%) of the Random Error
Component in Centralized Reading of BMD (g/cm²) Scans

	All Data	Winsorized	With Deletion
Mean			
Reader 1	1.0773	1.0773	1.0761
Reader 2	1.0753	1.0746	1.0733
Reader 3	1.0739	1.0765	1.0755
S.D.			
Reader 1	0.00451	0.00298	0.00302
Reader 2	0.00917	0.00467	0.00463
Reader 3	0.02295	0.00577	0.00578
CV			
Reader 1	0.42	0.28	0.28
Reader 2	0.85	0.43	0.43
Reader 3	2.14	0.54	0.54

at the centralized reading session were: 0.42% (reader 1), 0.85% (reader 2), and 2.14% (reader 3). The coefficients inherent to the centralized readers based on the Winsorized estimates were: 0.28% (reader 1), 0.43% (reader 2), and 0.54% (reader 3). Thus, all three readers had high precision levels in general, with a coefficient of variation averaging to 0.42%. Reader 1 offered the highest precision, and reader 3 the lowest, among the three centralized readers. The variation among the three centralized readers suggested that the precisions would vary somewhat in a decentralized setting even if the individual centers had personnel and facilities as ideal as those in the centralized setting.

4.2   Cross-Validation and Individual Center Performance

Given all three centralized readers were in agreement, Table 5 shows the results of the cross-validations and the evaluations of the individual center performances for the six combinations of choices of the roles of the centralized readers. The analyses were based on the original data, as they represent the results from the centralized reading session where the three centralized readers were shown to be in agreement. An example of the resulting regression analysis and the 95% confidence, 90% tolerance band is shown in Figure 2, with reader 3 as the future monitor and reader 1 as the concording reader. Data from the individual centers are also plotted. The six cross-validations resulted in a maximum of 7.4% of the 68 sample scan readings outside the tolerance limits. This was well within the 10% level specified in construction of the tolerance bands. All six monitoring procedures were therefore cross-validated.

In the assessment of the participating center performance, each center had at most one scan result outside the tolerance limits of each analysis. Centers 2 and 5 had 10 sample scans; the percentage of readings outside the tolerance limits was therefore within the expected for each of these centers. Center 4 had nine

Table 5   Cross-Validation and Center Performances: Readings outside the 95% Confidence 90% BMD Tolerance Limits

Future Monitor Reader:	1	1	2	2	3	3
Concording Reader:	2	3	3	1	1	2
Cross-Validation on Reader:	3	2	1	3	2	1
Cross-validation results						
Number outside limits	3	1	1	5	2	1
Percent outside limits	4.4	1.5	1.5	7.4	2.9	1.5
Center performance						
Number outside limits						
Center 1	0	0	0	0	0	0
Center 2	0	0	0	1	0	0
Center 3	0	0	0	0	0	0
Center 4	1	0	0	1	1	0
Center 5	1	0	0	1	0	0
Center 6	0	0	0	0	0	0
Center 7	0	0	0	0	0	0
Center 8	0	0	0	1	1	1
Percent outside limits, overall	2.9	0.0	0.0	5.9	2.9	1.5

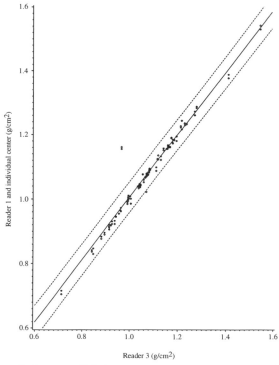

Figure 2. Tolerance limits set at 90% for BMD measurements: reader 1 (*), individual center (◇).

sample scans resulting in 11.1% of the readings outside the tolerance limits in three of the six monitoring procedures. Center 8 also had one sample scan (out of seven, 14.3%) outside the tolerance limits in three of the six procedures, but the reasons appeared to be coming from the outlier readings of centralized readers 2 and 3 rather than being related to the performance of the center (see Section 4.3). The percentages of readings outside the tolerance limits were not excessive. Further, the overall percentage of readings outside the tolerance limits was smaller than the percentage in the cross-validation for all six monitoring procedures. The individual centers were therefore comparable in performance to those of the centralized readers.

4.3 Investigations of the Scans outside the Tolerance Limits

The scans outside the tolerance limits were reviewed. Table 6 shows the details of these scans and the reader(s) or center(s) for which the readings were outside the tolerance limits of the six monitoring procedures. Some scans appeared to be more problematic to read. It was found that three patients had scans showing spinal abnormalities: a scoliotic curve appeared in scan 2210, an extra vertebra in scan 1007, and a scoliotic curve and an extra vertebra appeared in scan 1008, leading to a mislabeling of the vertebrae to be analyzed. One scan (1209) was not of good quality.

Choice of good readers, both as the future monitor and as the concording reader in the construction of the quality limits, was vital to the success of the monitoring procedure. Centralized reader 3 was noted as having an outlier reading for scan 2210, explaining why the extra reader and the center had readings

Table 6 Details of Scans outside the 95% Confidence 90% BMD Tolerance Limits[a]

Future Monitor Reader :	1	1	2	2	3	3
Concording Reader:	2	3	3	1	1	2
Cross-Validation on Reader:	3	2	1	3	2	1

Scan Description	Reader no. (i) or Center no. (C_i) with Scan Reading outside Limits					
Center 8 (2210,S)	3	2, C8	1, C8	3	—	—
Center 8 (2204)	3, C8	2	—	—	2	1
Center 4 (1007,X)	3	—	—	—	—	—
Center 5 (1209,Q)	3	—	—	3	—	—
Center 7 (2005)	3	—	—	3	—	—
Center 2 (505)	C2	—	—	—	—	—
Center 4 (1008,S,X)	C4	C4	—	C4	—	—
Center 5 (1211)	C5	—	—	C5	—	—

[a] C_i center i; S, scoliotic curve; X, extra vertebra; Q, inadequate quality.

outside the limits when reader 3 was the concording reader. Similarly, the reading was outside the limits if readers 1 and 2 (in either role) were used to construct the tolerance limits. The same applied to centralized reader 2 having an outlier reading for scan 2204. Precisionwise, centralized reader 1 was noted before as having the highest, and reader 3 the least, precision among the centralized readers. Similar findings were noted here. Tolerance limits based on readers 1 and 2 (especially with reader 1 as the concording reader) had higher percentages of scans outside the quality limits in both the cross-validation and the center performance evaluations, representing more stringent quality limits. Centralized reader 3 appeared to have more problems in reading the scans, with the readings outside the limits for scans 2210, 1007, 1209, and 2205 (three of which were more difficult to read) when cross-validated by tolerance limits constructed from readers 1 and 2. Similarly, monitoring procedures with tolerance limits based on centralized reader 3 had fewer percentages of scans outside the limits, representing less stringent quality limits.

5   CONCLUSIONS

The results of this study demonstrate that after a teaching session, BMD measurements of the lumbar spine are highly reliable in a centralized reading. In the current multicenter trial, lumbar spine BMD was determined on a population with relatively young subjects with little spinal pathology (fractures or lumbar disc degeneration). With stringent quality assurance measures done on each bone densitometer during the study and a teaching session of all participating technicians at the start of the study, BMD readings at the individual centers can also be reliable and reproducible. The decentralized operation maintains its control, and a centralized reading is not necessary in this trial.

In a study involving older populations, more difficulties are expected in the lumbar spine scan analysis phase of the BMD determinations, and thus the reproducibility of the scan analysis may be expected to decline. For osteoporosis trials or other studies on BMD in which patients may have more abnormalities, the methodology offered in this study provides a third alternative (i.e., that of using a monitoring program to do quality control in the decentralized readings). The program would combine the advantage of a centralized operation where readings are expected to be more homogeneous with that of a decentralized operation where the reading can be done with convenience.

A factor analytic framework was used here. Lin (1989) proposed a concordance correlation coefficient (ρ_c) to evaluate reliability. The coefficient gives an index for the degree in which multidimensional observations fall on the diagonal concordance line. This model is a special case of the model in this study, namely, $\mathbf{Y} = \mathbf{\Theta} + (\mathbf{E} + \mathbf{\Lambda F})$, in which the random error component, the scale shift component, and the random scan component are not differentiated. A re-derivation of Lin's extension to the multivariate case gives $\rho_c = 2$ (sum of off-diagonal elements of $\mathbf{\Sigma}$)/[sum of squares of differences between all possible pairs of θ's + $2(p - 1)$ (sum of diagonal elements of Σ)]. The concordance coefficient among the three centralized readers was $\rho_c = 0.9877$, confirming high concordance among the centralized readers. The advantage with the concordance coefficient is that it may eliminate situations in which the variability is so small that practically insignificant departures from the diagonal line would reach statistical significance level when the hypotheses for compatibility to the diagonal line were tested. However, further work is needed to construct a confidence interval for ρ_c under the multivariate extension for hypothesis-testing purposes. The factor analytic framework differentiates the components of the underlying structures in its model (i.e., the location, scale, and precision characteristics of each reader), providing individual estimates for further examination should the readers not be in agreement. The estimates of the precision of the centralized readers also provide information for choice of the future monitor.

SOFTWARE NOTES AND REFERENCES

The principal component solution was obtained using the PRINCOMP procedure in SAS with the COV option. The principal factor analysis with one factor was obtained using the FACTOR procedure in SAS with the PRINIT and COV options.

SAS Institute, Inc. (1988). *SAS Procedures Guide for Personal Computers*, 6th ed. Cary, N.C.: SAS Institute.

SAS Institute, Inc. (1987). *SAS/STAT Guide for Personal Computers*, 6th ed. Cary, N.C.: SAS Institute.

QUESTIONS AND PROBLEMS

1. The sample scans were randomly selected from the scans obtained in the multicenter clinical trial up to the time that this study was scheduled. Assuming that the patients enrolled thus far were representative of the patient populations, the readings would provide information about the BMD of the patients in the trial prior to receiving treatment. Suppose that you are part of the investigative team for this trial and you have the treatment regimen assignment and other information for each of these patients: What information can you get from the BMD data given? What methods would you use to answer your questions? How would different conclusions to your questions affect the remaining investigative efforts to evaluate the treatment regimens?

2. We have examined the individual centers only as to whether they conform to the standards of the centralized readers. Examine the data given. How do the readers at the individual centers compare to the centralized readers?

PART VI

Epidemiology, Toxicology

CHAPTER 18

Modeling the Precursors of Cervical Cancer

Alison J. Kirby and David J. Spiegelhalter

1 MOTIVATION AND BACKGROUND

To be able to plan the management of chronic diseases, some knowledge of their natural history is essential. There are many such diseases, with examples ranging from nonfatal myocardial infarctions to leukemia remissions and recurrences of asthma attacks. Prospective longitudinal studies are used increasingly to obtain information on such diseases, where the aim is not only to describe the outcomes but also to model the underlying disease process.

There has been a variety of recent developments in the statistical analysis of the data resulting from longitudinal studies. These "event history" data consist of the times and types of the observed events of interest, together with covariates, for each of the individuals in a study. For example, Clayton (1988a) gives a comprehensive review which links the epidemiologic person-years method for incidence rates derived from longitudinally observed cohort studies to partial likelihood methods and conditional logistic regression methods for case–control studies. If the data set is very good, with full information on covariates, disease states, and exact transition times, the extensions of the Cox proportional hazards model described by Aalen et al. (1980) and reviewed by Cuzick (1986) represent a sophisticated and flexible structure for analysis. However, data of such quality are not common, so alternative solutions are often required.

One possible and common imperfection in the data occurs when the exact transition times between states are not observed, resulting in interval censored data. This will typically be the case in follow-up of conditions such as diabetes or thyroid disease and in any context in which follow-up is based on routine appointments. In the past Markov models in discrete time have often been used,

Case Studies in Biometry, Edited by Nicholas Lange, Louise Ryan, Lynne Billard, David Brillinger, Loveday Conquest, and Joel Greenhouse. ISBN 0-471-58885-7 © 1994 John Wiley & Sons, Inc.

with failure to keep an appointment treated as a missing value within a framework of fixed time intervals between observations.

A second problem with data concerns errors in the measurement of the current state of the disease, which will generally be the case when a change in state is not immediately apparent and it is infeasible routinely to carry out full invasive tests. This leads to proxy measures of disease status being adopted. If independent repeated measures are available, latent class methods (Kaldor and Clayton, 1985) can be used to make inferences concerning the true underlying state. Independent studies where the common measure and a full invasive test are both carried out can be used to give information on error rates, but this can lead to a wide range of possible values. An alternative approach is to assume only certain types of error (e.g., not permit false positive measurements), but the appropriateness of this depends very much on the application.

A possible solution to these and other problems is to take a Bayesian approach, in which missing covariates, parameters, and observables are all treated as random quantities whose interdependencies are summarized by a graphical model; inference on quantities of interest may then be obtained by a computationally intense technique known as *Gibbs sampling*. This technique is one variant of numerous Monte Carlo Markov chain methods. It originates in the image processing field but its use in mainstream statistics has been suggested by both Gelfand and Smith (1990) and Clayton (1988b), and its applicability to a wide variety of problems has been shown (e.g., Gelfand et al., 1990; Smith and Roberts, 1992; Lange et al., 1992; Lange, 1992; Smith and Roberts, 1993; Gilks et al., 1993; Dellaportas and Smith, 1993.)

The following case study describes data collected on a routine basis from a cervical smear screening program which has some of the difficulties described above. A graphical model of the data is given, and the use of Gibbs sampling in deriving parameter estimates for a model based on this graph is outlined. Before the data set is described, some background medical information is given.

Medical Background

Cervical cancer is the second most common female cancer worldwide. However, unlike many other forms of cancer, the disease can be detected before it becomes invasive using a *cervical smear* or *Pap test* (Ginsberg, 1991), which shows cell changes which are precursors to the invasive disease. In the United Kingdom the smear-taking procedure is performed by doctors or nurses with wide ranges of expertise and training. The glass slide on which the cells are smeared is sent to a cytology laboratory, where it is stained and read. Depending on the protocol of an individual laboratory, the reading may be done with or without prior knowledge of the woman's previous smear results.

The smear is categorized (Table 1) according to the type of cell changes observed and the number of cells affected. The grades from 1 to 6 represent increasing severity of abnormalities. The categories are poorly defined and sub-

Table 1 Cytology Grades: Surface Level

Category	Grade
0	Missing or inadequate
1	Negative/normal
2	Inflammatory
3	Mild dyskaryosis
4	Moderate dyskaryosis
5	Severe dyskaryosis
6	Malignant
7	Viral changes[a]

[a]Indicates presence of human papillomavirus; this grade is used primarily in addition to one of categories 1–6.

jective, with only broad agreement among cytologists on what the classifications mean, despite national guidelines for the United Kingdom (Evans et al., 1986). The difficulty in definition is due partly to categorizing what is in effect a disease continuum.

Depending on the severity of the abnormalities, the results of any previous smears, and the local policy, the woman may be referred for a decision on treatment or asked to return for another smear a few months later. The treatment used will depend on the severity of disease but will result in the removal of tissue, which can be cross-sectioned and examined and histologically graded by pathologists. These biopsy grades (Table 2) are also subjective, although the consensus is that they are a more accurate indication of the "true" biological state.

Although it is known that the cell changes revealed by a smear test may be precursors to cervical cancer (Paul, 1988), estimates of the rate at which they progress to invasive disease vary considerably. In addition, it is possible for the cell changes to regress spontaneously. There is great interest in knowing what these rates are, as a sensible treatment policy should not unnecessarily

Table 2 Histology Grades: Tissue Cross-Section

Category	Grade[a]
0	Missing or inadequate
1	Negative/normal
2	CIN I
3	CIN II
4	CIN III
5	Microinvasive
6	Invasive

[a]CIN, cervical intraepithelial neoplasia.

treat women who will recover without intervention, yet must not allow women at high risk of progression to cancer to remain untreated.

In the past, modeling of the precursors and invasive stages has been done either by using incidence and prevalence data with rates of progression and regression chosen to give the observed incidences in a population (Knox, 1988) or by simple Markov chain modeling in discrete time of the smear categories observed (Coppleson and Brown, 1975). The former has the disadvantage that it makes no use of the actual smear histories of women, and in complex models the rates are often not uniquely defined. Simple Markov chains assume that the smear category is correct, whereas in reality it is merely a surrogate measure of the underlying state and is subject to errors.

2 DATA

The data set discussed in this case study is from a project carried out by the Harris Birthright Research Unit in the University of Aberdeen, which was set up to look at the natural history of cervical cytopathology in women whose smears showed minor abnormalities. The study chose 1000 previously untreated women from the local screening program, of whom 500 had a normal smear in 1978 (the controls) and 500 had a smear showing minor cellular abnormalities (the patients). The smear histories and any subsequent treatments for these women up to 1988 were obtained and recorded. A more complete description of this study may be found in Kirby et al. (1992). The sequences of smears for these 1000 women provide the data set used in the following analysis.

A representative sample of the data is shown in Table 3. The data have two separate components, one corresponding to each individual woman, and the second corresponding to each separate smear. The individual-specific component includes the patient/control code, her study number, number of smears, biopsy result (where "9" denotes no treatment), and time interval (in days) from the last smear to biopsy (where "−1" denotes no treatment). The smear-specific component includes the patient/control code, study number, smear number, current smear grade (reduced to a two-point scale for this analysis), and time (in days) from the previous smear. It will be noted that only 998 women are included, as two of the patients were found to have had a biopsy prior to 1978 and so were excluded from the study.

The individual smear histories of women may be plotted through time to show the variations that occur and to indicate possible difficulties in modeling the data. For many controls the history consists of a series of negative (smear grade 1) or perhaps inflammatory (smear grade 2) smears. There is little information on possible progression and regression rates in such histories, but they give a baseline for normality.

Figure 1 shows a smear history that is typical of that of a control. For some controls and many patients, however, the picture is (literally) very different.

Table 3 Sample of the Data

0	491	3	9	−1	0	500	1	0	0
0	492	6	9	−1	0	500	2	0	361
0	493	6	1	48	0	500	3	0	721
0	494	2	9	−1	0	500	4	0	1058
0	495	5	9	−1	1	1	1	1	0
0	496	4	9	−1	1	1	2	0	213
0	497	2	9	−1	1	1	3	0	1338
0	498	4	9	−1	1	1	4	0	1814
0	499	3	9	−1	1	1	5	0	236
0	500	4	9	−1	1	1	6	0	295
1	1	6	9	−1	1	2	1	1	0
1	2	2	9	−1	1	2	2	0	273
1	3	8	1	0	1	3	1	1	0
1	4	2	9	−1	1	3	2	1	21
1	5	7	9	−1	1	3	3	1	70
1	6	5	1	0	1	3	4	0	273
1	7	3	0	0	1	3	5	1	95
1	8	3	1	0	1	3	6	1	199
1	9	3	1	0	1	3	7	1	14
1	10	3	1	0	1	3	8	1	42

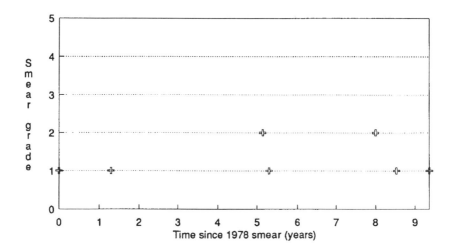

Figure 1. Example of a *normal* smear history.

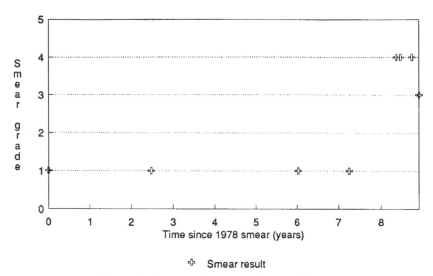

Figure 2. Example of a *progressive* smear history.

Figure 2 shows the history of control 490, which although it begins with negative smears, shows a progression through to more serious grades. This history is unusual only in that the woman has not yet been biopsied. On the other hand, the smear history of patient 56 (Figure 3) illustrates a dramatic regression. These histories show only some of the possibilities. Even though in Aberdeen a smear is read with knowledge of previous ones, there is a lot of variability in the grades assigned. The smear histories provide imperfectly observed "snapshots" of a discrete state process which is taking place through time, with unobserved transitions between states.

3   METHODS AND MODELS

The main methods used in dealing with the cervical smear data will be those of graphical modeling (Whittaker, 1990) for models of the disease process, data and parameter dependencies, and Gibbs sampling for estimating both model and natural history parameters.

3.1   Gibbs Sampling

Gibbs sampling is a technique widely used in image processing for the restoration of blurred or distorted pictures. It was developed from a Monte Carlo integration algorithm which Metropolis et al. (1953) originally described in the

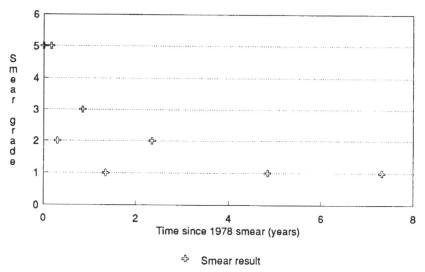

Figure 3. Example of a *regressive* smear history.

context of molecular modeling. The method was discussed in the context of conventional statistics by Hastings (1970), but it was Geman and Geman who extended it in image analysis into what is now known as Gibbs sampling. They described the method in detail (Geman and Geman, 1984), setting up a hierarchical stochastic model for the original image and giving an algorithm for computing the maximum a posteriori (MAP) estimate of the original image, which was essentially an annealing procedure applied to a generalization of the Metropolis algorithm.

In 1988, both Gelfand and Smith (1990) and Clayton (1988b) considered the use of the Gibbs sampler for calculating numerical estimates of marginal probability densities. This estimation problem arises frequently when a Bayesian approach is used and had previously required complex numerical methods, such as Laplace approximations and adaptive quadrature, which additionally often needed tailoring to a given problem (Smith, 1992).

The notation of Gelfand and Smith will be used here. Densities are denoted by square brackets so, for example, $[X, Y], [X|Y]$, and $[X]$ denote joint, conditional, and marginal forms. The notation "~" will be used to denote "is distributed as". It is assumed in the following that the random variables are real and possibly vector valued, having a joint density function that is strictly positive over the product sample space. This is to ensure that the full set of conditional distributions uniquely defines the full joint density. Densities for continuous variables are assumed to exist with respect to Lebesgue measure, while for discrete variables a density with respect to counting measure is assumed.

In relation to $U_1, \ldots, U_r$, a collection of random variables, suppose that for $p = 1, \ldots, r$, the conditional distributions $U_p|U_q$, $q \neq p$, are available, with possibly also the reduced forms $U_p|U_q$, $q \in S_p \subset \{1, \ldots, r\}$, where variables have local rather than global influence. Consider starting from $U_1^{(0)}, \ldots, U_r^{(0)}$, a set of arbitrary values.

$$\text{Draw } U_1^{(1)} \sim [U_1|U_2^{(0)}, \ldots, U_r^{(0)}],$$
$$\text{then } U_2^{(1)} \sim [U_2|U_1^{(1)}, U_3^{(0)}, \ldots, U_r^{(0)}],$$
$$\text{up to } U_r^{(1)} \sim [U_r|U_1^{(1)}, U_2^{(1)}, \ldots, U_{r-1}^{(1)}],$$

so each variable is visited once in the natural order. After i iterations through the r variables as above, the result is $(U_1^{(i)}, \ldots, U_r^{(i)})$. If the i iterations are repeated n times, this gives n independently and identically distributed r-tuples $(U_{1_j}^{(i)}, \ldots, U_{r_j}^{(i)})$, $j = 1, \ldots, n$. For each p, $1 \leq p \leq r$, the values of $U_p^{(q)}$ form a Markov chain as q ranges from 1 to i, which, under mild conditions, converges to an equilibrium distribution. Geman and Geman showed that:

1. *Convergence.* $U_p^{(q)} \xrightarrow{d} U_p \sim [U_p]$ as $q \longrightarrow \infty$, whatever the starting configuration and provided that all the variables are each visited infinitely often, under a defined visiting scheme.

2. *Ergodic Theorem.* From any initial configuration and for any measurable function T of $U_1, \ldots, U_r$ whose expectation exists,

$$\lim_{q \to \infty} \frac{1}{q} \sum_{l=1}^{q} T(U_1^{(l)}, \ldots, U_r^{(l)}) \xrightarrow{\text{a.s.}} E[T(U_1, \ldots, U_r)].$$

Hence, the marginal densities $[U_p]$, $p = 1, \ldots, r$, can be estimated by, for example, using the individual sampled points after the ith iteration from the n runs in a kernel density estimator or by averaging the densities these samples came from, that is,

$$[\hat{U}_p]_i = \frac{1}{n} \sum_{j=1}^{n} [U_p|U_q = U_{q_j}^{(i)}, q \neq p].$$

In practice, to be able to implement the Gibbs sampling mechanism means that it must be possible to evaluate and sample from $[U_p|U_q, q \neq p]$, the conditional distributions.

Several issues arise in the implementation of Gibbs sampling which will be mentioned briefly here. The results on convergence hold asymptotically and this raises the question of how to assess convergence in practice and whether convergence can be speeded up by, for example, reparameterizing the problem. The answer to the latter is that in certain cases using a parameterization where the parameters are "orthogonal" or independent can both speed up convergence and aid random variate generation (Wakefield et al., 1991). A wide variety of diagnostics has been suggested for assessing convergence, ranging from monitoring averages of certain scalar quantities, to examining the Markov chain properties of the output values for each variable from a long run of the sampler. The issue of whether to use a single long run or multiple shorter ones has raised much discussion. In the former, values from the initial iterations are discarded and the sample is formed of equally spaced outcomes from the remainder of the run, while in the latter the final values from each run form the sample. The merits of each are discussed in Smith and Roberts (1993) and Gelman and Rubin (1992). In the application discussed below, a single long run is used to give an idea of likely convergence properties and then multiple short runs are used for parameter estimation.

3.2 Graphical Models

Graphical models are an extension of graph theory where the nodes of the graph represent known data or unknown random variables, and the links between nodes are used to show the assumed dependencies between the variables and data. Figure 4 shows a simple directed graph where the three variables X_1, X_2, and X_3 are associated with observable quantities and X_4 represents an unknown latent variable which underlies the other three.

A comprehensive review of such models is contained in Whittaker (1990). The advantage of using such models is that the results of graph theory can be used to give additional information on the relationships between the variables. For example, in a directed graph the joint density of both the variables and parameters can be written as

$$[\mathbf{U}] = \prod_{U \in \mathbf{U}} [U|\ \text{parent}(U)], \tag{1}$$

where U is used to represent any node in the graph and parent(U) denotes

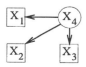

Figure 4. Simple directed graphical model, which represents X_1, X_2, and X_3 conditionally independent given X_4.

the "parents" or direct influences on U. This property essentially localizes the influences on a given node. It can be used directly within the Gibbs sampling context as, by Bayes theorem, the conditional distribution of any variable in the graph given that the rest is proportional to the joint distribution of all the variables, that is,

$$[U_p | U_q, \; q \neq p] \propto [U_p, U_q, \; q \neq p]$$
$$\propto [\text{terms containing } U_p],$$

which is proportional to the product of all component terms of the joint distribution containing U_p, that is, by equation (1), a "prior" term comprising the conditional distribution of U_p given its parents, and a "likelihood" term derived from the conditional probability of variables for which U_p is a parent (i.e., the children of U_p).

3.3 Models

Two models are used with the screening data. First, there is a model for the disease process that hypothesizes which disease states may exist and which transitions are allowed between these states. This will be taken to be a simple time-homogeneous Markov model in continuous time, with exact transition times between discrete states being unknown. Although a Markov assumption for the smear data for each woman may be unrealistic, since the timing and result of the next screening depend on previous test results, it seems reasonable to assume that the biological process may be Markovian.

The second model is graphical, showing the assumed relationships between the data and parameters. The properties implied by this graphical structure are then used in the estimation of parameters. Consider the data available for woman i. This consists of n_i smear grades, y_{ij} for $1 \leq j \leq n_i$, at known time intervals apart. Let t_{ij} be the time from the $(j-1)$st smear to the jth smear with $t_{i1} = 0$. Each smear grade will take one of m possible values. If the woman has been treated, there will also be the time this occurred, $t_{n_{i+1}}$, together with the biopsy result, $y_{n_{i+1}}$. Other covariate information, such as age at smear, may additionally be known.

The smear result provides an estimate of the underlying "true" state, X_{ij}. The errors in the cervical smear process can be represented by α, an $m \times m$ matrix, whose (r, s) entry is $\alpha_{rs} = \Pr(Y_{ij} = s | X_{ij} = r)$ [i.e., $\Pr$ (observed state is $s|$ true state is r)]. Since the row entries of this matrix must sum to 1, the (r, r) entry is conventionally taken as $1 - \sum_{s \neq r} \alpha_{rs}$. There may also be $X_{in_{i+1}}$, a state underlying the biopsy, but in the following the biopsy will be assumed to be a perfect observation (i.e., $X_{in_{i+1}} = Y_{in_{i+1}}$).

The transitions between states for the X's are assumed to follow a continuous-time Markov process. In contrast to a discrete-state, discrete-time Markov process, where transitions are governed by a probability transition matrix with the (k, l) entry corresponding to the probability that the next state is l conditional on the present state being k, in continuous time the process may usually be represented by a transition intensity matrix, $\mathbf{Q}(t)$, with (k, l) entry $q_{kl}(t)$, is defined by

$$q_{kl}(t) = \lim_{\Delta t \to 0} \Pr[X(t + \Delta t) = l \mid X(t) = k], \qquad k \neq l,$$

with

$$q_{kk}(t) = -\sum_{l \neq k} q_{kl}(t), \qquad k = 1, \ldots, m.$$

However, it is the probability of moving between two states at a given time which is usually of interest rather than the intensities. By using $P_{l_1 l_2}(s, t)$ to denote the probability of being in state l_2 at time t conditional on being in state l_1 at time s, the Markov assumption means that

$$P_{l_1 l_2}(s, t) = \sum_{k=1}^{m} P_{l_1 k}(s, u) P_{k l_2}(u, t),$$

$$\text{for } l_1, l_2 \in \{1, 2, \ldots, m\} \quad \text{and} \quad s < u < t, \qquad (2)$$

(the Chapman–Kolmogorov equation) holds. This may be used to derive two systems of differential equations for the transition probabilities (Cox and Miller, 1965). In matrix notation, the solution of equation (2) in the time-homogeneous case $[\mathbf{Q}(t) = \mathbf{Q}]$ is

$$\mathbf{P}(t) = \exp(\mathbf{Q}t), \qquad (3)$$

which, on diagonalizing the matrix $\mathbf{Q}$, reduces to

$$\mathbf{P}(t) = \mathbf{E}\mathbf{D}(t)\mathbf{E}^{-1}, \qquad (4)$$

where $\mathbf{E}$ is a matrix consisting of the normalized eigenvectors of $\mathbf{Q}$ and $\mathbf{D}$ is a diagonal matrix with (i, i) entry $\exp(\lambda_i t)$, with λ_i the ith eigenvalue of $\mathbf{Q}$. Hence the likelihood of a sequence of X's can be written down in terms of the entries of the transition intensity matrix. The derivation above is covered in more detail in Cox and Miller (1965). A graphical model for the data is given in Figure 5. Nodes associated with variables that are known (such as the smear results) are represented by rectangles, and nodes associated with unknowns have a circle or ellipse.

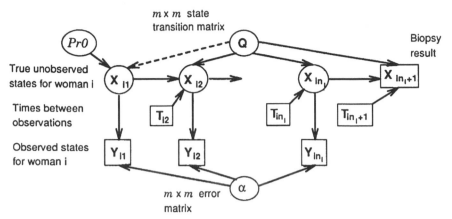

Figure 5. Graphical model of cervical smear data for one woman.

There are certain implications in the structure shown. The graph has an extra "X," X_{in_i+1}, representing a biopsy result. This node is present only if the woman has been treated. The biopsy grade is assumed to be the same as the underlying state and so has a rectangle. In a more complex model there would be a separate error matrix associated with treatment. A single error matrix is used to represent the uncertainty in the smear grade, although it is in fact a compound measure of all errors in the process, from the taking through to the grading. If it was required to attribute the error to the various sources, more detailed data would be needed.

The node $Pr0$ is used to model the prior probabilities of the states for the first smear. If the women in the study were a random sample from the population, the first smear result would be the incidence of the various states in the population and as such would depend on the transition intensity matrix (as the incidence in the population is the equilibrium distribution of the matrix). Then the dashed line from the Q matrix to X_{i1} would be a solid line and the node $Pr0$ would not be necessary. To account for the selection involved in this study, the smear which brought a woman into the study is modeled explicitly and separately for the patients and controls.

The graph is for one woman. For the many women in the study a stack of such graphs can be imagined. The error and transition matrices can initially be assumed to be common to all women, so there will be one node for each of these, linked to all women.

If there were no errors in the smear-taking and smear-reading process, the model would reduce to a simple discrete-state Markov chain in continuous time, and standard maximum likelihood methods could be used to obtain estimates of the rate parameters Q. Kalbfleisch and Prentice (1980) showed ways that standard errors for these estimates could be obtained in the case of equally spaced observations, although they admitted that the computation required when this was not the case could be high. If errors are allowed and the unobserved true states are regarded as nuisance parameters, estimation of the main rate parameters might be possible if the graph were collapsed down over the X's. This is the conventional way of proceeding with graphical models, but, as each X node may take one of m values, the computation would be prohibitive if every possible combination of these had to be summed over. Fortunately, Gibbs sampling offers an alternative way of estimating the parameters in the model using the structure of the graph.

Consider using Gibbs sampling to estimate the parameters in the graphical model where instead of the original six-point scale for the smears, this is reduced to a two-point scale. The choice of boundary between the states could be made in several ways, but in the following only one is described in detail. Define "0" to be a smear reading of 1 (negative) or 2 (inflammation); these are both readings which indicate that no dyskaryotic cells (those with characteristically abnormal nuclei) were found. Similarly, define "1" to be a smear reading of 3 (mild dyskaryosis) or greater. This encompasses a wide range of smears, but they all contain cells showing some degree of dyskaryosis, and this was the boundary used in determining whether a woman was a patient or a control. The biopsy grades may also be reduced to a two-point scale, which is comparable to that for the smears by taking 0 to correspond to an histology grade of negative and 1 to correspond to a grade of cervical intraepithelial neoplasia (CIN) I or worse.

For N women, the smear results $\{y_{ij}, 1 \leq i \leq N, 1 \leq j \leq n_i\}$ and the times between smears $\{t_{ij}, 1 \leq i \leq N, 1 \leq j \leq n_i\}$ are known. There are only two parameters in the **Q** matrix (q_0 and q_1), and the error matrix may be written as

$$\begin{pmatrix} 1 - \alpha & \alpha \\ \beta & 1 - \beta \end{pmatrix}, \qquad 0 \leq \alpha, \quad \beta \leq 1,$$

where the (i, j) entry in the matrix is $\Pr(Y = j \mid X = i)$.

In order to apply Gibbs sampling to this graphical model, it must be possible to sample from various conditional distributions (i.e., the distribution of each of the X's, q's, α, β, and $Pr0$) given the rest of the variables. For each unobserved node, the decomposition of the joint distribution expressed by the graphical structure determines the variables whose sampling distributions are required. From further inspection, these various sampling distributions may be determined. Specifically:

1. Each of the X's depend on the current values of the q's, the neighboring X's and t's, the corresponding y, α, and β (and $Pr0$ if the X is the first for a woman).
2. The q's depend on the X's and t's.
3. α and β depend on the X's and y's.
4. $Pr0$ depends on the X's that are first for each woman.

Denote the entries in the probability matrix $\mathbf{P}$ [cf. equation (4)] by p_{ij}, $i, j \in \{0, 1\}$. It follows that:

1. For the X's:

$$\Pr(x_{i1} \mid \text{other variables}) \propto \Pr(x_{i1} \mid Pr0) \Pr(x_{i2} \mid x_{i1}, q_0, q_1, t_{i2})$$
$$\cdot \Pr(y_{i1} \mid x_{i1}, \alpha, \beta), \qquad (5)$$

that is,

$$\Pr(x_{i1} \mid \text{other variables}) \propto \Pr(x_{i1} = 0) p_{01}^{x_{i2}} p_{00}^{(1-x_{i2})} (1 - \alpha)^{(1-y_{i1})} \alpha^{y_{i1}}$$

or

$$\Pr(x_{i1} \mid \text{other variables}) \propto \Pr(x_{i1} = 1) p_{11}^{x_{i2}} p_{10}^{(1-x_{i2})} \beta^{(1-y_{i1})} (1 - \beta)^{y_{i1}}.$$
$$\Pr(x_{ij} \mid \text{other variables}) \propto \Pr(x_{ij} \mid x_{ij-1}, q_0, q_1, t_{ij}) \Pr(y_{ij} \mid x_{ij}, \alpha, \beta)$$
$$\cdot \Pr(x_{ij+1} \mid x_{ij}, q_0, q_1, t_{ij+1}), \qquad (6)$$

where $2 \leq j \leq n_i - 1$, and

$$\Pr(x_{in_i} \mid \text{other variables}) \propto \Pr(x_{in_i} \mid x_{in_{i-1}}, q_0, q_1, t_{in_i})$$
$$\cdot \Pr(y_{in_i} \mid x_{in_i}, \alpha, \beta). \qquad (7)$$

2. For the q's:

$$f(q_0 \mid \text{other variables}) \propto f(q_0) \prod_{i=1}^{N} \prod_{j=2}^{n_i} \Pr(x_{ij} \mid x_{ij-1}, t_{ij}, q_0, q_1),$$

and

$$f(q_1 \mid \text{other variables}) \propto f(q_1) \prod_{i=1}^{N} \prod_{j=2}^{n_i} \Pr(x_{ij} \mid x_{ij-1}, t_{ij}, q_0, q_1).$$

Note that both $f(q_0 \mid \text{other variables})$ and $f(q_1 \mid \text{other variables})$ are proportional to

$$\prod_{i=1}^{N} \prod_{j \in S_{00}} p_{00} \prod_{j \in S_{01}} p_{01} \prod_{j \in S_{10}} p_{10} \prod_{j \in S_{11}} p_{11},$$

where S_{mn} is the set of transitions between states m and n.

3. For α:

$$f(\alpha | \text{other variables}) \propto f(\alpha) \prod_{i=1}^{N} \prod_{j=1}^{n_i} \Pr(y_{ij} | x_{ij}, \alpha, \beta)$$

$$\propto f(\alpha) \prod_{i=1}^{N} \prod_{j=1}^{n_i} [(1 - \alpha)^{1-y_{ij}} \alpha^{y_{ij}}]^{1-x_{ij}}. \qquad (8)$$

4. For β:

$$f(\beta | \text{other variables}) \propto f(\beta) \prod_{i=1}^{N} \prod_{j=1}^{n_i} \Pr(y_{ij} | x_{ij}, \alpha, \beta)$$

$$\propto f(\beta) \prod_{i=1}^{N} \prod_{j=1}^{n_i} [\beta^{1-y_{ij}} (1 - \beta)^{y_{ij}}]^{x_{ij}}. \qquad (9)$$

5. For the state prior to the first smear:

$$f(Pr0 | \text{other variables}) \propto f(Pr0) \prod_{i=1}^{N} \Pr(x_{i1} | Pr0). \qquad (10)$$

Since in this simplified case the X's are binary variables, one samples Bernoulli distributions with probabilities given by equations of the form of (5), (6), and (7) above (suitably normalized). For α and β, the terms in the product are simply of the form α and $1 - \alpha$ or β and $1 - \beta$, respectively, so the posterior conditional is a beta distribution. Similarly for $Pr0$, the distribution to sample is a product of terms of the form p and $1 - p$, again leading to a beta distribution.

The distributions for the q's, however, are not conjugate and hence not so easily sampled. Several approaches are possible here. If a suitable envelope function was known, the ratio of uniforms method (Ripley, 1987) could be used; while if the expressions were log-concave in the q parameters, the approach of Gilks and Wild (1992) could be used. As a starting point that requires few assumptions, the distributions may be sampled from using a brute force and rather inelegant technique based on the fact that for a random variable Z with continuous distribution function $F, U = F(Z)$ is distributed uniformly on the interval $U[0, 1]$, so F can be sampled from $Z = F^{-1}(U)$ provided that the inverse exists. (This result can be extended to any F provided that the inverse is carefully defined.)

4 RESULTS

The algorithm was first tested on the two-state model under the assumption of no error in the observations (i.e., $\alpha = \beta = 0$ and $X = Y$) using a uniform prior on the q's. The only parameters to be estimated are q_0 and q_1 and the methods of conventional maximum likelihood can be used and compared with the results from Gibbs sampling. This showed that parameterizing the problem by q_0 and q_1 produced marginal likelihoods which were difficult to sample. When the log-likelihood is plotted out over a grid of values (Figure 6), it is seen that this choice of parameterization is poor, with high correlation between the q's, especially near the maximum and a steep edge to the log-likelihood as q_0 approaches 0. This makes sampling very slow, if not impossible.

Several alternative reparameterizations are possible. The one used here is given in terms of r_0 and r_1, where

$$r_0 = \ln\frac{q_0}{q_1} \quad \text{and} \quad r_1 = \ln(q_0 q_1)$$

(so $q_0 = \exp[(r_0 + r_1)/2]$ and $q_1 = \exp[(r_1 - r_0)/2]$). The r's can be thought of as the relative rate of progression compared with regression and the overall rate of movement, respectively. If the log-likelihood surface is again plotted (Figure 7), it can be seen that r_0 and r_1 are slightly more orthogonal, especially around the maximum, which is the area where sampling will be concentrated since the contours are on a log scale. Overall the surface is better behaved, and the r's are not bounded below by 0.

The ideal reparameterization would choose variables that were in some sense orthogonal, but as the likelihood surface varies with the X's once errors are

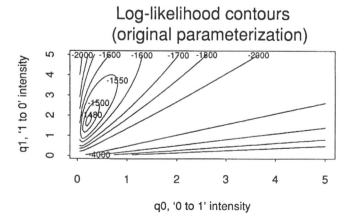

Figure 6. Log-likelihood contours parameterizing with q_1 and q_1, transition intensities.

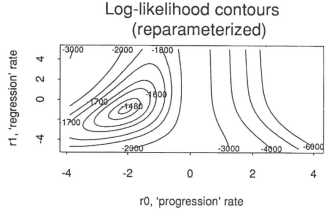

Figure 7. Log-likelihood following reparameterization.

allowed, it will change at each iteration, so a choice which is reasonable over a range of X's is needed. Another approach would be to sample directly from the two-dimensional distribution (or a reparameterization of it), perhaps using a bivariate normal distribution as an envelope function, but this is not pursued here.

As the "no error" case produced results that agreed with the maximum likelihood methods, the Gibbs sampler was implemented to allow errors in the smears (i.e., $\alpha, \beta \neq 0$). A uniform prior was used for each error parameter and for the first X node of each woman. An initial single run of 3000 iterations was used to give some idea of the convergence properties of the series. Figure 8 shows the results for the parameters r_0 and r_1.

These runs were used to obtain kernel density estimators (Silverman, 1986) for the posterior distribution of each of the four parameters. The r's were sampled by inverting their cumulative distribution function numerically. It would thus be quite space consuming to save and average these to estimate their distribution. However, the error parameters were drawn from simple beta distributions with two parameters defining each, and in this case, the distribution from which the samples were drawn may be averaged and compared with the kernel estimator. Figure 9 shows the kernel density estimators for the r's, and Figure 10 compares the kernel and averaged densities for the error parameters. The method of Raftery and Lewis (1991) was used to assess convergence, and based on the result, the Gibbs sampler was then run for 50 iterations, each of 300 iterations, with different random starting points for the parameters in each run.

The estimators for the r's appear reasonable, with r_1 having a wider posterior distribution than r_0. The values of the parameters after 300 and 250 iterations in each run were used in the estimators instead of those after 300, since the extra iterations allowed smoother density estimators without having to simulate an additional 50 runs. The gap of 50 between the values used ensures that

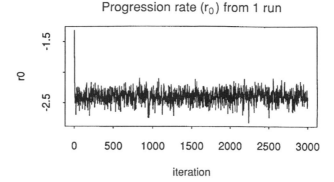

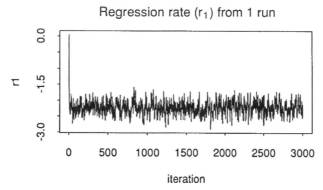

Figure 8. Sequences of r_0 and r_1, process parameters, from a single long run.

they are essentially independent. Although the error density estimates obtained by averaging the beta densities are more regular, the kernel estimators give a reasonable approximation. The values of α and β are both low, with $\alpha \simeq 0.02$ and $\beta \simeq 0.085$. It seems reasonable that the false positive rate should be smallest (since if the underlying disease is absent we would not expect a positive smear), and both are within the ranges of values found in other studies.

One of the advantages of the Gibbs sampling technique is that the estimation of posterior distributions is not restricted to those sampled during the iterations. Although the distribution of the main parameters in the model may be estimated most efficiently by averaging the sampled distributions, the kernel density method enables the estimation of the probability density functions of functions of the sampled parameters. For example, the probability that the first passage from state 1 to state 0 occurs before time T is $1 - \exp(-q_0 T)$. Thus, the sampled values of the r's can be transformed into samples of this probability and kernel methods used to give density estimates. In this case the probability of leaving state 0 within a year is roughly 0.09 and of leaving state 1 is roughly 0.66, showing high regression rates in the study.

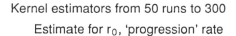

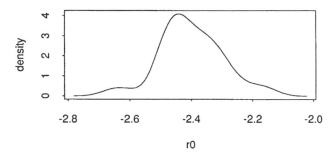

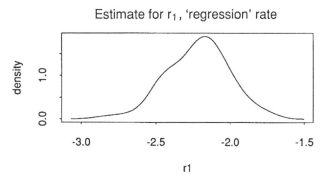

Figure 9. Kernel density estimators for r_0 and r_1, process parameters.

Given the two-state model, one of the questions of interest is how well it fits the data and how this can be measured. Recall that the model needs to estimate the X's at each iteration, for these are the underlying and unknown states and not actually observed. To get the fitted values, the Y's must be predicted back from the model. For $1 \leq i \leq 998$ and $1 \leq j \leq n_i$, the fitted value at each iteration is

$$
\begin{aligned}
E(Y_{ij}|\boldsymbol{\theta}) &= \sum_{y_{ij}} y_{ij} f(y_{ij}|\boldsymbol{\theta}) \\
&= 0 \cdot \Pr(Y_{ij} = 0|\boldsymbol{\theta}) + 1 \cdot \Pr(Y_{ij} = 1|\boldsymbol{\theta}) \\
&= \alpha \, \mathrm{I}(x_{ij} = 0) + (1 - \beta) \, \mathrm{I}(x_{ij} = 1),
\end{aligned}
$$

where α, β, and the X's are given by $\boldsymbol{\theta}$ and I is the usual indicator function. Since $\boldsymbol{\theta}$ is unknown, the overall fitted value is $E(Y_{ij}) = \int_{\boldsymbol{\theta}} \Pr(Y_{ij} = 1|\boldsymbol{\theta}) f(\boldsymbol{\theta}) \, d\boldsymbol{\theta}$. This integral can therefore be estimated by averaging the value of $\Pr(Y_{ij} = 1|\boldsymbol{\theta})$

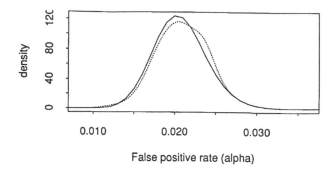

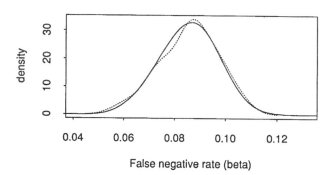

Figure 10. Comparison of averaged and kernel densities for α and β, error parameters.

over, for example, the 300th iteration of each of the 50 runs. This will amount to averaging a series of α's and $1 - \beta$'s, depending on the current value of the x_{ij} and the two error parameters. In a similar way, $E(Y_{ij}^2|\theta)$ can be estimated, allowing a standard error for the Y_{ij}'s to be found. This gives an idea of how sure the model is of a particular X_{ij}.

Figures 11 and 12 show the fitted values for two of the women whose histories were illustrated earlier, with the observed smears shown by "O"s and the fitted values by "f"s. In general the model appears to be able to predict the Y's well, which is perhaps surprising considering that the model is so simple.

Related to the issue of fitted values is the question of residuals. These can be defined in a number of ways for binary variables as discussed in McCullagh and Nelder (1989). Pearson residuals are defined by $e_{ij} = (y_{ij} - \hat{p}_{ij})/[\hat{p}_{ij}(1 - \hat{p}_{ij})]^{1/2}$, where $\hat{p}_{ij}$ is the expected value of Y_{ij} under the model. Deviance residuals are defined as $\text{sign}(y_{ij} - \hat{p}_{ij})d_{ij}^{1/2}$, where the overall deviance, $D = \sum_{i,j} d_{ij}$. In this case, $d_{ij} = -\ln[\Pr(y_{ij})]$, which, depending on the value of x_{ij} and y_{ij}, is the logarithm of one of $\alpha, 1 - \alpha, \beta,$ or $1 - \beta$. These residuals may be calculated at each iteration using the current parameter values. Since like the fitted values, these residuals depend on the unknown parameters in the model, an overall

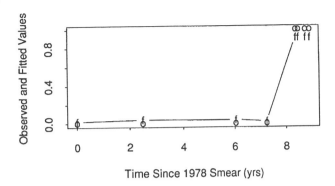

Figure 11. Fitted values for the smear history of control 490.

residual may be obtained by averaging the residuals at chosen iterations (using the parameter values at those iterations) in the same way as for the fitted values. As well as looking at the residuals for each smear, the residuals may be averaged for each woman, so that someone who has a series of unusual smears which the model is not able to fit well can be detected.

If the absolute values of the residuals are averaged over individual women, 10 of the 100 women for whom residuals were saved have an average Pearson residual value over 0.7, and only three have an average deviance residual over 0.7. If the histories of these women are examined, one finds that they correspond to situations where the history is not regressive or progressive but oscillates between the two states, or where the final smear result is close to treatment but is not reflected in the biopsy result, for example, control 468 and patient 20.

Since in the two-state model the positive state encompasses a range of cell abnormalities a three-state model was created, where only transitions between adjacent states were permitted. In this case, the transition matrix **Q** is

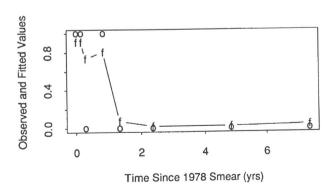

Figure 12. Fitted values for the smear history of patient 56.

$$\begin{pmatrix} -q_1 & q_1 & 0 \\ q_2 & -(q_2 + q_3) & q_3 \\ 0 & q_4 & -q_4 \end{pmatrix}, \tag{11}$$

and the expressions for the likelihood become more complex. The choice of reparameterization is not clear in this four-dimensional case, but by using a similar choice to the two-state one, the Gibbs sampler can be run. This shows both the lack of information about transitions between higher states and the difficulty in distinguishing between varying levels of cell abnormalities. For example, if the states are defined as "0," corresponding to a negative or inflammatory smear, "1," corresponding to a mildly or moderately dyskaryotic smear, and "2," corresponding to a smear grade of severe dyskaryosis or invasive, the first passage probabilities after one year show the relative stability of state 0 (with high probabilities of not having left this state), the greater transience of state 1 (with transitions either way possible and equally likely), and that although transitions from 2 to 1 are possible, so are transitions from 2 to 0. Also, the error rates for state 2 are high, with 81% of the smears of state 2 and 33% of the smears of state 1 assigned a true state of 2, although the error parameters associated with the first two states are all very low, ranging from $\simeq 0.006$ to $\simeq 0.04$. This shows the difficulty in accurately assigning women to positive states with an apparently blurred boundary between moderate and severe grades. This problem remains if the state boundaries are chosen differently.

5   CONCLUSIONS

This case study has looked at modeling data on the precursors of cervical cancer using Gibbs sampling within a graphical model. From such a model, the interactions between parameters are clearly shown and the structure may be exploited within the Gibbs sampling framework. Sampling in the case of underlying discrete-state Markov chains in continuous time results in conditional distributions difficult to sample in some cases, yet if the problem is simplified to assume no errors in the smear readings, the methods reassuringly give the same results as do maximum likelihood methods. The choice of parameterization is important for making the conditional distributions easier to handle. The sampling technique readily yields measures of the fit of the model, such as residuals and fitted values. The only disadvantage of using these is that they require additional storage.

Although Gibbs sampling has been the method used above, there are other Markov chain Monte Carlo methods, such as the Metropolis–Hastings algorithm, that can be used independently or in conjunction with the sampler, depending on the particular structure of the individual problem.

The estimates of error rates from this study are applicable to the general screening population. The false negative rate ($\beta \simeq 0.085$) seems reasonable compared with that in other studies. Brookmeyer et al. (1986) estimated an upper bound of 4%, while in a different project Day and Moss (1986) found a value of approximately 40%. The three-state model and the use of different boundaries in a two-state model both show that the current six-point scale for cervical cell abnormalities is unrealistic: a simpler scale is being investigated. The observed smear histories could be explained as either a relatively stable underlying process observed with error or a rapidly changing one observed with little error. The results of modeling suggest that the former is the case, which is in accord with current medical thought. The selection of women into the study means that the rate parameters are specific to the study. To obtain population rates the model would need to be applied to a random sample of screening histories. Once model parameters are obtained they can be used to simulate the effect of different screening and treatment policies in planning trials or alternative intervention studies.

Although the data relate to cervical cancer screening, they have a generic structure, being longitudinal in form, with irregularly spaced observations which are a surrogate measure for the underlying biological state, so the methodology could be applied to data from other areas.

The graphical model shown in Figure 5 may be viewed in more general terms as that shown in Figure 13. This is a very simple model but one that applies to many chronic diseases. It can itself be made more complex with the incorporation of covariates. Figure 14 shows such a graph. Instead of every woman having the same parameters governing state transitions, each woman is given a personal set of parameters particular to her, which set is drawn from some distribution for the whole population. The use of covariates influences the choice from the population distribution. In the current case, covariates such as "age at smear" or risk factors such as smoking could be used to individualize the rate parameters and highlight women at increased risk.

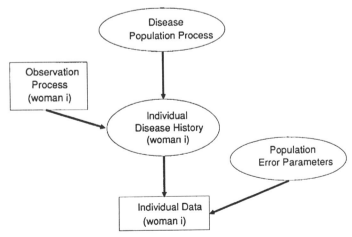

Figure 13. Simple graphical model of chronic disease data.

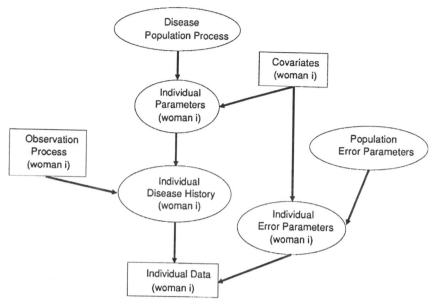

Figure 14. Generalized graphical model of chronic disease data.

SOFTWARE NOTES AND REFERENCES

Programming of the Gibbs sampling was implemented in FORTRAN using NAG libraries for random number and variate generation.

NAG Fortran Library Manual (Mark 14, 1990), Numerical Algorithms Group Ltd., Wilkinson House, Jordan Hill Road, Oxford, OX2 8DR, U.K.

QUESTIONS AND PROBLEMS

1. *Exploratory Data Analysis.*

    (a) Using the smear-specific data set, find the proportion of smears categorized as 0 that are followed by another 0, and the proportion of 1's that are followed by 1's. Repeat this for the patients and controls separately and comment.

    (b) From the same data set calculate the mean (and standard deviation) of the time following a smear for each category. Does this time seem to depend on the result of the following smear?

2. *Likelihood Function for Two-State Model.* Taking the transition intensity matrix, **Q**, as

$$\begin{pmatrix} -q_0 & q_0 \\ q_1 & -q_1 \end{pmatrix}, \qquad 0 \le q_0, q_1,$$

find (a) the eigenvectors and (b) the normalized eigenvalues of this matrix. Use equation (4) to find the entries in **P**, the probability transition matrix, and hence write down an expression for the likelihood of the data if there are assumed to be no errors in the process.

3. *Sampling from Distributions.* In the following it may be assumed that random samples from the uniform distribution on $[0, 1]$ are available.

   (a) Describe a method for producing a random sample from a distribution with two states where the first state has a probability of p and the second of $1 - p$ $(0 \le p \le 1)$.

   (b) Describe a method for producing a random sample from a beta distribution with probability density function $\propto p^{m-1}(1 - p)^{n-1}$.

4. *Gibbs Sampling.* In the following assume that the times between smears are all 1 unit and that q_0 and q_1 are fixed (at 0.1 and 1.2, for example). Use a uniform prior for α and β (the error parameters), for each of the X's, and for $Pr0$ (the prior on the first node). This latter should be split into two nodes, $Pr0c$ and $Pr0p$ for the control and patient groups, respectively, to model the selection into the study. Use the smear grades but not the treatment results.

   (a) Generate random starting points for each of the unknown quantities: the X's, $\alpha, \beta, Pr0c$, and $Pr0p$.

   (b) Use equations (5), (6), and (7) to derive expressions for the probability of each of the two states for the X's.

   (c) Use equations (8), (9), and (10) to derive the probability density functions (up to a constant) for the error parameters and the priors for the first smear in the two groups.

   (d) Starting with the priors on the first smear (using the randomly generated X's), the X's (where the error parameters and all other X's apart from the current one are assumed known) and following with the error parameters (where the X's are taken as fixed) perform a single iteration of the Gibbs sampler. Using the results from this, continue and repeat the iterations 500 times to give a single long run. Check that the order of visiting the variables does not affect the results.

5. *Density Estimation.* Use the results from a single long run derived in Problem 4 to obtain a kernel density estimator for α and β, the error parameters.

CHAPTER 19

Patterns of Lung Cancer Risk in Ex-Smokers

Brenda W. Gillespie, Michael T. Halpern, and Kenneth E. Warner

1 MOTIVATION AND BACKGROUND

Numerous studies have shown that compared with continuing smokers, the risk of death from lung cancer decreases following smoking cessation. Some studies have suggested that the risk for former smokers returns to the level of a never smoker several years after quitting; other studies have suggested that the risk remains constant at the level attained when the person stops smoking. While the patterns of risk for continuing and never smokers are well established, a variety of results on the magnitude and rapidity of risk reduction following smoking cessation has been reported in the literature. Figure 1 illustrates the known patterns of lung cancer death risk between ages 40 and 80 for continuing (solid line) and never (dotted line) smokers, as well as three possible patterns of risk for someone who quit smoking at age 65 (dashed lines). Although attempts have been made to incorporate relevant covariates in most studies of ex-smokers, sample sizes and available data have not often allowed for sufficient adjustment.

Most studies have reported relative risk by years since quitting for former smokers compared to either current or never smokers. These studies assume that the relative risk is constant for all ages of quitting. Given the variety of results obtained, it seems likely that this assumption does not hold. The 1990 Report of the Surgeon General (U.S. Department of Health and Human Services, 1990, p. 118) mentions that the patterns of declining risk have not been fully characterized, suggesting reasons such as small sample size and lack of adjustment for cumulative smoking exposure, age at initiation, years of smoking, number

Case Studies in Biometry, Edited by Nicholas Lange, Louise Ryan, Lynne Billard, David Brillinger, Loveday Conquest, and Joel Greenhouse.
ISBN 0-471-58885-7 © 1994 John Wiley & Sons, Inc.

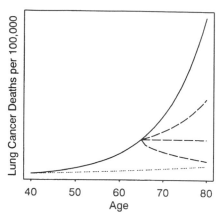

Figure 1. Possible patterns of lung cancer risk following smoking cessation at age 65 (dashed lines). Lung cancer risk for continuing smokers (solid line) and never smokers (dotted line) are given for reference.

of cigarettes smoked per day, inhalation practices, types of cigarettes, age at smoking cessation, and the reason for stopping. Many of these cited problems are overcome in the current analysis.

Since lung cancer, even among smokers, is a relatively rare event, a large data set was necessary to estimate lung cancer death risk while adjusting for covariates. The goal was to model lung cancer death risk as a function of age for current, former, and never smokers. The data set analyzed included mostly censored observations (i.e., observations in which the outcome, lung cancer death, did not occur), so methods of survival analysis were required. Logistic regression methods for survival data were employed. Since lung cancer death risk appeared to be a smooth function of age, the logit hazard as a function of age was modeled parametrically using polynomials and polynomial splines. Absolute rather than relative risks are reported, which allow easy comparison of many risks simultaneously, such as the risks by age for several different ages of quitting. Although some questions remain, this study represents a significant step forward in the understanding of patterns of risk after smoking cessation. The results from a medical perspective are given in Halpern et al. (1993). The statistical analysis behind the modeling of these patterns is the subject of this chapter.

2 DATA

The Cancer Prevention Study II (CPS-II) was a prospective cohort study of over 1 million people carried out between 1982 and 1988 by the American Cancer Society (ACS). This study has been described by Stellman et al. (1988) and

Stellman and Garfinkel (1989). In 1982, ACS volunteers enrolled over 1 million participants in all 50 states, the District of Columbia, and Puerto Rico to participate in this six-year prospective study. Participants completed a confidential four-page questionnaire focusing on health habits and history of cancer and other diseases.

Follow-up of all participants occurred every other year through 1988. For the six-year follow-up period, 98.2% of the participants were traced (dead or alive). A total of 79,820 deaths were reported, and death certificates were obtained for 94% of that number. Causes of death were coded using the International Classification of Diseases, volume 9 (ICD9). Lung cancer death for the present study included death due to cancer of the trachea, bronchi, and/or lungs.

The data set obtained for this analysis provided information on survival status, cause of death, age, gender, race, education, and several variables related to smoking status and history, including number of cigarettes smoked per day, number of years smoked, and years since quitting for former smokers. A listing of 15 records is given in Table 1. The first five are never smokers, followed by five current smokers, and five former smokers. The data are condensed by giving the frequency of occurrence for each unique covariate pattern. Table 2 shows descriptive statistics for the 852,789 subjects who were included in the

Table 1 Data Listing for a Few Records[a]

Age	Gender	Education	Smoker	Cigarettes/ Day	Years Smoked	Years Quit	Follow-up Time	Death	Frequency
41	1	1	1	0	0	0	6	0	2006
50	1	0	1	0	0	0	6	0	5160
62	0	1	1	0	0	0	4	2	3
69	0	1	1	0	0	0	3	1	15
53	1	0	1	0	0	0	6	0	2014
45	1	1	3	30	25	0	6	0	31
52	0	0	3	40	36	0	6	0	69
56	1	1	3	15	20	0	5	2	1
61	1	0	3	40	29	0	5	1	1
72	1	0	3	20	32	0	6	0	3
47	0	1	2	30	28	2	6	0	1
53	0	1	2	20	14	23	6	0	11
58	1	1	2	15	15	6	6	0	1
68	0	0	2	30	29	19	6	0	2
73	1	0	2	20	36	0	6	0	1

[a]Data codes: Age: age on January 1, 1982; Gender: 0, male, 1, female; Education: 0, no college, 1, some college; Smoker: 1, never, 2, former, 3, current; Cigarettes/day: values rounded up to the nearest 5; Years smoked: number of years smoked as of January 1, 1982; Years quit: number of years since smoking cessation as of January 1, 1982 (zero indicates less than one year); Follow-up time: years from January 1, 1982 until death or last interview; Death codes: 0, alive, 1, death from other causes, 2, lung cancer death.

Table 2   Descriptive Statistics

	Never Smokers		Current Smokers		Former Smokers	
	Male	Female	Male	Female	Male	Female
N	117,455	326,755	91,994	104,535	136,072	75,978
Mean age	57.2	57.4	55.3	53.9	59.0	56.4
Minority (%)	5.6	6.3	6.2	5.6	3.2	3.7
College (%)	62.9	47.4	51.0	49.6	58.8	60.0
Mean cigarettes/day	—	—	25.7	20.8	26.7	18.9
Mean years smoked	—	—	36.5	32.0	26.4	24.0
Mean age quit	—	—	—	—	45.1	44.8
Lung cancer deaths						
Number	109	273	1783	941	1028	248
Percent	0.09	0.08	1.94	0.90	0.76	0.33

Source : Halpern et al. (1993).

analysis. Being volunteer selected, the participants of this study are not representative of the entire U.S. population. However, CPS-II involved 1.5% of all Americans aged 45 and older and is therefore an important subgroup for study. The majority of subjects were female, and approximately half the subjects had never smoked. The other subjects were divided into roughly equal numbers of current and former smokers. The study included primarily older adults, with the mean participant age being 57. Minority representation was low compared to the general population. Raw lung cancer death rates were highest for current smokers, lowest for never smokers, and intermediate for former smokers. The rates for males in each category were higher than for females. Since study subjects were predominantly white and preliminary analysis indicated no significant differences in lung cancer mortality by race, all subjects were included in this analysis without regard to race. College attendance (any versus none) was included as a proxy for socioeconomic status and occupational exposure. Further, since the death rate from lung cancer is negligible before age 40 and the sample sizes were fairly small beyond age 80, the investigation was limited to ages 40 to 80. Thus, subjects who were between the ages of 40 and 80 at some point during the six years of the study were included.

Figure 2 gives the boxplot distribution of the number of cigarettes smoked per day (cigarettes/day) for current and former smokers grouped by gender. The figure illustrates that men tend to smoke more heavily than women, and that those who quit smoking are quite comparable to continuing smokers in terms of cigarette consumption. The median consumption for both men and women was 20 cigarettes/day (1 pack/day), an extremely common rate, with over a quarter of the smokers of both genders consuming this amount. Reporting bias toward rounding to the nearest 5 cigarettes/day is apparent. Consequently, values of cigarettes/day were rounded up to the nearest 5 for all participants. Because

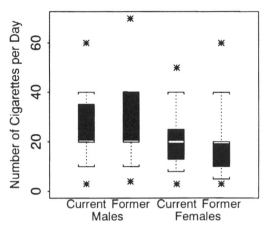

Figure 2. Boxplots of numbers of cigarettes smoked per day for current and former smokers by gender. The box encloses the 25th to 75th percentiles with a horizontal line at the median. The whiskers extend to the 10th and 90th percentiles, and asterisks indicate the 1st and 99th percentiles.

of the large range in numbers of cigarettes/day (3 to 95), this rounding should not have much effect on the analysis. Boxplot distributions of cigarettes/day by college attendance (not given) were virtually identical. Comparisons within deciles of age (or age at quitting) also revealed no differences.

3   METHODS AND MODELS

Data Exclusions
Out of 998,743 subjects available for analysis, 145,954 were excluded. Reasons for exclusion were missing data (44,547), outlying values including former smokers followed less than five years from quitting as discussed below (40,673), age under 40 or over 80 (31,586), or smoking cessation before age 30 or after age 75 (29,148), as discussed below. Because of the huge sample size and lack of access to the original data records, it was not possible to clean the data in the standard manner of investigating suspicious values. Instead, records with extremely large or small values for certain covariates were simply deleted. The variables cleaned in this manner were number of cigarettes smoked per day (acceptable range: 3 to 95), number of years of smoking (5 to 67), and age started smoking (8 to 52).

Age-at-Quitting Cohorts
To examine the effects on lung cancer risk of smoking cessation at different ages, former smokers were grouped into either 5- or 10-year age-at-quitting cohorts, which permitted independent examination of the effects of quitting at different ages. This strategy allowed for a more flexible model than one using a

single variable for years since quitting for all ex-smokers, regardless of the age when they quit. Table 3 gives the numbers of former smokers and lung cancer deaths for each age at quitting cohort: 30–39, 40–49, 50–54, 55–59, 60–64, 65–69 and 70–74. The younger age-at-quitting cohorts were grouped into 10-year intervals because of fewer lung cancer deaths; intervals smaller than five years were not feasible in any age range with the data available. As can be seen in Table 3, the numbers of smokers quitting after age 64 were marginal for analysis. Although the findings pertaining to these groups are summarized below, we do not include them in the graphical presentation of the results. Calculating mortality ratios from Table 3 values is not appropriate since those quitting at older ages are already older and thus at greater risk of lung cancer death.

"Quitting Ill" Effect

A recurring difficulty in studies involving smoking cessation is that smokers often quit smoking following the onset of disease symptoms or the diagnosis of a life-threatening disease. Therefore, an anomalous rise in lung cancer risk following smoking cessation relative to continuing smokers has been reported in several studies (Garfinkel and Stellman, 1988). This "quitting ill" effect has been seen for the first two to five years following cessation (Alderson et al., 1985; Brown and Chu, 1987; Higgins and Wynder, 1988; Ockene et al., 1990). In the current study population, those who quit had a greater risk of lung cancer death for one to four years following cessation, elevated over the risk for current smokers of the same age and gender. To avoid modeling the effects of quitting ill, which were not of interest, former smokers were not included in the analysis until five years after their reported quitting time.

Age–Period–Cohort Problem

Several authors have discussed the contributions to lung cancer risk of age, number of years of smoking, and age of starting smoking. All three factors are

Table 3 Numbers of Ex-Smokers and Lung Cancer Deaths by Age at Quitting

Age at Quitting	Number of Participants		Lung Cancer Deaths	
	Male	Female	Male	Female
30–39	42,323	25,621	79	23
40–49	47,790	25,283	221	66
50–54	19,691	10,629	178	40
55–59	13,374	7,062	215	39
60–64	8,160	4,624	201	50
65–69	3,577	2,077	105	24
70–74	1,157	682	29	6

Source : Halpern et al. (1993).

plausible contributors to lung cancer risk. Even in people who never smoked, lung cancer risk increases with age. Numerous studies have shown that lung cancer risk increases with number of years of smoking. More recently, some have conjectured that those who begin smoking in their teen years sustain more damage than those who start later since their bodies are still growing when the insult of smoking begins. Unfortunately, all three factors cannot be entered simultaneously into a model since they are collinear: age started smoking + years smoked = current age. The issue is the well-known age–period–cohort (APC) problem, referring to the similarly collinear effects of age, period of observation, and birth cohort. Vigorous attempts have been made by many authors to untangle these effects (e.g., Kupper et al., 1985; Holford, 1985). This problem appears not to have been mentioned in the smoking literature. Brown and Chu (1987) model the variables two at a time; however, as discussed in Kupper et al. (1985), the coefficients from such models cannot be interpreted as being free of effects of the third variable. In the current analysis, a decision was made to drop age started smoking from the model, and retain only age and years of smoking. The effect of age of starting is incorporated into the other effect estimates (in an unknown manner), so that all effects are included, even though the effect of each cannot be estimated separately.

Time Axis

When using survival analysis procedures, the time dimension is generally defined in the context of the problem. For example, in clinical trials the time axis usually begins with entry into the study. In prospective cohort studies such as this one, however, the time variable could be time-on-study, time since start-ing to smoke, or age, as discussed in Cox and Oakes (1984, pp. 2–4). Since the desired end result was to predict lung cancer mortality as a function of age, however, age was chosen as the time variable. This strategy is consistent with the analysis of Whittemore (1988), among others. Other time variables may be incorporated as covariates.

Relative versus Absolute Risk

Relative risk is defined as the ratio of incidence rates in exposed versus unex-posed groups, for some given exposure. In many studies relative risk is the parameter of interest. However, in settings where many factors are involved in a complex way, relative risks can be limiting since they always involve a pairwise comparison between two risks (e.g., former smokers versus current smokers). Absolute risks (i.e., incidence rates) allow comparison among any number of risk groups simultaneously. In particular, a comparison among the risks for current, former, and never smokers at various ages was desired here, so absolute risks are usually presented rather than relative risks.

Rate, Risk, and Hazard

In a prospective study, the incidence rate per year is defined as the proportion of incident disease cases in a year divided by the number of person-years at risk.

A distinction is often made between incidence rate per year and the probability of developing the disease during a year (Kahn and Sempos, 1989, p. 207). The difference is in the denominators of the respective estimates, where the denominator of the probability is the number of persons at risk at the beginning of the year, and the denominator of the rate is the same quantity (with units person-years instead of persons) diminished by the time after developing the disease for diseased persons, since those persons are no longer at risk. When the event rate per year is low, however, these two quantities will be nearly identical.

The probability of lung cancer death at various ages is considered here as an approximation to the incidence rate. Since the event rate for lung cancer death is very low (less than 0.05), this probability will be very close to the incidence rate.

The probability of death at a given age, t, can also be defined as the hazard of death at that age, $h(t)$. Formally, if age is considered to be a discrete variable in one-year units, and T is the random variable representing the age of lung cancer death, then $h(t) = \Pr(T = t \mid T \geq t)$ (i.e., the probability of lung cancer death at age t given survival to age t). This hazard will appear below in the discrete Cox model, and the equivalent probability will appear below as $\pi(t)$ in the logistic regression model. Interpretation of the hazard as a disease probability is straightforward in this case of equal time intervals of unit length but would need to be modified in other situations. In the sequel, the terms *risk* and *hazard* are used interchangeably.

Cox versus Logistic Regression

The design is a prospective cohort study with six years of follow-up, and the endpoint is lung cancer death. Since most observations are censored (i.e., the endpoint, lung cancer, is not necessarily observed during the study period), methods for censored survival analysis are required. A person who died of other causes was considered to be censored with respect to lung cancer death.

The goal was to estimate lung cancer risk as a function of age and other covariates. Several possible regression models were considered. The most natural choice was Cox's proportional hazards regression model, which is designed to model censored survival data as a function of covariates without parametric assumptions on the failure-time distribution. The hazard function is given by

$$h(t; \mathbf{x}) = h_0(t) \exp(\mathbf{x}\boldsymbol{\beta}), \tag{1}$$

where $h(t; \mathbf{x})$ is the hazard function at time t for an individual with row vector of covariates $\mathbf{x}$, $h_0(t)$ is the baseline hazard at time t for an individual with all covariates at the zero level, and $\boldsymbol{\beta}$ is the column vector of regression coefficients. The Cox model allows covariate parameters to be estimated without estimating the baseline hazard function, which in many situations is not of interest. The assumption is that the ratio of hazards of failure for any two levels of a covariate (say, male versus female) is constant over all time points.

Three issues made use of the Cox model difficult for the data set considered here. First, interest was in explicitly estimating the hazard function rather than treating it as a nuisance parameter. Second, the analysis would involve time-dependent covariates (i.e., covariates that change in value with increasing time, such as the variable, "years smoked," which will increase with age for continuing smokers). Third, the risk set (the set of subjects at risk for failure at any given age) would change over time. Changes in the risk set over time means that all subjects don't begin at time zero and continue in the study until censored or death. In the current study, the "time variable" is age and different six-year age windows were observed on each of thousands of people, which would mean that the risk set would be changing constantly as a function of age. While Cox regression can accommodate time-dependent variables and changes in the risk set, some programming finesse is necessary and the computer time required is often excessive.

Logistic regression, which is a regression method for the situation of dichotomous outcomes, can be used to approximate Cox regression when the time axis is divided into discrete periods, such as one-year intervals. The logistic model provides an excellent approximation to the Cox model when the rate of occurrence of the event of interest in each interval is low, as it is with lung cancer. The logistic regression model is given by

$$\text{logit}\,[\pi(\mathbf{x})] = \log\left[\frac{\pi(\mathbf{x})}{1 - \pi(\mathbf{x})}\right] = \mathbf{x}\boldsymbol{\beta}, \tag{2}$$

where $\pi(\mathbf{x})$ is the probability of lung cancer death in a one-year interval given the row vector of covariates $\mathbf{x}$, and $\boldsymbol{\beta}$ is the column vector of regression coefficients. Age is included among the covariates, and thus $\pi(\mathbf{x})$ can be considered as the probability of death at a certain age, given that the person is alive at that age and has certain other covariates. This probability is simply the discrete hazard as a function of age, gender, college attendance, and smoking covariates, as seen above. Given estimates of the β's (denoted by $\hat{\beta}$), $\pi(\mathbf{x})$ can be estimated by inverting the logit function: $\hat{\pi}(\mathbf{x}) = \exp[\mathbf{x}\hat{\boldsymbol{\beta}}]/[1 + \exp(\mathbf{x}\hat{\boldsymbol{\beta}})]$.

Two advantages of the logistic approximation are: time-dependent covariates, including changes in the risk set, are easily handled; and the baseline hazard function can be modeled parametrically (i.e., smoothed), leading to hazard estimates with much smaller variance, if the parametric function is an appropriate one, than the nonparametric estimates which can be computed based on life table methods. Although the analysis is then parametric, the family of possible distributions based on fitting the logit hazard with polynomials or polynomial splines is much richer than the usual parametric alternatives of Weibull, log-normal, log-logistic or gamma.

The method of using logistic regression to analyze survival data was discussed in the early biometric literature by Brown (1975), Thompson (1977) and Mantel and Hankey (1978), and has been referred to as a "person-time" (Ingram and Kleinman, 1989), "partial" (Efron, 1988), or "pooled" (D'Agostino et al., 1990) logistic model. Hosmer and Lemeshow (1989, pp. 238–245) provide a clear description of the mechanics of this method. Allison and Yamaguchi describe the same method from a sociological viewpoint, Allison in a very readable monograph (Allison, 1984) and chapter (Allison, 1982), and Yamaguchi in a more recent monograph (Yamaguchi, 1991). Lawless (1982) describes this method as a generalization of life tables to include covariates. [Poisson regression and complementary log-log link models have also been proposed for this situation (Prentice and Gloeckler, 1978; Holford, 1980; Whitehead, 1980; Laird and Olivier, 1981; Abbott, 1985; Whittemore, 1985). In cases where the event rate in each interval is low, all these models will give almost identical results.]

To use logistic regression with survival data, one must first expand the data so that each subject has a separate record for each year of enrollment in the study. Since the current study spans six years, a person who was alive and observed for all six years would contribute six observations to the analysis, one for each age of life in which he or she was enrolled. Someone who died in the third year of the study would contribute three observations. The outcome variable is dichotomous, corresponding to whether the person died of lung cancer in the interval. Covariates may have different values for each year of entry; therefore, "time-dependent covariates" do not require special treatment. For example, someone aged 65 in 1982 was 66 in 1983, and the yearly observations can reflect these changes in age. A standard logistic regression analysis with the time variable, age, included among the covariates, is performed using the expanded data. The dependence between multiple observations per person does not cause problems for estimating either the parameters or standard errors (Allison, 1982), in the same sense that hazard estimates in each interval of a life table are (at least approximately) uncorrelated.

The basic idea behind the approximation of Cox regression by logistic regression is as follows. Since time is discrete in any fixed unit of measurement, it is reasonable to approximate a continuous Cox model with a discrete one. If t is considered as a discrete time variable, then in the Cox regression model given by (1), consider $h(t; x)$ to be the discrete hazard function for an individual with covariates x, and $h_0(t)$ to be the discrete baseline hazard for an individual with all covariates at the zero level. Since the discrete hazard is defined as the probability of failure at time t, given survival to time t, the hazard of failure in any interval for a given set of covariates is the same as $\pi(t, x)$, or simply $\pi(x)$, the probability from the logistic model given in (2), where t is included among the covariates x. Thus, the Cox model can be written with $\pi(t, x)$ replacing the $h(t; x)$. Further, the discrete baseline hazard function, $h_0(t)$ in (1), can be replaced by $\exp(\beta_{0j})$ without loss of flexibility in the model, where β_{0j} is the hazard in the jth interval. Then $h_0(t) = \exp(\beta_{0j})$ can be put into the exponential term, $\exp(x\beta)$, by incorporating an additional set of covariates that are indicator functions for each time interval. Taking the log of both sides yields $\log \pi(x) = x\beta$, which is very similar to the logistic model (2). If the event rate in each interval is near zero, then $1 - \pi(x)$ from (2) is approximately 1, so that $\pi(\mathbf{x})/[1 - \pi(\mathbf{x})] \approx \pi(\mathbf{x})$. Thus, the logistic and Cox models will have approximately the same form.

As mentioned above, incorporating a set of covariates that are indicators for each time interval gives the same flexibility as the unspecified baseline hazard of the discrete Cox model. The hazard, although discrete, can be thought of as a step function taking different values in each age interval (similar to piecewise exponential). There are other possibilities for modeling the hazard as a function of time which may be useful in some circumstances. A constant hazard, $h(t) = \alpha$, yields an exponential distribution of failures over time. A log hazard that is linear in t, $\log h(t) = \alpha_0 + \alpha_1 t$, leads to the Gompertz distribution, and a log hazard that is linear in $\log t$, $\log h(t) = \alpha_0 + \alpha_1 \log t$, yields a Weibull distribution of failures. In general, specifying a function $h(t)$ is equivalent to specifying a probability distribution for failures over time. Using logistic regression, the logit hazard (which approximates the log hazard when the event rate is low) is most easily modeled as a polynomial or polynomial spline in t or $\log t$. Alternatively, nonparametric smoothing techniques could be employed to smooth the logit hazard, leading to a much larger class of underlying probability distributions. Most such hazard functions do not yield density functions with simple forms, but that is usually of little concern. While a completely flexible step function may seem ideal, true hazard functions are likely to be smooth. Thus, smoothing the hazard function, if a reasonable function can be found, is a good idea when the hazard function itself is of interest. There is no obvious advantage in forcing a known distribution (e.g., a Weibull or lognormal) and much to be gained by investigating various possibilities. Efron (1988) found that a cubic-linear spline provided a good fit to the logit hazard function in a cancer data set and suggested that a flexible specification of the hazard function can also allow for incomplete survival fractions (i.e., distributions for which there is some probability of never failing).

For the CPS-II data set, smoothing the logit hazard function using polynomials worked well. In general, parsimonious estimation of the hazard function does not improve the estimates or standard errors of the β values for other covariates (Efron, 1977). Focusing on estimation of the hazard function and momentarily ignoring covariates, however, if the smoothing function is appropriate, the variance of the resulting hazard estimate will be reduced, on average, by p/N compared with the variance of the hazard estimate using life table methods, where p is the number of parameters and N is the number of discrete time intervals (Efron, 1988). When each interval has a separate hazard estimate, then $p = N$, and the baseline hazard is estimated as in the discrete Cox model. Fitting the hazard function with a simple polynomial or polynomial spline function can reduce considerably the variance of the hazard estimate. In the current study, $N = 41$ and $p \leq 4$ (see Section 4), so the variance of the estimated hazard from logistic regression will be less than 10% of the variance of the estimated hazard that would have been obtained from life table methods.

The proportional hazards assumption of the Cox model is replaced in the logistic model by the assumption of proportional odds, as can be seen from the model statements. When the event rate is low, however, these assumptions will be nearly the same because the ratio of hazards will be approximately equal to the ratio of odds.

When using the Cox model, one checks the proportional hazards assumption relative to the time axis (i.e., the assumption that all covariates have the same multiplicative effect on the hazard at all time points). For deviation from the proportional hazards assumption in the Cox model, a stratified Cox model is often recommended, where a separate baseline hazard function is estimated within each level of some covariate. Alternatively, a time-dependent covariate can be incorporated. Both of these methods are ways to model an interaction between time and some covariate; stratification models the most general form of interaction, whereas a time-dependent covariate can model a specific form of an interaction. When using the logistic model with survival data, an interaction between time and another covariate can be included in the model as an ordinary interaction term. Thus, nonproportional odds can be tested or modeled by including interaction terms between the time variable(s) and other covariates. Interactions with other variables should be checked similarly. For example, if the gender-by-number-of-cigarettes-per-day interaction is not included in the model, the assumption is that the hazard ratio (or odds ratio) for males to females is constant for any numbers of cigarettes smoked per day.

Model Building
Prior to model building, the data were converted into the person-years format, with one record per subject per year on study. For each subject, each successive record was updated for age, number of years of smoking (for current smokers) and number of years since quitting (for former smokers).

The ultimate model-building goal was to build a comprehensive model which included current, former, and never smokers. Initially, however, a model was fitted for current and never smokers only, to explore interactions and find the important covariates for these two groups. Since the effects of smoking variables were expected to dampen but not change in form with years since quitting, smoking and demographic variables were included in the comprehensive model based on this initial model of current and never smokers. Some researchers have used pack-years as a measure of cumulative tobacco exposure, but it was felt that using the more complete information of two separate variables (cigarettes/day and number of years smoked) would provide a better model fit.

For all continuous variables, linear, quadratic and cubic terms were investigated. Log transformations were tried for the age and years smoked variables. Although it seemed unlikely that cohort effects could be observed in a span as short as six years, a variable for year-of-study (two-year intervals) was initially included to check for this effect. This variable was not significant ($p = 0.30$) and was not considered further. For interactions involving continuous variables, both linear and quadratic interaction terms were investigated. All plausible interactions were checked, and significant terms were retained in the model. Hierarchical models were tested using the likelihood ratio test. Because of multicollinearity between variables such as age and years smoked, some interactions would change substantially in importance (based on *p*-values) from model to model. The overall strategy was to prefer lower-order interactions to higher-order terms and to find the most parsimonious model possible. For quadratic, cubic, and interaction terms, each continuous factor was centered by subtracting the sample mean value before multiplying.

The effects of covariates on lung cancer mortality were expected to be complex, and the size of the data set allowed for lots of data analysis exploration. However, the size of most models was near the edge of the limits imposed by software and the University of Michigan mainframe computer. Often, one model would run, but adding one more variable would exceed the computer limits. One key factor was the number of covariate patterns generated. Grouping the number of cigarettes/day by 5's was done midway through the modeling and allowed the final modeling to proceed. A full step-down model was impossible; the general strategy was first to include the main effects and introduce higher-order terms a few at a time, retaining the significant ones and deleting the insignificant ones. Since some variables are correlated (e.g., age and years smoked), the variables and interactions included in the final model may not form the unique best model but will do approximately as well at prediction as other models based on these variables.

For former smokers, years since quitting smoking was included in the model, multiplied by an indicator variable for the appropriate age-at-quitting cohort. Initially, linear, quadratic, and cubic terms were included for each cohort, allowing independent cubic polynomial functions in years since quitting to be fitted. Cubic terms were dropped from the earlier cohorts when not significant, but the quadratic terms were retained, even when insignificant, to maintain flexibility. Cubic terms were retained in the older age-at-quitting cohorts, even though not significant, because the functions for the various cohorts showed a consistent cubic pattern which seemed plausible. A method of regression splines, discussed below, was used to force the ex-smoker curves to match the current smoker curves at the point of quitting. To investigate the possibility that patterns of cancer risks after quitting smoking differ by gender, the interaction terms gender × (years quit), gender × (years quit)^2, and gender × (years quit)^3 were included for the 55–59 and 60–64 age-at-quitting cohorts, where the sample size and numbers of deaths were felt to be sufficient for investigating this question. These terms were not significant ($p > 0.5$ in all cases) and were dropped from the model. Differences in risk patterns for ex-smokers by daily cigarette consumption were investigated similarly, with interactions involving cigarettes/day dichotomized as ≥1 pack/day and < 1 pack/day. Significant differences were found for one of the cohorts (55–59) but not the other. However, a plot of the hazard estimates for the two consumption groups in this cohort showed crossing risk curves which were difficult to interpret. Thus, these terms were dropped from the model. Although the power to detect differences by cigarette consumption in the risk patterns for former smokers was marginal, no evidence of strong differences was found.

The attempt in modeling the risk for former smokers was not to verify any theoretical model, such as a multistage model of cancer pathogenesis, but simply to fit the data to appropriate smooth curves from which hypotheses about cancer mechanisms can be generated.

Hazard estimates, $\hat{\pi}(\mathbf{x})$, for a given covariate pattern x were calculated using the inverse logit function (i.e., the logistic transform): $\hat{\pi}(\mathbf{x}) = \exp(\mathbf{x}\hat{\boldsymbol{\beta}})/[1 + \exp(\mathbf{x}\hat{\boldsymbol{\beta}})]$. One-standard-error intervals for $\pi(\mathbf{x})$ were calculated by applying the logistic transform to one-standard-error intervals for the linear predictor, $\mathbf{x}\boldsymbol{\beta}$, for various values of $\mathbf{x}$: Let $[\eta_L(\mathbf{x}), \eta_U(\mathbf{x})] = \mathbf{x}\hat{\boldsymbol{\beta}} \pm \{\mathbf{x}[\mathrm{Var}(\hat{\boldsymbol{\beta}})]\mathbf{x}^T\}^{1/2}$. Then one-standard-error limits for $\pi(\mathbf{x})$ are given as $\pi_L(\mathbf{x}) = \exp[\eta_L(\mathbf{x})]/\{1 + \exp(\eta_L(\mathbf{x}))\}$, and $\pi_U(\mathbf{x}) = \exp[\eta_U(\mathbf{x})]/\{1 + \exp[\eta_u(\mathbf{x})]\}$. The one-standard-error intervals can be interpreted as approximate pointwise 68% confidence intervals for $\pi(\mathbf{x})$.

Difficulty was encountered initially in obtaining a positive-definite estimate of the covariance matrix of the $\hat{\beta}$'s, which led to negative variance estimates of the linear predictor, $\mathbf{x}\boldsymbol{\beta}$, for some values of $\mathbf{x}$. This problem arose because the covariate scales were widely different, accentuated by quadratic and cubic terms in the model. The problem was solved by scaling (dividing) the jth continuous covariate by $c_j = [\Sigma x_i^2/n]^{0.5}$. The effect of this scaling on $\hat{\beta}_j$ is to multiply it by c_j; to facilitate interpretation, however, the β's appropriate for the unscaled data are presented.

Spline Method for Fitting Ex-smokers

A simple method of regression splines was used to force a knot in the hazard functions for former smokers at the age of quitting. Regression splines are piecewise polynomial functions, and the join points are called knots. The functions are usually constrained to match at the knots, as well as to satisfy some condition of smoothness at the knots, defined by equality of derivatives of the functions on either side of the join. Using the "+ function" notation common in the regression spline literature, define $u_+ = u$ if $u > 0$ and $u_+ = 0$ if $u \leq 0$. Consider the situation of a single knot at $x = t$, with a quadratic function on either side of the knot. As explained in Smith's (1979) paper on regression splines, the function

$$f(x) = \beta_{00} + \beta_{01}x + \beta_{02}x^2 + \beta_{10}(x - t)_+^0 + \beta_{11}(x - t)_+^1 + \beta_{12}(x - t)_+^2 + \epsilon$$

yields a completely separate quadratic function on either side of the knot at t. The $\beta_{10}(x - t)_+^0$ term allows the functions to be disjoint at t. Dropping $(x - t)_+^0$ from the model (i.e., $\beta_{10} = 0$) forces the functions to join at t, but without restrictions on smoothness of the join. Dropping $(x - t)_+^1$ as well (i.e., $\beta_{10} = 0$ and $\beta_{11} = 0$) forces the functions not only to join but also to have equal first derivatives at t. In most spline applications smooth joins are desired, but in this case, the hazard of lung cancer death might change abruptly at the point of quitting smoking. For this reason, the functions were forced to join at the age of quitting without requiring any other continuity restrictions, so that terms of the form $(x - t)^1_+, (x - t)^2_+$, and $(x - t)^3_+$ were included in the model, but not $(x-t)^0_+$ (i.e., there is no simple indicator of the age-of-quitting cohort). The knot t is the age of quitting, so that $(x - t)_+$ is the number of years since quitting. By multiplying each such term by an indicator for the respective cohort, all age-at-quitting cohorts could be fitted in the same model.

Checking Goodness of Fit

Since several data records are generated from a single subject, Hosmer and Lemeshow (1989, p. 244) express concern about the use of logistic regression diagnostics to assess the fit of the model when using logistic regression with survival data. However, because the hazard estimates in separate intervals of a life table (which are analogous to the hazard estimates for each age in the logistic regression) are approximately uncorrelated, it was felt that regression diagnostics should have, at least approximately, the usual properties. The usual goodness-of-fit tests and residuals plots were done, as well as a plot of observed versus expected values.

Goodness-of-fit tests can be problematic even in the standard logistic regression setting, and this situation was particularly sticky. The Pearson or likelihood-ratio chi-squared tests work well if the expected number of observations per cell is, say, five or more. In this case, assuming that the observed values roughly reflect the expected values, there are 307,262 (56%) covariate patterns with a single observation, and 84% of covariate cells with fewer than four observations. As would be expected from the enormous number of degrees of freedom, the Pearson chi-square indicates highly significant lack of fit. On the other hand, the Hosmer–Lemeshow statistic was developed for the case when the number of covariate patterns is approximately equal to the sample size (roughly one observation per cell). On the other end of the very skewed distribution of numbers of observations per covariate cell in this data set, however, there are hundreds of high-frequency cells, almost 100 with frequencies from 10,000 to nearly 37,000. The Hosmer–Lemeshow test indicates that the fit is quite good ($p = 0.52, \hat{C} = 7.19$, 8 d.f.), but this result should not be taken as conclusive evidence of a good model fit since the χ^2 distribution of the test statistic has not been verified in the case of such a mix of sparse and high-frequency cells.

Observed versus expected values were also plotted by age and smoking category, pooled over other covariates. Some grouping was necessary for calculating observed lung cancer death rates. Yearly mortality proportions were fairly noisy, so the data were grouped by five-year intervals, which provided enough smoothing to assess the model reasonably. (Intervals at the end of the age scale for ex-smokers included more than five years when the entire time period was not divisible by 5.) The observed rates are simply the number of lung cancer deaths during the five-year period divided by the number of person-years at risk. These are equivalent to life-table hazard rates, unadjusted for covariates.

The expected lung cancer death risks were computed by first calculating an estimated risk for each observation in the data set [i.e., $\hat{\pi}(\mathbf{x})$, given the person's covariate vector $\mathbf{x}$], then summing the risks for each age and smoking category and dividing by the number of observations. The plot of expected values by age is not completely smooth, since the covariate values are changing with the risk set at each age. Such a plot of observed versus expected values is possible only with a large data set, since observed rates with smaller samples are often too variable to assess the model fit visually. Since the expected value of a function of variables is not necessarily equal to the function of the expected values of those variables (Casella and Berger, 1990), expected hazard values were *not* computed by calculating the estimated risk for the mean values of covariates in the data set.

Birth Cohort Effects

One limitation of this analysis is that patterns observed at different ages may be partially the result of a birth cohort effect. For example, people in their 70s at the time of the study have different smoking histories than those in their 50s: on average the former started smoking later in life and were more likely to smoke unfiltered cigarettes (U.S. Department of Health and Human Services, 1989b). Hence, if those in their fifties could be followed for the next 20 years, they might not have the identical lung cancer risk as those in their seventies at the time of the study. Such birth cohort effects could not be examined without more data on smoking histories and without a wider study period.

4   RESULTS

Figures 3 and 4 show model estimates of the risk of lung cancer death (number of deaths per 100,000 per year) by age for males and females, respectively. In these figures, the solid line represents current smokers and the dotted line represents never smokers. A symbol is present on the current smoker line at the mean age of each age-at-quitting cohort, representing the absolute risk of lung cancer death at the mean age of smoking cessation for that cohort. The line for each cohort is dotted for the first five years, reflecting the period which the model does not predict because of the quitting-ill effect. Following this five-year period, a dashed line traces the absolute risk of lung cancer death with increasing age. One-standard-error bars are shown at several points. To make the figures relevant to contemporary young adult smokers, the estimates were based on the average smoking characteristics of participants in the CPS-II aged 30 to 39 at the onset of the study in 1982. On average, male smokers in this group began smoking at age 17.5 and reported smoking 26 cigarettes/day, while females started at age 18.5 and reported smoking 22 cigarettes/day. College attendance proportions were 60% for males and 54% for females, and these proportions were used as the college covariate values instead of zero or 1. The difference in the scale of lung cancer death rates in the two figures reflects

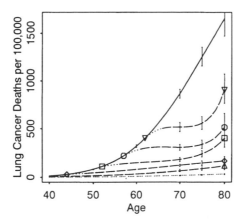

Figure 3. Model estimates of lung cancer death rates by age for male current, former, and never smokers, based on smokers who started at age 17.5 and smoked 26 cigarettes/day. Estimates are plotted for current smokers (solid line), never smokers (dotted line), and former smokers (dashed lines). The five age-at-quitting cohorts are distinguished by the following symbols on the graph at the age of quitting and also at age 80: (△) 30–39, (◇) 40–49, (□) 50–54, (○) 55–59, (▽) 60–64 (from Halpern et al., 1993).

differences in male and female smoking histories, as discussed by the Surgeon General (U.S. Department of Health and Human Services, 1989b).

Both figures illustrate the dramatic rise in lung cancer death risk with age for continuing smokers compared with never smokers. Lung cancer death risks following smoking cessation follow a similar pattern for all age-at-quit-

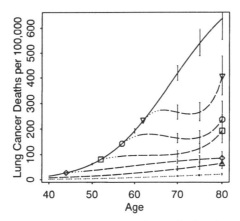

Figure 4. Model estimates of lung cancer death rates by age for female current, former, and never smokers, based on smokers who started at age 18.5 and smoked 22 cigarettes/day. Estimates are plotted for current smokers (solid line), never smokers (dotted line), and former smokers (dashed lines). The five age-at-quitting cohorts are distinguished by the following symbols on the graph at the age of quitting and also at age 80: (△) 30–39, (◇) 40–49, (□) 50–54, (○) 55–59, (▽) 60–64 (from Halpern et al., 1993).

ting cohorts. A slight rise is observed between lung cancer risk at the age of quitting and the risk five years later. For those quitting between ages 30 and 49, the risk following the five-year gap gradually increases with age at a rate slightly but persistently greater than that for never smokers. For those quitting between ages 50 and 65, the risk plateaus near the five-year post-quitting level for the next 10 to 20 years. However, starting around age 75, the risk for these cohorts again increases at rates well in excess of those for the younger age-at-quitting cohorts; the rate of increase is steepest for the older age-at-quitting cohorts.

As expected, smokers who quit after age 65 showed lung cancer risks below those of current smokers. However, a sharp decline in risk with age was observed in this group, which led to predicted risk at age 80 below the predicted risk of earlier age-at-quitting cohorts. Such anomalous patterns can probably be attributed to small sample sizes in these groups and possible competing risk effects because those quitting late in life are perhaps more likely to quit for other health reasons. Thus, these groups were dropped from Figures 2 and 3.

Estimated regression coefficients are presented in Table 4. Although the number of interactions and higher-order terms makes the model look complex, interpretation of most model terms is straightforward. Risk factors include gender, college attendance, age, number of cigarettes smoked per day, and number of years as a smoker. For dichotomous variables, $\exp(\hat{\beta})$ approximates the relative risk (RR) for the variable at level $x = 1$ versus the variable at level $x = 0$. The gender factor (RR = 0.70, indicating lower risk for females) probably reflects both less occupational exposure and differences in nonmeasured smoking habits (depth of inhalation, tendency to smoke filtered cigarettes, smoking the whole or just part of the cigarette, etc.), but may also represent biological differences. College attendance effects (RR = 0.71, indicating lower risk for those attending some college) may reflect similar differences in occupational exposure or smoking habits as well as other effects of socioeconomic status. For continuous variables, $\exp(\hat{\beta})$ approximates the relative risk for a 1-unit increase in the variable value, and $\exp(10\hat{\beta})$ approximates the relative risk for a 10-unit increase. Age and years smoked are both strong predictors of lung cancer death risk (RR = 2.34 and RR = 1.73, respectively, for a 10-year increase, based on the linear term only). The negative coefficients of the squared terms of age and years smoked indicate a damping of the approximately linear function of logit(risk) with increasing age (i.e., the risk increases almost but not quite exponentially with age). For the number of cigarettes smoked per day, however, the risk function reaches a maximum at around 55 cigarettes per day and then decreases. It is likely that the true risk function levels off beyond 55 cigarettes per day, and that a quadratic function could not fit such a pattern. The nonsignificant variable "smoking status," which equals 1 for current or former smokers and zero for never smokers, was retained in the model. Lack of significance of this variable indicates that overall increases in lung cancer mortality of smokers and ex-smokers over never smokers has been explained with the other variables included in the model.

Table 4   Logistic Model for Lung Cancer in Never, Current and Former Smokers

Variable	$\hat{\beta}$	p-Value
Intercept	-9.87	0.000
Gender (0 = male, 1 = female)	-0.35	0.000
College (0 = no, 1 = yes)	-0.34	0.000
Gender × college	0.24	0.000
Age[a]	8.5×10^{-2}	0.000
Gender × age	-1.5×10^{-2}	0.001
Age^2	-7.9×10^{-4}	0.002
No. cigarettes/day	2.5×10^{-2}	0.000
Gender × No. cigarettes/day	7.8×10^{-3}	0.004
College × No. cigarettes/day	4.2×10^{-3}	0.049
(No. cigarettes/day)^2	-4.0×10^{-4}	0.000
Years smoked	5.5×10^{-2}	0.000
Gender × years smoked	-8.8×10^{-3}	0.001
Age × years smoked	-6.0×10^{-4}	0.001
(Years smoked)^2	-3.7×10^{-4}	0.026
Smoking status[b]	-0.29	0.306
Years quit, 30–39 quit cohort	-4.4×10^{-2}	0.006
(Years quit)^2, 30–39 quit cohort	4.6×10^{-4}	0.330
Years quit, 40–49 quit cohort	-3.8×10^{-2}	0.002
(Years quit)^2, 40–49 quit cohort	1.6×10^{-4}	0.732
Years quit, 50–54 quit cohort	-2.7×10^{-2}	0.474
(Years quit)^2, 50–54 quit cohort	-3.6×10^{-3}	0.386
(Years quit)^3, 50–54 quit cohort	1.4×10^{-4}	0.214
Years quit, 55–59 quit cohort	2.1×10^{-2}	0.620
(Years quit)^2, 55–59 quit cohort	-8.9×10^{-3}	0.120
(Years quit)^3, 55–59 quit cohort	3.0×10^{-4}	0.100
Years quit, 60–64 quit cohort	2.8×10^{-2}	0.611
(Years quit)^2, 60–64 quit cohort	-1.2×10^{-2}	0.187
(Years quit)^3, 60–64 quit cohort	5.4×10^{-4}	0.110

Source: Halpern et al. (1993).
[a]Adjusted age (age − 40).
[b]Smoking status equals 0 for never smokers, 1 for current or former smokers.

Interaction effects in the model include gender by college, gender by age, gender by number of cigarettes per day, college by number of cigarettes per day, gender by years smoked, and age by years smoked. The positive coefficient for the gender by college interaction indicates that risks for females (coded 1) with some college (coded 1) are too low when estimated with multiplicative effects and should be adjusted upward. This interaction effect probably reflects occupational exposures leading to higher lung cancer risk in males without college.

The gender by age interaction (which is significant even among never smokers, as verified by a separate model) indicates a protective effect for females with increasing age. This effect could reflect a biological difference between men and women in lung cancer rates, but environmental or occupational factors related to gender are more likely to explain this interaction. A plot of the gender by years-smoked interaction is given in Figure 5. This plot shows model-based estimates of risk [$\hat{\pi}(\mathbf{x})$], for males and females by years of smoking, with all other covariates equal. Risk is plotted on a logit scale so that interaction can be detected as nonparallelism in the two lines. If females differ from males in their smoking habits or occupational exposure, as mentioned, the effect of smoking more years may have a different effect on females than it does on males. Although the explanation is conjectural, such a pattern can be seen in the plot, with males incurring increasingly greater risk than females with additional years of smoking. The protective effect of being female is reversed, however, when considering the interaction of gender with number of cigarettes smoked per day. Higher cigarette consumption appears to be more harmful in women than men. Surprisingly, higher cigarette consumption also appears to be more harmful to those attending college, as indicated by the positive coefficient of the college × cigarettes/day interaction. The age × (years smoked) interaction has a negative coefficient of the same order of magnitude as the coefficients of age^2 and (years smoked)^2, and years smoked is highly correlated with age in current (but not former) smokers. Since the quadratic terms for age and years smoked represent a damping of the linear relationship of these variables with

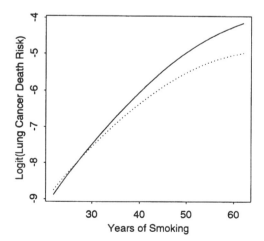

Figure 5. Interaction of gender and number of years of smoking indicated by the nonparallelism of logit(lung cancer risk) for males (solid line) and females (dotted line) over years of smoking. Curves are based on smokers with no college attendance, with the average age 57.5, and the average daily cigarette consumption 23.56/day.

the logit risk, the age × (years smoked) interaction may represent differential damping among current and former smokers.

Slightly different model formulations resulted in essentially the same curves, indicating that although the covariates may not provide a unique characterization of lung cancer risk, the model is fairly robust to small changes in model structure.

To examine the fit of the model, Figure 6 plots the observed lung cancer risks (grouped by five-year intervals) versus the summed expected risks calculated from the model for all individuals in the study. Perhaps more reassuring than any other goodness-of-fit measure, this plot shows that the model provides a good fit to the data.

Standard error bars in Figures 3 and 4 illustrate that the lung cancer risk of all cohorts of quitters remains above that of never smokers; even those quitting in their thirties have a risk approximately twice that of never smokers, a difference that does not decrease with age. However, for all age-at-quitting cohorts examined, lung cancer risk is well below that of current smokers. The curves for each age-at-quitting cohort are for the most part distinct (i.e., standard error bars do not overlap) until near age 80 and reflect a clear pattern of increasing risk with increasing age of quitting.

Table 5 converts the estimates of absolute risk for never and former smokers into relative risks with respect to current smokers at three time points (ages 55, 65, and 75). Predictably, relative risk increases with age at quitting and decreases with years since quitting.

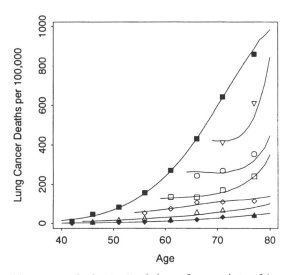

Figure 6. Observed lung cancer death rates (pooled over five-year intervals) versus expected rates generated from the model for the participants in the study (solid lines). Symbols for observed death rates: (■) current smokers, (♦) never smokers, and age-at-quitting cohorts (△) 30–39, (◇) 40–49, (□) 50–54, (○) 55–59, and (▽) 60–64. (from Halpern et al., 1993).

Table 5 Relative Risk of Lung Cancer Death Following Smoking Cessation: Never and Former Smokers, as Compared to Current Smokers

Cohort	Relative Risk		
	Age 55	Age 65	Age 75
Males:			
Never smokers	0.05	0.03	0.03
Quit 30–39	0.14	0.09	0.07
Quit 40–49	0.36	0.18	0.12
Quit 50–54	—	0.29	0.19
Quit 55–59	—	0.56	0.27
Quit 60–64	—	—	0.45
Current smokers	1.0	1.0	1.0
Females:			
Never smokers	0.07	0.05	0.04
Quit 30–39	0.17	0.11	0.10
Quit 40–49	0.40	0.22	0.15
Quit 50–54	—	0.33	0.23
Quit 55–59	—	0.60	0.31
Quit 60–64	—	—	0.49
Current smokers	1.0	1.0	1.0

Source: Halpern et al. (1993)

5 CONCLUSIONS

Although many studies have demonstrated that quitting smoking is beneficial, the patterns of risk following cessation had not previously been well characterized. The main reason for the variability seen among earlier study results is very possibly the lack of adjustment for age of quitting, an adjustment that this study has demonstrated to be an important factor. Lubin et al. (1984) adjusted for the number of years of smoking, which should be roughly equivalent to adjusting for age of quitting, but he did not plot the absolute risk curves. To see the importance of this effect, note in Table 5 the relative risks approximately two decades after quitting for the age at quitting cohorts 30–39, 40–49, and 55–59. The respective relative risks are 0.14, 0.18, and 0.27 for males, and 0.17, 0.22, and 0.31 for females, indicating a near doubling of relative risk from quitting in the thirties to quitting in the late fifties. Thus, relative risks calculated for various years since quitting without adjusting for the age of quitting will depend on the mix of subjects under study.

   Some limitations of this study deserve mention. Data were not available on reasons for quitting, depth of inhalation, type of cigarettes smoked, and occupational exposure, which are probably important covariates. Birth cohort effects almost certainly have some effect on the estimates; a longer-term study would allow those effects to be estimated. Finally, although it is difficult to complain too much about sample size with such an enormous study, the sample size required to study former smokers is much greater than that necessary to study current smokers if separate functions are estimated for each age of quitting. Consequently, larger sample sizes of former smokers would allow more precise estimation of the risk functions for those groups and allow more complete testing of interactions between risk patterns and covariates such as daily cigarette consumption.

In conclusion, an effective way to model lung cancer mortality following smoking cessation has been demonstrated, a method that can be applied in more general situations. The use of logistic regression to approximate Cox regression is a useful tool whenever hazard smoothing is appropriate or covariates are time dependent. The method of modeling two or more curves simultaneously with a join point can be performed in any regression setting. Employing absolute rather than relative risk was found to be helpful in displaying patterns of risk as a function of several other variables.

ACKNOWLEDGMENTS

We thank the American Cancer Society for the use of the CPS-II data set. Useful comments were provided by Lawrence Garfinkel, Clark Heath, Jr., and Michael Thun of ACS, and by Mark Becker, Marcia Feingold, Dana Flanders, Andrzej Galecki, John Gillespie, David W. Hosmer, Daniel Normolle, Roy St. Laurent, Thomas TenHave, and Robert Wolfe. We are grateful to Jewel Johanns for producing the graphs. Funding for computing was provided through the University of Michigan Information Technology Division, Computer Allocation for the Computational Sciences.

SOFTWARE NOTES AND REFERENCES

All modeling was done using SAS © Proc Logistic (SAS/STAT User's Guide, 1989). The events/trials syntax was used, in which a single record is entered for each covariate pattern, with the numbers of deaths and subjects at risk as summary variables. This method is computer-efficient and was necessary with the large data set of this study.

SAS Institute, Inc. (1989). *SAS/STAT User's Guide, Version 6,* 4th ed., Vol. 2. Cary, N.C.: SAS Institute.

QUESTIONS AND PROBLEMS

1. Discuss how the patterns of risk after quitting smoking observed here could be partially explained by a birth cohort effect.

2. Discuss the added flexibility which logistic regression provides over Cox regression. What are the possible disadvantages?

3. The modeling used here was based entirely on polynomial functions of age in the logistic model. Would nonlinear forms be more appropriate and more consistent with current theories of cancer pathogenesis? Alternatively, non-parametric smoothing techniques would give more flexibility than the cubic model. Try other functions and evaluate the fit.

4. Joining the curves for ex-smokers to the smoker curve at the age of quitting assumes that those who quit are no different (at the point of quitting) in terms of lung cancer risk than continuing smokers with the same other covariates (i.e., that a "random sample" of smokers with given covariates has chosen to quit smoking). Is this a plausible assumption? Is there any way to check this assumption?

5. The observed values in Figure 6 were obtained from the ratios of five-year observed lung cancer deaths to the total number of subject-years observed in the interval. These values are somewhat arbitrary, since using different five-year windows (or using windows of size other than five years) will result in different values. Try redrawing this plot with different intervals for the observed values. (The movement of points as the windows are changed should make clear that the plot should be used for overall model evaluation and not for interpretation of specific points.)

6. The quadratic function for cigarettes/day was found to peak at 55 cigarettes/day. Since risk should plausibly be a monotone function of cigarettes/day, this functional form appears to be misspecified. Discuss possible alternatives, including transformations, nonlinear functions, threshold functions, and categorical variables.

CHAPTER 20

Two-Stage Sampling Designs for Adolescent Depression Studies

Cheryl L. Addy, Kirby L. Jackson, Robert E. McKeown, Jennifer L. Waller, and Carol Z. Garrison

1 MOTIVATION AND BACKGROUND

Study of the assessment, frequency, and correlates of depressive symptoms and disorders in community populations of young adolescents is a developing area of epidemiologic research. The study of adolescent depression in this chapter has two main goals: to estimate the prevalence of adolescent depression in a community-based setting and to identify risk factors for the condition. Existing studies have provided important new information but are generally limited by an inadequate or nonrepresentative sample, diagnosis of overall impairment rather than specific clinical entities, or incomplete or otherwise inadequate data collection procedures. Also, the random sample required to yield a sufficient number of cases can be prohibitively expensive. An alternative design strategy is needed.

One such strategy is the two-phase survey design, also called the double sampling design. Two-phase designs have been discussed by Neyman (1938), Tenenbein (1970), Cochran (1977), Deming (1977), and Shrout and Newman (1989). In this design, a random sample is evaluated with a simple and inexpensive screening tool. Second-phase individuals are then sampled based on the first-phase results. Issues affecting the optimal design of a two-phase survey include the expected prevalence of the disorder, the sensitivity and specificity of the screening tool, the cost of the screening relative to the cost of a complete diagnostic evaluation, and the costs of both false negatives and false positives from the screen.

In this chapter we discuss the application of such a two-stage design in a study of adolescent depression (see Garrison et al., 1991, 1992). In addition to

Case Studies in Biometry, Edited by Nicholas Lange, Louise Ryan, Lynne Billard, David Brillinger, Loveday Conquest, and Joel Greenhouse.
ISBN 0-471-58885-7 © 1994 John Wiley & Sons, Inc.

estimating prevalence and identifying risk factors, we also sought to establish psychometric properties of a depression screening tool in a community population of adolescents. We evaluate the efficiency of the design that was used and discuss its implications for the analysis of the study results.

2   DATA

The first-stage sample consisted of seventh and eighth graders enrolled in four public middle schools in a single southeastern school district. Students were followed as they progressed into high school, and the new classes of seventh graders and new eighth and ninth graders in the school district were added to the sample for assessment and follow-up in successive years. Data have been organized into baseline and follow-up data sets. The baseline data include information from the first screening and evaluation of students regardless of the year in which the initial assessment occurred.

In the first stage of the study all students were screened in classroom settings utilizing self-administered questionnaires. The questionnaires included (1) the Center for Epidemiologic Studies Depression Scale (CES-D; Radloff, 1977); (2) the Family Adaptability and Cohesion Evaluation Scales (FACES-II; Olson et al., 1982); and (3) demographic and general information.

The CES-D is a 20-item, self-report symptom rating scale developed to measure depressive symptomatology in community adult populations. The respondent is asked to report on his or her feelings during the preceding week. The total score (range 0 to 60) is obtained by summing the 20 depression items; the individual's item mean is substituted for any missing items if at least 17 items had valid responses. Since screening cutpoints for adolescents had not been established when the study began, a cutpoint of 30, reflecting the top decile of scores, was used to indicate probable cases.

The FACES-II includes 16 items measuring the emotional bonding which family members had toward one another, as well as the individual autonomy experienced within the family system. The possible range of scores for the family cohesion dimension was 16 to 80, with scores greater than 64 denoting extreme closeness and limited autonomy in the family (enmeshment), scores less than 48 denoting low emotional bonding and high individual autonomy (disengagement), and midrange scores (48 to 64) indicating a balance between bonding and autonomy. The individual's item mean was substituted for missing items if at least 14 items had valid responses.

In the second stage of the study, a stratified sample of students selected for interviews based on the screening results was evaluated. The first stratum includes all students presumed to be at higher risk of major depression, consisting primarily of students obtaining CES-D scores in the highest decile (≥30). The second and third strata consist of a random sample of all remaining students; the third stratum is distinguished by an oversampling of black stu-

Table 1   Variables in Adolescent Depression Data Set[a]

id	clinical	stratum	race	gender	rparents	cesdtot	cohtot	mdd	weight
1	0	3	1	1	0	3.0	80.0	9	2332
2	0	3	1	1	0	17.0	57.1	9	2332
3	0	3	1	1	1	17.0	36.3	9	2332
6	0	1	1	2	0	31.0	40.0	9	417
7	0	3	1	2	0	26.0	60.0	9	2332
8	0	3	1	1	1	2.0	64.0	9	2332
13	1	3	1	1	1	3.0	72.0	0	2332
18	0	2	2	2	1	12.0	63.0	9	4421
162	1	1	1	2	1	28.0	61.0	0	417

[a]Variable   definitions:

id	Subject identifier
clinical	Indicator for selection into clinical sample: 1, in clinical sample; 0, not in clinical sample
stratum	Stratum membership: 1, high screen; 2, low-screen blacks; 3, low-screen whites
race	Subject's self-reported race: 1, white; 2, black
gender	Subject's gender: 1, male; 2, female
rparents	Subject's guardian status: 1, does not live with both natural parents; 0, lives with both natural parents
cesdtot	Subject's total CES-D score (range 0–60)
cohtot	Subject's total cohesion score (range 16–80)
mdd	Clinical diagnosis of major depression: 1, positive diagnosis; 0, negative diagnosis; 9, missing
weight	Defined as number of subjects in screening sample in each stratum

dents. Each subject and one parent were interviewed separately in the home utilizing the Present Episode Version of the Schedule for Affective Disorders and Schizophrenia in School Age Children (K-SADS; Chambers et al., 1985). *Diagnostic and Statistical Manual of Mental Disorders*, 3rd edition (DSM-III, 1980), decision rules were applied to reported symptoms to assign diagnoses. To be considered a case, subjects had both to meet the DSM-III criteria for a specific diagnosis and to have significant impairment as indicated by a score ≤60 on the Children's Global Assessment Scale (Shaffer et al., 1983).

Results are based on students having complete data on select demographic variables, the CES-D, and cohesion. The variables used in the analyses and a sample of the data are listed in Table 1.

3   METHODS AND MODELS

Issues are discussed relative to selection of a sampling design that allows valid estimation of prevalence and other psychometric measures and identifies enough cases of depression to allow assessment of correlates. A subject of debate is whether and how to incorporate such a complex sampling scheme into any analysis. Methodology is presented that accounts for the two-stage design and demonstrates the impact of the design on the results. The specific techniques are estimation of a confidence interval for a weighted prevalence, estimation of sensitivity and specificity utilizing complete screening data, and multivariable modeling using logistic regression with sampling weights. An implicit goal in developing and presenting this methodology is to demonstrate techniques that can be implemented in conjunction with existing software by relatively simple programming (see the Software Notes and References section for this chapter).

3.1   Comparison of Two-Stage Sampling Designs

Design was a major issue in planning the adolescent depression study. Diagnosis of the primary outcome of interest, major depressive disorder, requires a relatively lengthy clinical interview (K-SADS; Chambers et al., 1985) of both the adolescent and a parent and thus is expensive and demanding. However, the self-administered CES-D measures depressive symptoms highly associated with major depression, and is administered easily and inexpensively. In this section we investigate several two-stage sampling designs in which selection of a second-stage sample of individuals is based on the screening scores in the complete population. Primary issues in evaluating possible designs are detection of a maximum number of cases and valid parametric and nonparametric estimation of the prevalence.

The structure of the two-stage sampling procedure can be characterized by three random variables X, R, and G. At the first stage, the variable X is measured on a sample of N individuals. Further samples are then taken, depending on the value of X. The variable R indicates whether ($R = 1$) or not ($R = 0$) an individual is sampled at the second stage. The variable G indicates whether ($G = 1$) or not ($G = 0$) an individual has the disorder of interest, and will be known only for individuals evaluated at the second stage. For the purpose of study design, the variable X is assumed to be normally distributed, with parameters depending on group membership G. The prevalence of the disorder of interest [i.e., $\Pr(G = 1)$] can thus be thought of as a parameter in a mixture of two normal distributions. This formulation has been discussed by other investigators, including Hosmer (1973) and Aitkin and Wilson (1980), although these authors did not consider a second-stage sample based on an initial screening variable.

For the present study, the screening variable X corresponds to the outcome of the self-administered CES-D. Maximum likelihood can be used to estimate five parameters: the means and variances of the CES-D for the major depression group (μ_1, σ_1^2) and for the not depressed group (μ_2, σ_2^2), and the prevalence p. Let f_1 and f_2 denote the densities of X, the CES-D scores, in the two populations:

$$f_1 \sim N(\mu_1, \sigma_1^2) \quad \text{and} \quad f_2 \sim N(\mu_2, \sigma_2^2).$$

Then the mixture distribution is $f_3 = pf_1 + (1-p)f_2$. The likelihood is proportional to

$$\prod_{i=1}^{m_1} pf_1(x_i) \prod_{j=1}^{m_2} (1-p)f_2(x_j) \prod_{k=1}^{m_3} f_3(x_k),$$

where m_1 is the number of individuals evaluated at the second stage and identified as $G = 1$, m_2 is the number evaluated at the second stage and found with $G = 0$, and m_3 is the number of individuals screened only at the first stage and hence with G unknown. Explicit solutions to the likelihood equations are not possible, but iterative solutions are straightfoward.

During the planning stages of the present study, and prior to data collection, a simulation study investigated various sampling schemes (Kemmerlin, 1986; Kemmerlin and Jackson, 1987). Sample sizes of 1000 individuals in the total screening population and 190 in the second-stage sample were specified a priori to reflect limited resources and the relative costs of screening and diagnostic evaluation. The expected prevalence was chosen as 0.05, and the mean and variance for each group were identified from previous studies (Garrison et al., 1989). Results assuming equal variance in the two groups are presented here. Four study designs were chosen to represent a wide range of possibilities:

Design A is a random sample of size 190.

Design B selects for diagnostic interview those individuals with the top 100 scores and a random sample of size 90 of the remaining scores.

Design C includes only those individuals with the top 190 screening scores.

Design D selects the individuals with the top 50 scores, a random sample of size 50 of the next 100, and a second random sample of size 90 of the remaining.

Although these designs are not optimal according to Shrout and Newman (1989), they are consistent with the multiple goals of the study and practical details of administration. The cost of screening all students rather than a random sample is minimal relative to the administrative cost of selecting a sample. For design A, standard binomial models can be used to estimate prevalence. For design C, the maximum likelihood techniques described previously can be applied. For designs B and D, modifications are needed to account for the fact that the second-stage samples include two (design B) or three (design D) different strata.

3.2 Weighted Prevalence Estimates and Confidence Intervals

Prevalence can be estimated using a weighted average of the stratum-specific prevalences. Symbolically, the weighted prevalence is

$$\hat{p} = \sum_{i=1}^{L} w_i \hat{p}_i, \tag{1}$$

where $\hat{p}_i$ is the stratum-specific prevalence, w_i the weight assigned to the ith stratum, and L the number of strata; the weights are defined to sum to 1.

Numerous possible methods used to construct the overall confidence interval were investigated using simulation procedures; three with stronger theoretical justification and better performance are presented here: (1) combining stratum-specific binomial variances, (2) combining stratum-specific confidence intervals based on the F-distribution (F) approximation to the cumulative binomial, and (3) combining the binomial variance method and the F-distribution method when a zero prevalence occurs in any stratum. These methods are evaluated in terms of coverage probability and bias.

The simplest method of confidence interval estimation involves combining stratum-specific binomial variances for proportions. A weighted average of the stratum-specific variances is calculated and used with the overall weighted prevalence estimate $\hat{p}$ to find an overall confidence interval

$$\hat{p} \pm z_{1-\alpha/2} \left[\sum_{i=1}^{L} \frac{w_i^2 \hat{p}_i(1 - \hat{p}_i)}{n_i} \right]^{1/2}.$$

The weights are comparable to the proportions screening positive or negative (Shrout and Newman, 1989); however, since the entire population is screened, the weights are regarded as being constant.

If the event is rare, the normal distribution might be an inadequate approximation of the skewed binomial distribution; the lower limit of the confidence interval could be negative. If the estimated prevalence within a particular stratum is zero, the variance is incorrectly estimated to be zero.

Using the F approximation to the cumulative binomial (Fisher and Yates, 1963; Brownlee, 1965; Bliss, 1967), the confidence limits are found by using a weighted average of the stratum-specific confidence limits. Lower and upper confidence limits are, respectively,

$$\sum_{i=1}^{L} \frac{w_i y_i}{y_i + (n_i - y_i + 1)F_{1-\alpha/2}[2(n_i - y_i + 1), 2y_i]}$$

and

$$\sum_{i=1}^{L} \frac{w_i(y_i + 1)F_{1-\alpha/2}[2(y_i + 1), 2(n_i - y_i)]}{(n_i - y_i) + (y_i + 1)F_{1-\alpha/2}[2(y_i + 1), 2(n_i - y_i)]},$$

where y_i is the number of events and n_i is the sample size in the ith stratum. The F method estimates a nonzero upper limit when a zero prevalence occurs in any stratum and gives an asymmetric confidence interval. However, in contrast to using a summary variance estimate, any method combining stratum-specific confidence intervals is inherently conservative.

To overcome the problem of zero prevalences in some strata, a hybrid method of confidence interval estimation combines the F and binomial variance methods. For strata which do not have a zero prevalence, an interval is constructed by combining the stratum-specific binomial variances. In strata with zero prevalence, confidence intervals are constructed by combining the stratum-specific confidence intervals based on F. The overall confidence interval is found by combining these confidence intervals with the appropriate weights. For example, using three strata with stratum three having a zero prevalence, the overall lower confidence limit is

$$(w_1 + w_2)\left[\frac{(w_1\hat{p}_1 + w_2\hat{p}_2)}{w_1 + w_2}\right.$$

$$\left. - z_{1-\alpha/2}\left(\frac{1}{(w_1 + w_2)^2}\sum_{i=1}^{2}\frac{w_i^2\hat{p}_i(1 - \hat{p}_i)}{n_i}\right)^{1/2}\right] + w_3 \cdot 0$$

and the overall upper confidence limit is

$$(w_1 + w_2)\left[\frac{(w_1\hat{p}_1 + w_2\hat{p}_2)}{w_1 + w_2}\right.$$

$$\left. + z_{1-\alpha/2}\left(\frac{1}{(w_1 + w_2)^2}\sum_{i=1}^{2}\frac{w_i^2\hat{p}_i(1 - \hat{p}_i)}{n_i}\right)^{1/2}\right]$$

$$+ \frac{w_3 F_{1-\alpha/2}[2, 2n_3]}{n_3 + F_{1-\alpha/2}[2, 2n_3]}.$$

The coverage probabilities and bias of the methods are determined using simulation procedures with three strata. Two different first-stage weighting schemes are defined; these parameters are necessary for the estimation of a confidence interval but are not directly used in the simulation. The first weighting scheme uses weights of 0.15, 0.15, and 0.70 in the three strata to represent use of a screening tool in the first stage of sampling. The second weighting scheme uses equal weights of one-third in each stratum to represent sampling by a demographic variable. Data are simulated for four different second-stage situations with two total second-stage sample sizes each (180 and 600, respectively), resulting in eight simulated data sets. Second-stage samples are defined by the cross-classification of two combinations of stratum-specific prevalences and equal or unequal strata. Stratum-specific prevalences are high, 9%; medium, 6%; and low, 3%. In each data set, 2000 replications are made. Methods are compared empirically with the adolescent depression data.

3.3 Stratified Estimates of Sensitivity and Specificity

Psychometric properties of the CES-D have been well established for adult but not young adolescent populations; thus another study goal is to validate the tool for use among adolescents. Evaluation of a screening tool's ability to identify individuals with a particular disorder requires estimation of sensitivity and specificity. An empirical receiver operating characteristic curve summarizes the sensitivity and specificity of the screening tool across the range of possible values.

The sensitivity of a screening tool is

$$\Pr(\text{high screen}|\text{disorder}) = \frac{\Pr(\text{high screen, disorder})}{\Pr(\text{disorder})}.$$

To allow for different strata, sensitivity can be calculated as

$$\text{sensitivity} = \frac{\sum_{i=1}^{L}\Pr(i)\Pr(\text{high screen, disorder}|i)}{\sum_{i=1}^{L}\Pr(i)\Pr(\text{disorder}|i)}.$$

This expression still does not use all of the information available: screening data are available on a much larger sample than the second-stage sample. A more efficient estimate of the sensitivity would use these data, decomposing the probabilities above into high-screen and low-screen prevalences as

$$\Pr(\text{disorder}) = \Pr(\text{disorder}|\text{high screen})\Pr(\text{high screen})$$
$$+ \Pr(\text{disorder}|\text{low screen})\Pr(\text{low screen}).$$

The stratum-specific probabilities of disorder must still be weighted by the first-stage proportions, with the probability of high or low screen estimated from the complete first-stage data. Thus, the weighted averages of stratum-specific prevalences among high- and low-screen individuals are

$$\Pr(\text{disorder}|\text{high screen})$$

$$= \sum_{i=1}^{L} \Pr(i|\text{high screen}) \, \Pr(\text{disorder}|i, \text{high screen})$$

and

$$\Pr(\text{disorder}|\text{low screen})$$

$$= \sum_{i=1}^{L} \Pr(i|\text{low screen}) \, \Pr(\text{disorder}|i, \text{low screen}).$$

The estimate for $\Pr(\text{high screen, disorder})$ is modified similarly:

$$\Pr(\text{high screen, disorder}) = \Pr(\text{disorder}|\text{high screen}) \, \Pr(\text{high screen}),$$

where the conditional weighted prevalence is as defined previously and $\Pr(\text{high screen})$ is estimated from the complete screening data.

The specificity is calculated in a similar manner:

$$\Pr(\text{low screen}|\text{no disorder}) = \frac{\Pr(\text{low screen, no disorder})}{\Pr(\text{no disorder})}.$$

Application of this estimation procedure requires six frequencies for each stratum. Four of these are based on second-stage data: numbers of high-screen individuals with and without disorder and numbers of low-screen individuals with and without the disorder. The remaining two frequencies, numbers of high- and low-screen individuals, are based on first-stage data.

A receiver-operating characteristic (ROC) curve can be constructed from the sensitivity and specificity at values of the CES-D from 0 to 60. The ROC curve is a plot of the sensitivity against false positive rate (or 1-specificity) and demonstrates visually how the CES-D discriminates between depressed and nondepressed adolescents. The area under the ROC curve can be interpreted as the probability that from one depressed and one nondepressed individual, the depressed individual can be identified; the area under the diagonal corresponds to the probability of agreement being no better than a coin toss.

3.4 Logistic Regression Analysis

A final goal is to explore the relationship between major depression and risk factors. Epidemiologic studies are inconsistent in the use of design features. Some literature suggests that ignoring design effects is appropriate, especially if factors involved in the design are used as covariables in the analysis (Korn and Graubard, 1991). However, other studies find that ignoring design effects can cause substantial changes in the estimated covariate effects and inferences, especially when the variables related to the sampling are correlated with the outcome (Chambless and Boyle, 1985).

Logistic regression procedures or similar categorical procedures are appropriate here since the outcome is dichotomous and predictors are both continuous and categorical. Three logistic regression methods are considered: (1) analyzing unweighted data, effectively ignoring the sampling design; (2) analyzing unweighted data adjusting for design variables; and (3) using a logistic regression method and accompanying software that estimates correctly using survey data coefficients and variances. The first two methods have the advantage of working with existing logistic regression software: automated stepwise model selection procedures and general likelihood ratio tests are available. Method 1, however, ignores the study design. Method 2 has some major strengths for the analysis and should give appropriate estimates under certain conditions. Method 2 allows estimation of the relationship between a variable and the outcome within each stratum and then combines these stratum-specific estimates to obtain an overall estimate. If the effect of this variable is the same across strata, a point estimate from an analysis that adjusts for stratum effects should be unbiased. However, there may be interactions between variables defining the strata and variables of interest, which if not included in the model could result in inappropriate individual point estimates. Since the second-stage sample does not represent the original population, parameter estimates ignoring interactions do not represent an average population effect. However, including interactions of design and other variables of interest is not a solution, as interpreting the individual parameters becomes difficult and parameter estimates may be unstable even in a relatively simple model.

The third method, although more difficult to implement, has the advantage of truly incorporating the sample design into the analysis. If G_i is the dependent variable, g_i its observed value, and $\mathbf{x}_i$ is a vector of independent variables, the weighted likelihood equations are

$$\sum_{i \in S} w_i^* \mathbf{x}_i^\mathrm{T} p_i(\hat{\boldsymbol{\beta}}) = \sum_{i \in S} w_i^* \mathbf{x}_i^\mathrm{T} g_i,$$

where $w_i^* = N_i/w_i$ is the sampling weight applied to each subject and

$$p_i(\hat{\boldsymbol{\beta}}) = \Pr[g_i = 1 | \mathbf{x}, \hat{\boldsymbol{\beta}}] = [1 + \exp(-\mathbf{x}_i\hat{\boldsymbol{\beta}})]^{-1}.$$

The Newton–Raphson recursion formula for the parameters is

$$\hat{\boldsymbol{\beta}}_k = \hat{\boldsymbol{\beta}}_{k-1} + \left(\sum_{i \in S} w_i^* \mathbf{x}_i^T \mathbf{x}_i \hat{d}_{i,k-1} \right)^{-1} \left[\sum_{i \in S} w_i^* \mathbf{x}_i^T (g_i - \hat{p}_{i,k-1}) \right]$$

where

$$\hat{p}_{i,k-1} = p_i(\hat{\boldsymbol{\beta}}_{k-1})$$

and

$$\hat{d}_{i,k-1} = \hat{p}_{i,k-1}(1 - \hat{p}_{i,k-1}).$$

The weighted covariance matrix is calculated using linearized variable vectors based on a Taylor expansion. These covariances are used to construct Wald tests of hypotheses about the parameters.

4 RESULTS

4.1 Selection of Study Design

Table 2 shows the results of the simulation procedure to evaluate possible study designs. These results indicate that the stratified designs (designs B and D) are substantially better than the other designs and that the nonparametric estimates have reasonable efficiencies. Design B, which selects the highest 100 scores and a random sample of the remaining 90, was selected for three reasons: (1) there were reservations about the assumption of normality necessary for the

Table 2 Relative Efficiencies of the Maximum Likelihood Estimates and Nonparametric Estimates of the Prevalence of Major Depression and Expected Numbers of Cases Detected for Different Sampling Designs

	Relative Efficiency		
Sampling Design	Maximum Likelihood	Nonparametric	Expected Number of Cases
A: Simple random sample	0.76	0.49	9.5
B: Top 100 + random 90	0.90	0.71	26.9
C: Top 190	0.89	0.15[a]	32.8
D: Top 50 + 50 of next 100 + random 90	1.00	0.66	24.9

[a]Point estimate is biased since no sample taken from lower stratum.

MLE procedures; (2) design C (selecting the top 190 scores) would not allow nonparametric estimation of the prevalence; and, (3) design B yielded more cases and the best relative efficiency. The similarity of the two stratified designs suggests that this general strategy may be robust to minor modifications in the sampling plan. In practice, the high-risk group was selected using the CES-D profile, including the top decile of total scores and other high-risk individuals.

The utility of this two-stage sampling procedure is seen by comparing the actual number of cases detected to the corresponding prevalence and confidence interval to those expected from a random sample. The observed weighted prevalence was 8.79%, with 95% confidence limits (5.82, 11.75), based on 73 cases among 459 individuals interviewed. Using this observed prevalence under simple random sampling assumptions yields only 40 expected cases with a 95% confidence interval of (6.20, 11.37). Although some precision is lost in estimating the prevalence with the stratified design, almost twice as many cases are detected. This finding demonstrates the importance of investigating the procedure in view of research goals before implementation of the design.

4.2   Comparison of Weighted Prevalences and Confidence Intervals

Simulation results for the two second-stage sample sizes are similar. Results for the smaller sample size of 180 and a confidence level of 95% are presented in Table 3. Coverage probabilities are influenced by prevalence for all methods. The method that performs best is the one that combines the binomial variance and the F methods when a zero prevalence occurs in any stratum. The resulting coverage probability does not attain the nominal confidence level in general, yet is closest. Combining stratum-specific binomial variances gives coverage probabilities that are too low, while the coverage probabilities using the F method are very conservative.

The bias for each method is examined by comparing the confidence limits to the true prevalence. True prevalence is known from first-stage weights and specified stratum-specific prevalences. When the upper, right-hand endpoint of the confidence interval is less than the true prevalence, the method is said herein to be biased downward. When the lower, left-hand endpoint of the confidence interval is greater than the true prevalence, the method is said herein to be biased upward. Table 3 shows that confidence intervals using the binomial variance, regardless of use of F for any zero stratum-specific prevalence, are more likely to be biased downward. Confidence intervals found when combining the stratum-specific confidence intervals based on F alone are more likely to be biased upward.

Each method of interval estimation was used to construct a 95% confidence interval for the prevalence of major depression among adolescents. Intermedi-

Table 3   Coverage Probabilities and Bias for the Three Methods of Confidence Interval Estimation Using a Confidence Level of 95%, $N = 180$

	Second-Stage Proportions			
	$\frac{1}{3}, \frac{1}{3}, \frac{1}{3}$		$\frac{1}{2}, \frac{1}{6}, \frac{1}{3}$	
	Second Stage Prevalences			
Method	H, L, M	H, L, L	H, L, M	H, L, L
	Unequal First-Stage Weights			
Combining stratum-specific				
	$100 \times$ coverage probability			
(a) Binomial	89.0	85.1	90.7	86.1
(b) F	99.4	100.0	99.5	99.7
(a) and (b) combined	90.9	96.7	94.8	92.5
	$100 \times$ probability of underestimation			
(a) Binomial	10.1	14.4	8.7	13.2
(b) F	0.0	0.0	0.0	0.0
(a) and (b) combined	8.2	2.8	4.6	6.8
	$100 \times$ probability of overestimation			
(a) Binomial	0.9	0.5	0.6	0.7
(b) F	0.6	0.0	0.5	0.3
(a) and (b) combined	0.9	0.5	0.6	0.7
	Equal First-Stage Weights			
Combining stratum-specific				
	$100 \times$ coverage probability			
(a) Binomial	90.3	93.7	92.7	90.7
(b) F	100.0	100.0	100.0	99.9
(a) and (b) combined	93.3	95.0	97.9	92.5
	$100 \times$ probability of underestimation			
(a) Binomial	8.5	5.7	6.5	8.7
(b) F	0.0	0.0	0.0	0.0
(a) and (b) combined	5.5	4.4	1.3	6.8
	$100 \times$ probability of overestimation			
(a) Binomial	1.2	0.6	0.8	0.6
(b) F	0.0	0.0	0.0	0.1
(a) and (b) combined	1.2	0.6	0.8	0.7

Table 4   Weighted Prevalence of Major Depression and Corresponding Confidence Intervals for Females

	High-Risk	Low-Risk Black	Low-Risk White
Screening sample	264	234	1119
Clinical sample	145	37	78
Depression diagnosis	47	0	4
First-stage weight	0.1633	0.1447	0.6920
Prevalence	0.3241	0.0000	0.0513
Variance $\times 10^4$	15.1085	0.0000	6.2375
F lower limit	0.2488	0.0000	0.0141
F upper limit	0.4068	0.0949	0.1261

ate calculations are presented in Table 4 for estimation among female students. First-stage weights are simple proportions [e.g., $0.1633 = 264/(264 + 234 + 1119)$], and prevalences are weighted averages as in (1), and so on. Resulting confidence intervals for the estimated prevalences (expressed as percents) are given in Table 5. The methods of combining the binomial variances, regardless of use of the F-distribution for any zero stratum-specific prevalence, yield the narrowest confidence intervals. The F method tends to have the widest confidence intervals, consistent with being the most conservative method. Also shown in Table 5 are the unweighted prevalences and confidence intervals; as expected given the sampling design, these rates are noticeably higher.

Table 5   95% Confidence Intervals for the Prevalence of Major Depression by Gender

	Gender	
	Males	Females
Weighted prevalence (%)	8.71	8.84
Confidence interval method		
(a) Binomial	(4.01, 13.41)	(5.23, 12.45)
(b) F	(3.55, 17.75)	(5.04, 16.74)
(a) and (b) combined	(4.01, 13.41)	(5.23, 13.82)
Unweighted prevalence (%)	11.06	19.62
Confidence interval method		
Binomial	(6.70, 15.41)	(14.79, 24.44)
F	(7.06, 16.26)	(14.97, 24.97)

**Table 6   Frequencies for Calculating Sensitivity and Specificity of
CES-D for Major Depression among Females at a Cutpoint of 16**

	High-Risk	Low-Risk Black	Low-Risk White
High-screen (CES-D ≥ 16)			
Screening	262	119	428
Clinical sample			
Major depression	47	0	3
No major depression	96	15	27
Low-screen (CES-D < 16)			
Screening	2	115	691
Clinical sample			
Major depression	0	0	1
No major depression	2	22	47

4.3   Validity of CES-D for Adolescent Depression

A primary reason for collecting extensive screening data was to establish the
validity of the CES-D in community adolescent populations. When used as a
screening tool for depression among adults, a CES-D cutpoint of 16 is chosen. Table 6 presents frequencies from which sensitivity and specificity at this
cutpoint can be calculated among females. These result in sensitivity and specificity of 0.90 and 0.54, respectively. The sensitivity and specificity at various
values of the CES-D are shown in Table 7. From these data, optimal cutpoints
of 14 for males and 20 for females result in sensitivity and specificity 0.81 and
0.59 for males and 0.90 and 0.71 for females, respectively.

**Table 7   Sensitivity and Specificity of CES-D for Major
Depression at Selected Cutpoints by Gender**

	Gender			
	Male		Female	
Cutpoint	Sensitivity	Specificity	Sensitivity	Specificity
≥10	0.90	0.38	0.90	0.28
≥12	0.90	0.49	0.90	0.38
≥14	0.81	0.59	0.89	0.46
≥16	0.70	0.67	0.90	0.54
≥18	0.30	0.72	0.90	0.63
≥20	0.24	0.78	0.90	0.71
≥30	0.12	0.94	0.56	0.91

From sensitivity and specificity at CES-D scores from 0 to 60, the ROC curves for males and females are constructed (see Figure 1). These graphs suggest that the CES-D is a better screen for females. The estimated areas under the curve based on stratified estimates are 0.66 for males and 0.81 for females. The ROC curves based on unweighted estimates (not shown) are visibly but not practically different from the stratified estimates.

4.4   Risk Factor Analysis in a Two-Stage Design

The effect of incorporating the sampling procedure into the actual estimation is evident when comparing the three methods for analysis of the same predictor variables. These predictor variables are race, gender, guardian status, and family cohesion. Table 8 shows the distribution of these variables by stratum membership. The stratification is most strongly related to race and CES-D; gender and guardian status also show noticeable differences across strata.

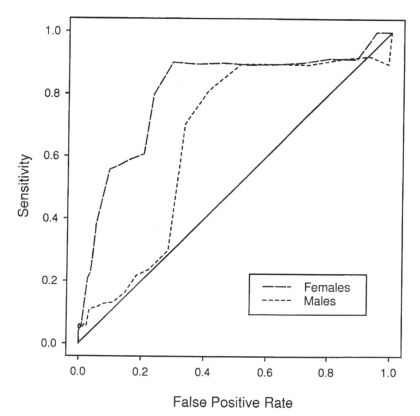

Figure 1. ROC curves of CES-D for major depression by gender.

Table 8 Description of Predictor Variables by Selection Stratum

	Stratum		
	High-Screen	Low-Screen Black	Low-Screen White
	N %	*N %*	*N %*
Race			
White	188 83	—	163 100
Black	39 17	69 100	—
Gender			
Male	82 36	32 46	85 52
Female	145 64	37 54	78 48
Guardian status			
Lives with both parents	102 45	26 37	98 60
Other	125 55	43 63	65 40
Cohesion score			
Mean (sd)	46.19 (12.99)	54.94 (13.08)	58.29 (11.29)
CES-D score			
Mean (sd)	33.13 (7.29)	14.33 (6.35)	12.19 (6.60)

Table 9 gives estimated odds ratios and corresponding confidence intervals for each of three different logistic regression models, with depression as the dependent variable. All three models used all of the covariates shown, yet in the different ways as indicated in the columns of Table 9. There are marked differences in the odds ratios for guardian status, race, and gender, while the

Table 9 Comparison of Odds Ratios and 95% Confidence Intervals for Three Methods of Logistic Regression Analysis of a Two-Stage Sample

	Analytic Approach		
	Unweighted	Unweighted with Strata Indicators	Weighted for Design Effects
Race	0.77	1.71	0.50
	(0.40, 1.48)	(0.77, 3.82)	(0.23, 1.07)
Gender	1.90	1.71	1.05
	(1.09, 3.32)	(0.96, 3.04)	(0.52, 2.13)
Cohesion score	0.96	0.97	0.94
	(0.94, 0.98)	(0.95, 0.99)	(0.91, 0.98)
Guardian status	2.06	2.12	3.22
	(1.18, 3.59)	(1.20, 3.74)	(1.53, 6.79)

odds ratio for cohesion changes less noticeably. The association of depression and race changes direction when strata indicators are used. The gender effect becomes weaker and insignificant when the design is incorporated by either strata indicators or weighted analysis. However, this may reflect differential response rates by males and females in the clinical evaluation. The effect of guardian status becomes much stronger when the design effects are used correctly. Results from other models (not shown) constructed to clarify the effect of the sampling design suggest that using race and a dichotomized CES-D indicator, rather than explicit stratum indicators, results in noticeably weaker associations for all variables. Also, models incorporating interactions between the stratum indicators and other predictor variables give evidence of effect homogeneity across the strata; however, this homogeneity does not imply that the second-stage sample represents the original population.

5   CONCLUSIONS

In the design of an epidemiologic study, competing goals of research interest and limited resources must be balanced. Alternatives to simple random sampling may achieve that balance. In this chapter we have presented a strategy to identify efficient sampling designs for planned analyses and suggest that analyses must appropriately account for design effects.

One simple analysis is prevalence estimation. Based on simulation studies, the recommended method of confidence interval estimation is a hybrid combination of binomial variance and F methods when a zero prevalence occurs. Although somewhat biased, as indeed were all methods considered here, this method gives better coverage probabilities, accounts for zero stratum-specific prevalences, and can yield asymmetric confidence intervals. This method gives relatively narrow confidence intervals for the prevalence of depression among adolescents. Comparison of unweighted and weighted prevalence estimates illustrates that the inclusion of design effects in this analysis is necessary.

Estimates of sensitivity and specificity are least influenced by the study design. One caveat of the estimation procedure that combines screening and clinical data is that the estimated ROC curve can show slight departures from monotonicity. This departure is negligible and occurs at extreme values of the screening tool, where the estimates are less stable and less informative.

Comparison of different estimation procedures for logistic regression shows the importance of including design effects. Researchers often ignore design effects at this level of analysis, due to the complexity of multivariable analysis incorporating the sampling design and the lesser availability of appropriate computer software. However, our results show that when the design variable is related to both the outcome and predictor variables under investigation in the study, incorporating the design can have a major impact on both estimation and statistical inferences. In many stratified study designs, the associations of the predictor variables with the stratification may be much weaker, and the unweighted analyses may give results more consistent with results incorporating design effects.

The techniques presented in this chapter are easily implemented with existing software or simple programming and thus are available to any researcher. Comparison of results with and without design effects suggests that improperly ignoring the design can lead to biased and misleading interpretations. Given the widespread availability of computer equipment, software, and expertise, the increased complexity of analyses should not be a deterrent to their proper execution.

SOFTWARE NOTES AND REFERENCES

The third logistic regression method is based on the LOGIST and RTILOGIT procedures in SAS. The LOGIST procedure estimates regression coefficients correctly by incorporating user-specified weights. The RTILOGIT procedure then computes the correct variance and covariances based on the sampling design. The theory is based on a Taylor series for estimating variances of nonlinear functions as described in Binder (1981). This procedure allows incorporation of very complicated multistage cluster designs into an analysis. As of this writing, RTILOGIT has been replaced by a procedure LOGISTIC within the general program SUDAAN, also available from the Research Triangle Institute. This program runs independently of SAS or can be called by SAS.

Harrell, F. E. (1983). *SUGI: Supplemental Library User's Guide*, Cary, N.C.: SAS Institute, pp. 181–202.

Shah, B. V., Folsom, R. E., Harrell, F. E., and Dillard, C. N. (1984). *Survey Data Analysis Software for Logistic Regression*. Research Triangle Park, N.C.: Research Triangle Institute.

QUESTIONS AND PROBLEMS

1. Propose at least one additional study design applicable for a community-based study of a condition such as depression, with the objectives of estimating prevalence and identifying risk factors of the condition. Discuss how this design might be evaluated by stating any necessary assumptions and presenting a strategy for a simulation study. What are potential limitations and biases of this design?

2. Using all males in the adolescent depression data, verify the confidence intervals calculated by each of the three proposed methods. What other methods can you propose for construction of a confidence interval for a weighted proportion?

3. Calculate unweighted sensitivity and specificity of the CES-D for major depression. What might account for the similarity of the weighted and unweighted estimates, in contrast to the differences noted for all other analyses? What considerations other than the actual sensitivity and specificity might be involved in identifying an appropriate cutpoint for the CES-D as a screening tool for depression?

4. Discuss issues related to the incorporation of study design effects in a statistical analysis. Are there circumstances in which the design effects can be ignored? Are there circumstances in which the design effects should be used in analysis? If analyses with and without design effects differ, how might the more correct analysis be identified? What are simple ways to incorporate design effects in a multivariable analysis, in contrast to the more complex weighted logistic analysis?

CHAPTER 21

Drug Interactions between Morphine and Marijuana

Chris Gennings, W. Hans Carter, Jr., and Billy R. Martin

1 MOTIVATION AND BACKGROUND

The use of combination drug therapy in the treatment of disease is increasing. Since most therapeutic drugs can be toxic at high doses, it is often advantageous to use a combination therapy. Doses of each of the two or more drugs given in combination may be lower than when given alone, yet the therapeutic response is the same. The ideal combination is one in which the drugs have a synergistic effect on the therapeutic response but an antagonistic effect on any toxic response.

The combination of two classes of compounds, opioids and cannabinoids, are of particular interest in the context of clinical pain management. An example of an opioid is morphine; an example of a cannabinoid is Δ^9-tetrahydrocannabinol (Δ^9-THC) which is the active ingredient in marijuana. Both of these compounds are analgesic (i.e., provide pain relief), but they are also associated with adverse side effects. Morphine is known to produce dependencies and respiratory depression, while Δ^9-THC is known to produce adverse behavioral side effects such as increased psychological activity (Noyes et al., 1975). The motivation behind using these two drugs in combination is that although they both produce analgesia, their associated side effects are different. Therefore, it is of interest to determine if combination doses exist that are associated with desired levels of pain relief without the associated side effects of each component.

The data considered in this chapter are from a mouse study where the primary endpoint was analgesia and the side-effect endpoints were chosen to address the behavioral effect of Δ^9-THC. In this study, the combination of morphine and marijuana produced an analgesic effect at lower doses than when either drug was used alone. In addition, these compounds in combination antagonized the

Case Studies in Biometry, Edited by Nicholas Lange, Louise Ryan, Lynne Billard,
David Brillinger, Loveday Conquest, and Joel Greenhouse.
ISBN 0-471-58885-7 © 1994 John Wiley & Sons, Inc.

associated toxic responses of hyperactivity and hypothermia (i.e., larger doses of either drug are required to surpass a safe level of the detrimental responses than when the drugs combine additively). Such a combination is said to have a wide "window of safety" since the doses that yield the desired therapeutic response are given at a reduced risk of toxic side effects. Therefore, by characterizing the interaction of a combination of drugs/compounds in terms of therapeutic and toxic responses, it is possible for investigators to choose treatment combinations with a wide window of safety.

Isobolograms have been used widely to detect graphically and to characterize the interactions among two jointly administered drugs or chemicals (Fraser, 1872; Loewe, 1957; Berenbaum, 1981; Wessinger, 1986). An isobologram is presented in Figure 1 for two hypothetical drugs, $drug_1$ and $drug_2$. The method involves comparing the isobol (i.e., the contour of constant response) to the "line of additivity" (i.e., the line connecting the single drug doses that yield the level of response associated with the contour). The interaction is described as synergistic, additive, or antagonistic according to whether the contour is below, coincident with, or above the line of additivity, respectively (see Loewe, 1957; Berenbaum, 1981). Berenbaum (1981) detected departure from additivity by use of an interaction index I that can be expressed as

$$I = \frac{x_1}{X_{1E}} + \frac{x_2}{X_{2E}},$$

where x_1 and x_2 are the doses in combination associated with a given level of

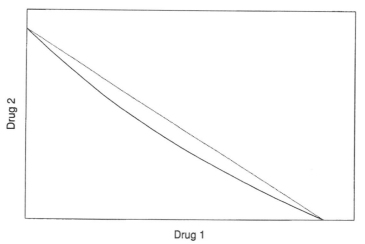

Figure 1. Example of an isobologram. The dashed line is the theoretical line of additivity (i.e., the contour of constant response under the hypothesis of additivity). The solid curve is the observed isobol (contour of constant response). Since the isobol bows below the line of additivity, a synergism is suggested between $drug_1$ and $drug_2$.

effect E, and X_{1E} and X_{2E} are the doses of the individual drugs that produce the same level of effect E. When the interaction index I is less than 1, the drugs are said to interact synergistically; when it is greater than 1, the drugs are said to interact antagonistically; and when it is equal to 1, the drugs are said to interact additively.

Both graphical and algebraic comparisons as described by Berenbaum (1981) fail to take into account the variability of the data. Carter et al. (1988) related the interaction index to the interaction parameter(s) of a statistical model. For example, consider the dose–response relationship of a combination of two drugs, $drug_1$ and $drug_2$, modeled as

$$E(Y) = \beta_0 + \beta_1 x_1 + \beta_2 x_2 + \beta_{12} x_1 x_2,$$

where x_1 is the dose of $drug_1$, x_2 the dose of $drug_2$, and $\beta_0, \beta_1, \beta_2$, and β_{12} are unknown regression coefficients. The dose of $drug_1$ alone that yields a specified response y_E is $X_{1E} = (y_E - \beta_0)/\beta_1$, and similarly for $drug_2$, $X_{2E} = (y_E - \beta_0)/\beta_2$. The equation of the contour of constant response (isobol), $y_E = \beta_0 + \beta_1 x_1 + \beta_2 x_2 + \beta_{12} x_1 x_2$, can be algebraically manipulated to the form

$$\frac{x_1}{(y_E - \beta_0)/\beta_1} + \frac{x_2}{(y_E - \beta_0)/\beta_2} = 1 - \frac{\beta_{12} x_1 x_2}{y_E - \beta_0},$$

such that the left-hand side is equivalent to Berenbaum's interaction index I. For increasing dose–response curves, the denominator on the right-hand side is positive since the response of interest y_E is greater than the background response β_0. If β_{12} is greater than zero, $I < 1$, indicating a synergistic relationship between the drugs; if β_{12} is less than zero, $I > 1$, indicating an antagonistic relationship between the drugs; and if β_{12} is not different from zero, $I = 1$, indicating that the drugs combine additively. The significance of β_{12} and its algebraic sign is thus indicative of the interaction between the drugs. Gennings et al. (1990) developed a graphical procedure for characterizing drug interaction, which allows the level of statistical significance to be determined for the interaction. Those authors construct a simultaneous confidence band about the isobol (contour of constant response). If the line of additivity falls outside this confidence band, departure from additivity is concluded.

An implicit assumption in both the construction of isobolograms and the interaction index is that the compounds in the combination have similar pharmacological profiles (i.e., they each are capable of producing the effect of interest either alone or are potentiators/antagonists to other compounds in the combination for producing the effect). The interaction of combinations that include compounds which have "opposite" effects on a response (e.g., one compound causes hypothermia and another causes hyperthermia), cannot be described adequately by isobolograms or the interaction index.

One way of describing the interaction between a pair of dissimilar compounds is through comparison of the slopes of the dose–response curves when the compounds are given alone to that when given in combination (see Figure 2). If the dose–response curve for $drug_1$ shifts to require either more or less of $drug_1$ in the presence of $drug_2$ to achieve the same response, but the slope remains the same (Figure 2a), it can be concluded that the combination is only additive. In other words, $drug_2$ in combination with $drug_1$ acts only like

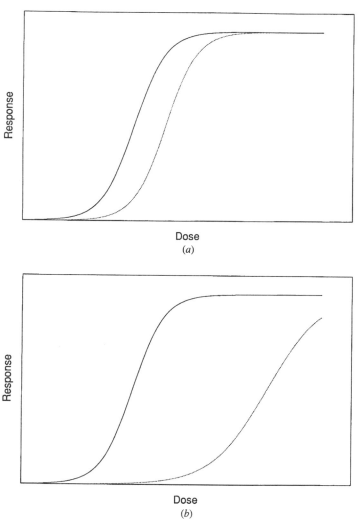

Figure 2. Example of dose–response curves in the absence (a) and presence (b) of interaction. When the dose–response curves of $drug_1$ alone (A: solid curve) and at a fixed dose of $drug_2$ (A: dashed curve) are parallel, $drug_2$ acts as a dilution of $drug_1$ indicating no interaction. If the presence of $drug_2$ (B: dashed curve) changes the slope of the dose–response curve of $drug_1$ alone (B: solid curve), an interaction is suggested.

a dilution of *drug*₁ in producing a parallel dose–response curve to that with *drug*₁ alone. On the other hand, if the slope of the dose–response curve for *drug*₁ changes in the presence of *drug*₂ (Figure 2*b*), the pair is said to interact. Statisticians use this definition for interaction in statistical models where both linear and cross-product terms are included in the model. If the cross-product term(s) is (are) significant, the combination is said to interact.

Many pharmacologists believe that the characterization of a drug interaction with respect to a response of interest may depend on the dose region (i.e. a combination may be synergistic in one region and antagonistic in another). Therefore, Carter et al. (1988) suggested fitting a model with higher-order interaction terms which can be used to describe the dose-related characterization of the interaction. The analysis presented here follows the graphical approach of Gennings et al. (1990) and uses statistical models with higher-order interaction terms. The characterization of the interaction is thus allowed to be dose related. A simultaneous test on the significance of all cross-product terms is a test for departure from additivity. If the hypothesis of no interaction is rejected, the characterization of the interaction is given using a graphical approach. A $100(1 - \alpha)\%$ simultaneous confidence band about the response surface is compared to a restricted response surface under the hypothesis of additivity. Dose combinations where the former is above (or below) the surface of additivity are concluded to be synergistic (or antagonistic). Such three-dimensional representations of departure from additivity are analogous to the work of Prichard and Shipman (1990) except that these authors compared observed responses to fitted surfaces of additivity which may possibly attribute random variation to drug interaction.

2 DATA

Studies were conducted in male mice to determine whether combinations of Δ^9-THC and morphine sulfate would produce additive, synergistic, or antagonistic antinociceptive (analgesic) effects with acceptable concomitant side effects, specifically hyperactivity as measured by spontaneous activity, and hypothermia as measured by rectal temperature (see Table 1). A stock solution of Δ^9-THC was prepared by dissolving 100 mg of the drug in 1 mL of a 1 : 1 mixture of emulphor, and appropriate dilutions were made with a solution containing emulphor/ethanol/saline (1 : 1 : 18). Morphine was dissolved in saline. Immediately before each experiment, equal volumes of the appropriate concentration of each drug were combined so that the drug combinations could be administered as a single injection.

For the spontaneous activity and rectal temperature responses, 35 groups of mice (six animals per group) from a 5×7 factorial experiment were randomly assigned to receive a single injection of one of the possible combinations of morphine sulfate (0, 2, 4, 6, 8 mg/kg) and Δ^9-THC (0, 0.5, 1.0, 2.5, 5.0, 10.0, 15.0 mg/kg). A second replication of the experiment was performed. For

Table 1   Sample of the Data

Data for Side-Effect Endpoints

Observation	Morphine (x_1)	Δ^9-THC (x_2)	Replication	Spontaneous Activity	Baseline Rectal Temp.	60-Minute Rectal Temp.
1	0	0.0	1	147	38.0	38.5
2	0	0.0	1	92	39.0	38.0
3	0	0.0	1	95	38.0	38.0
4	0	0.0	1	11	38.0	39.0
11	0	0.0	2	47	38.5	36.5
12	0	0.0	2	55	38.0	37.5
⋮	⋮	⋮	⋮	⋮	⋮	⋮
405	8	15	1	0	36.5	35.0
413	8	15	2	0	38.5	35.0
414	8	15	2	42	39.0	34.0
415	8	15	2	15	38.0	34.0
416	8	15	2	11	38.5	35.0

Data for Tail-Flick Latency

Observation	Replication	Morphine (x_1)	Δ^9-THC (x_2)	Control Flick Time	Test Flick Time
1	1	0.0	0.0	2.2	3.8
2	1	0.0	0.0	3.6	2.9
3	1	0.0	0.0	3.7	2.7
16	1	1.0	0.0	2.0	3.6
17	1	1.0	0.0	3.1	5.6
18	1	1.0	0.0	2.7	2.7
⋮	⋮	⋮	⋮	⋮	⋮
499	3	6	15	2.1	10.0
500	3	6	15	3.7	10.0
501	3	6	15	2.8	10.0
502	3	6	15	2.9	10.0
509	3	8	15	2.8	10.0
510	3	8	15	3.9	10.0

antinociceptive activity, a 5 × 5 factorial design (Δ^9-THC ranging from 0 to 5 mg/kg; morphine ranging from 0 to 8 mg/kg) and a 5 × 7 factorial design as described above were used.

The antinoceptive response was measured by the tail-flick procedure (Dewey et al., 1970). The assay is essentially a measure of the time required for an animal to flick its tail voluntarily from beneath a heat stimulus. A control reaction time was determined for each mouse, and those which did not flick away from the heat lamp within 2 to 4 seconds were not entered into the study. Following drug administration, the animals were retested and the tail-flick latency of each mouse was recorded. A maximum latency of 10 seconds was imposed to avoid tail damage. For the side-effect response studies, 5 minutes after receiving an intravenous injection of the drugs, the mice were placed individually into clear plastic rectangular cages (20 × 33 cm), each of which was situated between a single photocell beam and detector. The spontaneous activity response was measured as the number of interruptions of the photocell beams over a 10-minute period of time. The mice were acclimated in the laboratory (ambient temperature 21 to 24°C) overnight. Rectal temperature was recorded just before and again 60-minutes after the injection with a telethermometer and a thermistor probe. Change in rectal temperature was calculated as the 60-minute temperature minus the baseline temperature, thereby making a negative value correspond to a decrease in temperature.

3 METHODS AND MODELS

Two compounds are considered to be additive if the effect of the combination, $f(x_1, x_2)$, is equal to the sum of the effects of the individual compounds, $f_i(x_i), i = 1, 2$ [i.e., $f(x_1, x_2) = f_1(x_1) + f_2(x_2)$]. If the combination yields a response significantly greater than that expected under additivity, the combination is considered to be synergistic [i.e., $f(x_1, x_2) > f_1(x_1) + f_2(x_2)$ for increasing response functions]. If the combination yields a response significantly less than that expected under additivity, the combination is considered to be antagonistic [i.e., $f(x_1, x_2) < f_1(x_1) + f_2(x_2)$ for increasing response functions]. If the response is a decreasing function, the interpretation is reversed. When the response is binary (e.g., tail flick or no tail flick), the proportion p_x of subjects responding to a specified dose combination is modeled, for example, by using a logistic model. For increasing dose–response relationships, two compounds are considered to be additive if

$$\text{logit}(p_x) = \ln \frac{p_x}{1 - p_x} = f_1(x_1) + f_2(x_2).$$

If logit(p_x) is significantly greater than $f_1(x_1) + f_2(x_2)$, synergism is claimed; and if logit(p_x) is significantly less than $f_1(x_1) + f_2(x_2)$, antagonism is claimed (Ashford and Smith, 1964). For decreasing dose–response relationships, the interpretation is switched. A similar interpretation can be applied using a probit transformation.

3.1 Model and Test Statistic

For the data analyses presented in this chapter, a polynomial model is used to represent $f(x)$. For continuous responses assumed to be normally distributed, these polynomial models can be expressed in matrix notation as

$$\mathbf{Y}_{n \times 1} = \mathbf{X}_{n \times p} \boldsymbol{\beta}_{p \times 1} + \boldsymbol{\epsilon}_{n \times 1}$$

$$= [\mathbf{X}_{1_{(n \times q)}} \quad \mathbf{X}_{2_{(n \times p - q)}}] \begin{bmatrix} \boldsymbol{\beta}_{1_{(q \times 1)}} \\ \boldsymbol{\beta}_{2_{(p - q \times 1)}} \end{bmatrix} + \boldsymbol{\epsilon}_{n \times 1}, \tag{1}$$

where $\mathbf{X}_1$ is a matrix of the q cross-product terms; $\mathbf{X}_2$ is a matrix consisting of the $(p - q)$ terms in the additive model; $\boldsymbol{\beta}$ a vector of unknown parameters partitioned into $\boldsymbol{\beta}_1$ and $\boldsymbol{\beta}_2$, with $\boldsymbol{\beta}_1$ being a vector of unknown parameters associated with the cross-product terms and $\boldsymbol{\beta}_2$ a vector of unknown parameters associated with the pure terms; and $\boldsymbol{\epsilon}$ is a vector of unobservable independent normal random error terms with mean $\mathbf{0}$ and variance $\sigma^2 \mathbf{V}$, where $\mathbf{V}$ is assumed to be a known diagonal matrix and σ^2 is an unknown dispersion parameter. If the observations are assumed independent and identically distributed, $\mathbf{V}$ is an $n \times n$ identity matrix. The "full model" consists of cross-product terms (with coefficients in $\boldsymbol{\beta}_1$) and pure terms (with coefficients in $\boldsymbol{\beta}_2$) (i.e., linear terms, quadratic terms, etc.). The pure terms are included to describe adequately the single dose–response curves of each drug when given alone. The cross-product terms are included to allow for changes in the dose–response curve of a single compound as a function of the other compound, hence an interaction.

The motivation of the analysis is to compare the "full model," estimated from the data, to the model under the hypothesis of no interaction, H_0: $\boldsymbol{\beta}_1 = \mathbf{0}$. The null model corresponding to no interaction is

$$\mathbf{Y}_{n \times 1} = \mathbf{X}_{2_{(n \times p - q)}} \boldsymbol{\beta}_{2_{(p - q \times 1)}} + \boldsymbol{\epsilon}_{n \times 1}$$

and will be called the *additive model*. Let $\mathbf{W} = \text{diag}(\mathbf{V}^{-1})$. Then, the conditional weighted least-squares estimate for $\boldsymbol{\beta}$ is

$$\hat{\boldsymbol{\beta}} = (\mathbf{X}^T \mathbf{W} \mathbf{X})^{-1} \mathbf{X}^T \mathbf{W} \mathbf{Y}.$$

The statistic for testing the hypothesis H_0: $\boldsymbol{\beta}_1 = \mathbf{0}$ (e.g., Myers, 1990) is

$$F = \frac{\mathbf{Y}^T[\mathbf{W}\mathbf{X}(\mathbf{X}^T\mathbf{W}\mathbf{X})^{-1}\mathbf{X}^T - \mathbf{X}_2(\mathbf{X}_2^T\mathbf{W}\mathbf{X}_2)^{-1}\mathbf{X}_2^T\mathbf{W}]\mathbf{Y}}{q(\text{MSE})},$$

where $\mathbf{X}_1$ and $\mathbf{X}_2$ are defined in (1) and the mean-squared error is,

$$\text{MSE} = \frac{(\mathbf{Y} - \mathbf{X}\hat{\boldsymbol{\beta}})^T(\mathbf{Y} - \mathbf{X}\hat{\boldsymbol{\beta}})}{n - p}.$$

Conditional on the weights and under the null hypothesis, F follows a $\mathcal{F}(q, n -$

p) distribution. If $F \leq \mathscr{F}_{1-\alpha}(q, n - p)$, where $\mathscr{F}_{1-\alpha}(q, n - p)$ is the $100(1 - \alpha)$ percentile of the central $\mathscr{F}$ distribution with q and $n - p$ degrees of freedom, the hypothesis of additivity (or no interaction) cannot be rejected; if $F > \mathscr{F}_{1-\alpha}(q, n - p)$, the hypothesis of additivity is rejected.

To construct a suitable model of the form given in (1), it is critical to parameterize the model in such a way that the single-drug dose–response curves are adequately described and where the nature of the interaction is allowed sufficient flexibility. Using data from a factorial design allows the estimation of high-order interaction terms and therefore flexibility in the model. In Section 3 the procedure used to construct the models given in the example is described. In that case a 5×7 factorial design was completely replicated. One replication was used to describe the additive model, which was used in an algorithm to select which cross-product terms to include in the full model. The other replication was used to fit the final model. In this way the construction of the full model was not based on the data used in the final analysis.

3.2 Graphical Analysis

Response surfaces associated with the additive and full models can be examined to identify regions of synergy or antagonism. Following the notation defined at (1), let $\mathbf{Y} = \mathbf{X}_1\boldsymbol{\beta}_1 + \mathbf{X}_2\boldsymbol{\beta}_2 + \boldsymbol{\epsilon}$. A simultaneous $100(1 - \alpha)\%$ confidence band on the response $\mathbf{x}\boldsymbol{\beta}$ from the full model for all $\mathbf{x} \in R^p$ is (Carter et al., 1986; Graybill, 1976)

$$\mathbf{x}\hat{\boldsymbol{\beta}} \pm [\mathbf{x}(\mathbf{X}^T\mathbf{W}\mathbf{X})^{-1}\mathbf{x}^T \, \text{MSE} \, p\mathscr{F}_{1-\alpha}(p, n - p)]^{1/2}.$$

Over a fine grid of points (x_1, x_2),

$$K_{\text{low}} = \mathbf{x}\hat{\boldsymbol{\beta}} - [\mathbf{x}(\mathbf{X}^T\mathbf{W}\mathbf{X})^{-1}\mathbf{x}^T\text{MSE} \, p\mathscr{F}_{1-\alpha}(p, n - p)]^{1/2},$$
$$K_{\text{high}} = \mathbf{x}\hat{\boldsymbol{\beta}} + [\mathbf{x}(\mathbf{X}^T\mathbf{W}\mathbf{X})^{-1}\mathbf{x}^T \, \text{MSE} \, p\mathscr{F}_{1-\alpha}(p, n - p)]^{1/2}$$

and $Y_{\text{add}} = \mathbf{x}^{(2)}\hat{\boldsymbol{\beta}}_2$ are evaluated, where $\mathbf{x}^{(2)}$ is a $(p - q)$ row vector of the pure terms in $\mathbf{x}$ associated with $\boldsymbol{\beta}_2$. For increasing dose–response relationships (e.g., hyperactivity), $Y_{\text{add}} < K_{\text{Low}}$ implies synergism and $Y_{\text{add}} > K_{\text{High}}$ implies antagonism. Otherwise, additivity holds. For decreasing dose–response relationships (e.g., hypothermia), the interpretations are reversed. These points of synergism/antagonism can be plotted on a graph to indicate regions of interaction.

3.3 Analysis of Binary Data

For binary data, likelihood ratio tests based on logistic regression models can be used to test for synergy or antagonism. Suppose that the response of interest is whether a mouse initially flicked its tail more than 8 seconds after it was placed under a heat lamp. The response is binary: $Y = 1$ if the tail-flick latency is more than 8 seconds, and $Y = 0$ otherwise. Suppose that the probability of response is π and Y is a binomial random variable with parameters π and $n = 1$.

Let y_{ij} be the binary response of the jth mouse in the ith treatment group, $i = 1, \ldots, k; j = 1, \ldots, n_i$. Define $\mathbf{x}_i$ to be a p-dimensional row vector associated with the dose combination given the ith treatment group, $i = 1, \ldots, k$. Similar to equation (1), the elements in $\mathbf{x}_i$ can be partitioned into two components $\mathbf{x}_i = [\mathbf{x}_i^{(1)} \ \mathbf{x}_i^{(2)}]$ such that $\mathbf{x}_i^{(1)}$ is a q-dimensional row vector that includes cross-product terms and $\mathbf{x}_i^{(2)}$ is a $(p-q)$-dimensional row vector that includes the pure terms. Let π_i be the response probability after exposure to the hot pad given the ith treatment combination. The dose–response relationship can be modeled using a logistic function, that is,

$$\pi_i = \{1 + \exp[-(\mathbf{x}_i^{(1)}\boldsymbol{\beta}_1 + \mathbf{x}_i^{(2)}\boldsymbol{\beta}_2)]\}^{-1},$$

where $\boldsymbol{\beta}_1$ is a q-vector of unknown regression coefficients associated with cross-product terms and $\boldsymbol{\beta}_2$ is a $(p-q)$-dimensional vector of unknown regression coefficients associated with pure terms. Assuming mutually independent observations, the unrestricted likelihood is proportional to

$$\mathcal{L} = \prod_{i=1}^{k} \pi_i^{r_i}(1 - \pi_i)^{n_i-r_i},$$

where $r_i = \sum_{j=1}^{n_i} y_{ij}$. The probability of response under the hypothesis of additivity (i.e., $H_0: \boldsymbol{\beta}_1 = \mathbf{0}$), is given by $\pi_{i0} = [1 + \exp(-\mathbf{x}_i^{(2)}\boldsymbol{\beta}_2)]^{-1}$, and the restricted likelihood is given by

$$\mathcal{L}_0 = \prod_{i=1}^{k} \pi_{i0}^{r_i}(1 - \pi_{i0})^{n_i-r_i}.$$

The log-likelihood ratio statistic for testing the hypothesis of additivity, $2[\ln \mathcal{L} - \ln \mathcal{L}_0]$, thus follows a $\chi^2(q)$ distribution for large samples. A simultaneous $100(1 - \alpha)\%$ confidence band about the probability of response, $\pi = [1 + \exp(-\mathbf{x}_i\beta)]^{-1}$, is given by (Carter et al., 1986)

$$\Pr\{\hat{p}_L(\mathbf{x}) \leq [1 + \exp(-\mathbf{x}_i\beta)]^{-1} \leq \hat{p}_U(\mathbf{x}),$$
$$\text{simultaneously for all } \mathbf{x} \in R^p\} = 1 - \alpha,$$

where

$$\hat{p}_L(\mathbf{x}) = \{1 + \exp[-\mathbf{x}_i\boldsymbol{\beta} + \mathbf{x}\mathbf{J}\mathbf{x}^T\chi_{1-\alpha}^2(p)]\}^{-1},$$
$$\hat{p}_U(\mathbf{x}) = \{1 + \exp[-\mathbf{x}_i\boldsymbol{\beta} - \mathbf{x}\mathbf{J}\mathbf{x}^T\chi_{1-\alpha}^2(p)]\}^{-1},$$

and $\mathbf{J}$ is the sample information matrix. Define $\pi_{\text{add}} = [1 + \exp(-\mathbf{x}_i^{(2)}\hat{\boldsymbol{\beta}}_2)]^{-1}$. For increasing dose–response relationships, $\pi_{\text{add}} < \hat{p}_L(\mathbf{x})$ at the point (x_1, x_2) implies synergy, while $\pi_{\text{add}} > \hat{p}_U(\mathbf{x})$ implies antagonism.

4 RESULTS

4.1 Development of the Models

Using one replication of the data and taking advantage of the implicit balance in a factorial design, we determined a polynomial form of $f_i(x_i)$, by sequentially fitting polynomial models in x_i, until a goodness-of-fit test indicated that additional higher-order terms were not necessary. The additive model was then given by the sum of the two polynomials, $f_1(x_1) + f_2(x_2)$. For example, the relationship between change in body temperature and morphine sulfate (x_1) was considered to be well approximated by a linear function, and a cubic function was considered to describe adequately the Δ^9-THC (x_2) response curve. Therefore, the additive model for change in body temperature is given by

$$y = \beta_0 + \beta_1 x_1 + \beta_2 x_2 + \beta_3 x_2^2 + \beta_4 x_2^3 + \epsilon.$$

The form of the full model, which allowed for departure from additivity, was constructed by adding to the additive model additional terms which corresponded to cross-products of all the terms in $f_1(x_1)$ with the terms in $f_2(x_2)$. For example, for the change in body temperature response, the cross-product terms added were $\beta_5 x_1 x_2, \beta_6 x_1 x_2^2$, and $\beta_7 x_1 x_2^3$. These full models are given in equation (4) below.

Logistic regression was performed to assess the relationship between the proportion (p) of animals with a tail-flick latency greater than 8 seconds and the doses of the drugs. An additional term was added to the model to adjust for the pretreatment tail-flick latency. The full model was parameterized as

$$\ln \frac{p}{1-p} = \beta_0 + \theta t + \beta_1 x_1 + \beta_2 x_2 + \beta_3 x_2^2 + \beta_4 x_1 x_2 + \beta_5 x_1 x_2^2, \quad (2)$$

where x_1 and x_2 are the doses of morphine sulfate and Δ^9-THC, respectively; t is the pretreatment tail-flick latency centered at zero (i.e., t = pretreatment flick time – mean pretreatment flick time); $\beta_0, \beta_1, \beta_2, \beta_3, \beta_4$, and β_5 are the unknown parameters associated with the effect of morphine sulfate and Δ^9-THC; and θ is an unknown parameter associated with the association of the pre- and post-treatment tail-flick latency. Following the notation in equation (1), we write $\boldsymbol{\beta}_1 = [\beta_4, \beta_5]^T$ and $\boldsymbol{\beta}_2 = [\beta_0, \beta_1, \beta_2, \beta_3]^T$. The effect of the choice of the cut-off time point was investigated by also considering 7-, 9- and 10-second cutoff times. None of these analyses resulted in an indication of departure from additivity ($p = 0.82, p = 0.99$, and $p = 0.60$, respectively). This consistency in the analyses indicates that the loss of information due to switching from analysis of time-to-response data to binary data did not compromise the qualitative conclusion of additivity.

The relationship between spontaneous activity and the doses of morphine and Δ^9-THC was approximated by the model given in equation (1) parameterized as

$$
\begin{aligned}
y = \beta_0 &+ \beta_1 x_1 + \beta_2 x_2 + \beta_3 x_1^2 + \beta_4 x_2^2 \\
&+ \beta_5 x_1 x_2 + \beta_6 x_1 x_2^2 + \beta_7 x_1^2 x_2 + \beta_8 x_1^2 x_2^2 + \epsilon,
\end{aligned}
\tag{3}
$$

where y is a function of the number of interruptions of the photocell beam by each mouse, x_1 and x_2 are the doses of morphine sulfate and Δ^9-THC, respectively, and $\beta_j, j = 1, \ldots, 8$, are the unknown parameters. The square root of the spontaneous activity count was used in the analysis since this transformation on count data has desirable statistical properties. The method of weighted least squares was used to estimate the unknown parameters which are provided in Table 2 (see, e.g., Neter et al. 1990).

The dose–response relationship of change in rectal temperature from 60 minutes to baseline postinjection was approximated by the model in equation (1) parameterized as

$$
\begin{aligned}
y = \beta_0 &+ \beta_1 x_1 + \beta_2 x_2 + \beta_3 x_2^2 + \beta_4 x_2^3 \\
&+ \beta_5 x_1 x_2 + \beta_6 x_1 x_2^2 + \beta_7 x_1 x_2^3 + \epsilon,
\end{aligned}
\tag{4}
$$

where y is the change in body temperature at 60 minutes from baseline, x_1 and x_2 are the doses of morphine sulfate and Δ^9-THC, respectively, and $\beta_j, j = 1, \ldots, 7$, are the unknown parameters. The method of weighted least squares was used to estimate the unknown parameters which are given in Table 2.

Plots of the data indicated that the variance for neither the spontaneous activity (Figure 3a) nor the rectal temperature responses (Figure 3b) is constant across dose combinations. Therefore, the method of weighted least squares was used to estimate the parameters in models (3) and (4). The response used was the mean response from each treatment combination which was independent of the estimate for the variance of the same groups. The weight associated with each group was the inverse of the sample variance. Model adequacy was ascertained graphically for models (3) and (4) (Figures 3c and 3d, respectively) and by using the chi-squared goodness-of-fit test for model (2) ($p = 0.62$).

Table 2 Analysis of the Interaction of Morphine Sulfate and Δ^9-THC

Variable[a]	Parameter Estimate	Standard Error	p-Value
Tail-Flick Activity[b]			
Intercept	-2.17	0.615	<0.001
t	1.22	0.490	0.013
x_1	9.04	2.06	<0.001
x_2	4.86	3.22	0.132
x_2^2	-2.52	2.86	0.930
$x_1 x_2$	-2.61	14.28	0.855
$x_1 x_2^2$	0.899	15.4	0.953
Spontaneous Activity[c]			
Intercept	10.3	0.775	<0.001
x_1	1.52	5.04	0.765
x_2	-8.604	3.89	0.036
x_1^2	1.89	6.02	0.756
x_2^2	1.60	2.51	0.528
$x_1 x_2$	-47.4	21.2	0.034
$x_1 x_2^2$	29.7	13.47	0.036
$x_1^2 x_2$	57.2	27.3	0.046
$x_1^2 x_2^2$	-38.1	17.3	0.037
Rectal Temperature[c]			
Intercept	1.021	0.2508	<0.001
x_1	-0.600	0.471	0.214
x_2	-11.7	2.73	<0.001
x_2^2	4.76	5.20	0.368
x_2^3	0.593	2.417	0.808
$x_1 x_2$	-0.878	5.564	0.876
$x_1 x_2^2$	14.7	11.1	0.195
$x_1 x_2^3$	-8.70	5.25	0.109

[a]x_1 = associated with dose of morphine sulfate (cg/g); x_2 = associated with dose of Δ^9-THC (cg/g).
[b]Logistic regression based on equation (2).
[c]Regression analysis based on equations (3) and (4).

4.2 Comparison of Data

The estimated dose–response relationships of morphine sulfate and Δ^9-THC on spontaneous activity (hyperactivity), rectal temperature (hypothermia), and tail-flick latency (analgesia) are presented in Figure 4 using the parameter estimates provided in Table 2. The edges along the dose axes of these three-dimen-

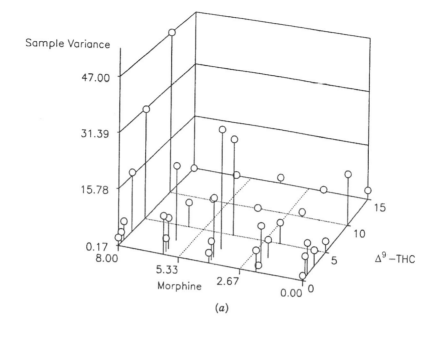

(a)

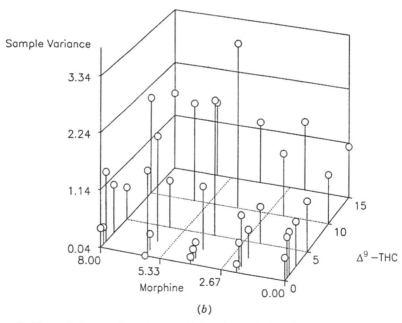

(b)

Figure 3. Plots of the sample variances of the observed data for the spontaneous activity (a) and change in rectal temperature (b) endpoints. Plots of observed and predicted responses for spontaneous activity (c) and change in rectal temperature (d) endpoints indicate adequate predictability by models (3) and (4).

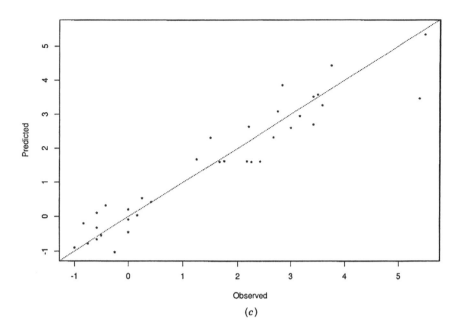

(c)

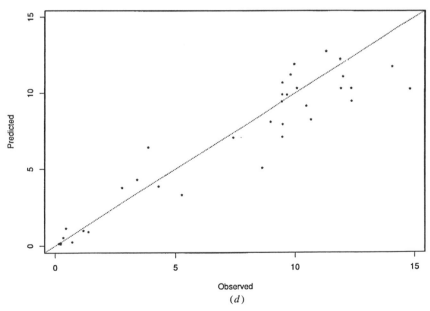

(d)

Figure 3. (*Continued*)

sional graphs represent the dose–response curves of the individual drugs when administered alone. Morphine sulfate and Δ^9-THC produced different effects on locomotor activity, with Δ^9-THC alone decreasing activity and morphine sulfate having no significant effect (Figure 4b). Similarly, Δ^9-THC alone tended to decrease body temperature (Figure 4c) by producing a rapid decrease at lower doses, which reached a plateau at higher doses. Morphine sulfate alone had no significant effect on body temperature. As for antinociceptive effects, both compounds increased tail-flick latency (Figure 4a). The antinociceptive response is presented as the proportion of animals exhibiting a tail-flick latency greater than 8 seconds. Since this response is positive and increases as a function of the dose of each compound, the proportion of animals with a tail-flick latency greater than 8 seconds increases with increasing doses of morphine sulfate and Δ^9-THC.

From Figure 4, the dose–response curve of each compound can also be visualized at fixed levels of the other compound by following an interior grid line in the same direction as either edge. If the change in the dose–response curve from the edge (where the dose of the other compound is zero) to that associated with a fixed dose of the other compound is only increased or decreased by a constant amount, and if it does not change shape, an additive effect of the combination is likely (e.g., Figure 4a). If the dose–response curve of one compound changes shape in the presence of different doses of the other compound, an interaction between the compounds is likely to have occurred (e.g., Figure 4b and c). However, it is difficult to determine the nature/direction of the inter-

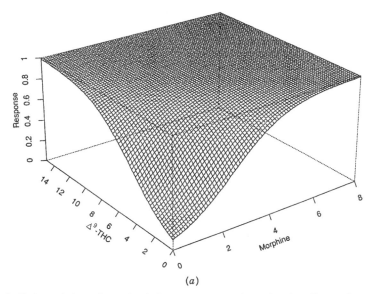

(a)

Figure 4. Estimated three-dimensional dose–response surfaces for the effects of the Δ^9-THC (mg/kg) and morphine sulfate (mg/kg) combination treatment on tail-flick latency (a), on spontaneous activity (b), on change in rectal temperature (c).

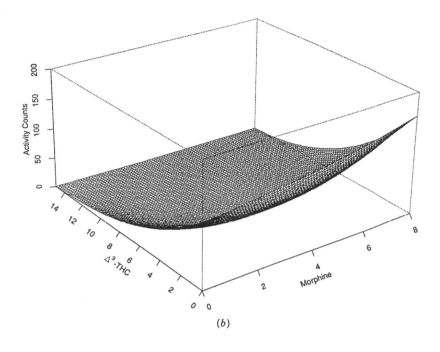

(b)

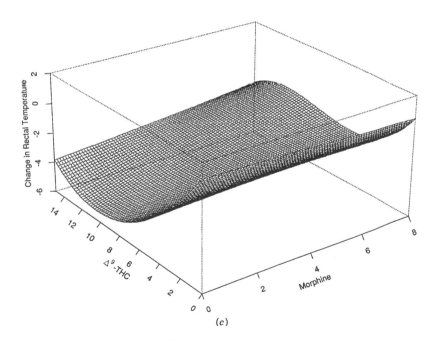

(c)

Figure 4. (*Continued*)

action using only this visual aid, especially when the number of components to the combination exceeds two.

To characterize the interaction, it is useful to consider a test of the model parameters. Under the definition that two compounds in combination interact additively if the effect of the combination is equal to the sum of the effects of the individual compounds, a test of additivity is given by a simultaneous test on the significance of the cross-product terms in the model. If the coefficients for the cross-product terms in models (3) and (4) are simultaneously zero, the remaining model is referred to as an *additive model* (Figure 5). For the spontaneous activity data, this simultaneous test on the significance of $\beta_5, \beta_6, \beta_7$, and β_8 was rejected at the 5% significance level ($p = 0.033$). For the rectal temperature data, this simultaneous test on β_5, β_6, and β_7 was also rejected ($p = 0.002$). In other words, the effects of the combination of Δ^9-THC and morphine sulfate on spontaneous activity and rectal temperature differed significantly from additivity. When the response is quantal, a test for interaction, namely the likelihood ratio test, is also based on the significance of cross-product terms. For the tail-flick data, this simultaneous test on β_4 and β_5 was not rejected ($p = 0.961$). It is therefore reasonable to conclude that morphine sulfate and Δ^9-THC have an additive antinociceptive effect.

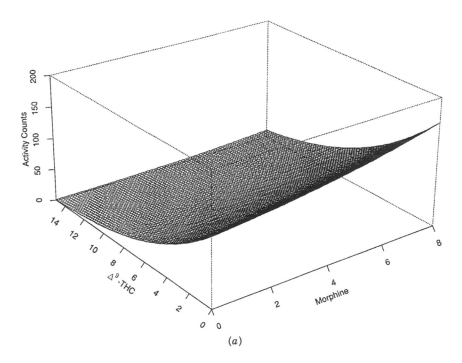

(a)

Figure 5. Surface for the additive model for the effects on spontaneous activity (a) and on change in rectal temperature (b). Additivity is represented in the model when the cross-product terms are zero.

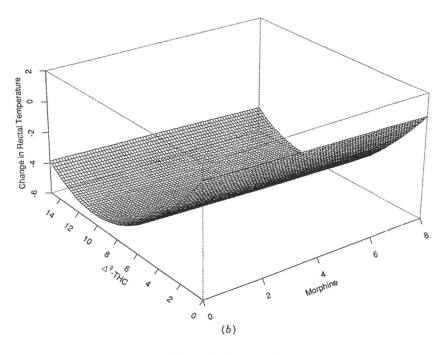

Figure 5. (*Continued*)

Following the logic of Gennings et al. (1990), a generalized isobologram (as described above) was constructed for both the spontaneous activity and rectal temperature data in order to characterize the nature of the interaction associated with the combination of these two drugs. Briefly, a 95% simultaneous confidence region was constructed about the response surface. The predicted response from the additive model (analogous to the line of additivity in the usual isobologram analysis), presented in Figure 5, was compared to the simultaneous confidence region about the response from the full model (analogous to the isobol in the usual analysis). For a given dose combination (e.g., the spontaneous activity response data), if the response from the additive model is greater than the upper confidence band on the response from the full model, the particular dose combination is antagonistic; if the response from the additive model is less than the lower confidence band on the response from the full model, the particular dose combination is synergistic; otherwise, it cannot be concluded that the combination is different from additive. For both the spontaneous activity and rectal temperature responses, the combination is concluded to be antagonistic (less than additive) in the shaded regions displayed in Figure 6. The combination doses associated with the nonshaded regions cannot be shown to differ from additivity.

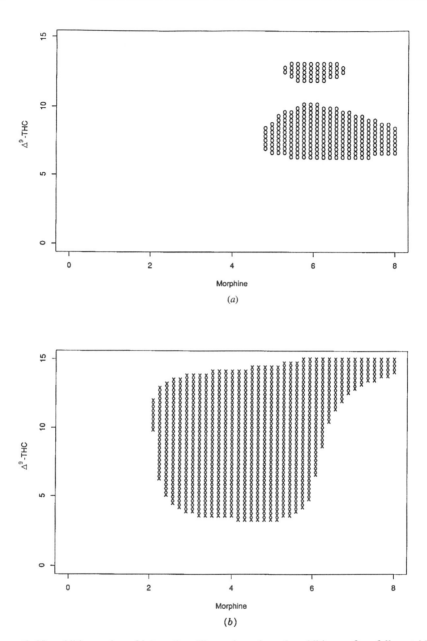

Figure 6. Nonadditive region of interaction. The region where the additive surface falls outside the 95% simultaneous confidence band on the full response surface is shaded. At each fixed dose combination in the shaded region, the response of the full model is less extreme than that under additivity, indicating that the combination is antagonistic within this region for both spontaneous activity (*a*) and change in body temperature (*b*). The shaded regions are plotted together in (*c*) to indicate dose regions where both side-effect endpoints are antagonistic. The dose scale for morphine sulfate and Δ^9-THC is in mg/kg.

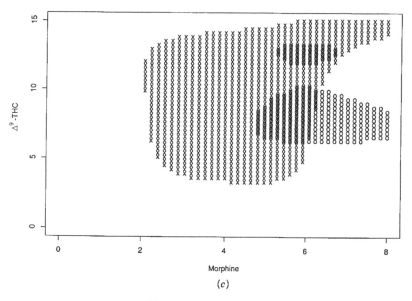

Figure 6. (*Continued*)

5   CONCLUSIONS

The methodology used in this chapter illustrates the isobologram technique of Gennings et al. (1990). The combination of some compounds may show evidence of regions of additivity and regions of departure from additivity in contrast to a global interaction relationship. The parameterization of the model used in Gennings et al. (1990) does not allow for identification of regional differences in the nature of the interaction since a single parameter is used to describe the interaction. In contrast, the generalization employed here allows for multiple parameters to describe departure from additivity, thereby allowing for characterization of regional changes. A nonlinear line of additivity can be constructed by using an effect-addition argument (i.e., arguing that a combination of two compounds is considered additive if the effect of the combination is the sum of the effects of the two compounds). The methodology used here allows for complex contours of additivity.

In bioassays the response of interest is often binary (i.e., either the experimental unit responds or it does not respond). For such data, the proportion of responders is modeled as a function of dose. Clearly, proportional data are constrained to be within the unit interval (i.e., [0,1]). An appropriate statistical model must also be constrained to this interval. By using the argument of Ashford and Smith (1964), the analysis of an interaction for such data should be performed on a continuous scale implicit to the constrained model. This can be interpreted as an implicit dose–effect surface for the tolerance distribution, where if the effect exceeds the tolerance level, the experimental unit will respond; otherwise, it will not. An example of such an analysis is that given in (2), where the logistic model (i.e., $p = \{1 + \exp[-t(x)]\}^{-1}$), is constrained to the unit interval and the logit (i.e., $\ln[p/(1-p)] = t(x)$) can be any real number. The analysis of interaction is performed on the logit scale.

Dose–response surface analysis is an informative technique for evaluating drug interactions. This method not only allows one to determine the type of interaction that results from drug combinations, it provides an indication of the dose combinations that are responsible for a particular interaction. It is entirely possible that different dose combinations of the same two agents could result in additive, antagonistic, and synergistic effects. As for the interactions between Δ^9-THC and morphine sulfate, the antinociceptive effects were additive, whereas the effects on locomotor activity and rectal temperature were less than additive in selected dose ranges. The less-than-additive effects for spontaneous activity were observed in the dose range of 2 to 6 mg/kg for morphine sulfate and at doses above 3 mg/kg for Δ^9-THC. The effects on rectal temperature were less than additive at doses above 4 and 6 mg/kg for morphine sulfate and Δ^9-THC, respectively.

Frequently, the effects produced by combinations of drugs serve as a basis for predicting whether they act through a common mechanism. Although parallelism of dose–response curves and additivity (effect addition) are expected of drugs which act through a single mechanism, these same characteristics may also occur with drugs acting through different mechanisms. There is ample evidence to demonstrate that the antinociceptive properties of morphine sulfate and Δ^9-THC are due to distinctively different mechanisms, as discussed earlier, and that the additivity of antinociception as defined by the dose–response surface analysis should be interpreted with care.

All antinociceptive agents exhibit serious adverse effects which hamper their acute and chronic use in controlling pain. Therefore, any improvement in the ratio of morphine's antinociceptive potency to side effects has clinical relevance. It may well be that the addition of a cannabinoid (such as Δ^9-THC) to an opioid (such as morphine sulfate) may increase analgesic potency without contributing to morphine's adverse effects. Of course, extrapolation of the results from the present mouse studies to a potential clinical situation must be done cautiously because it is not known how changes in spontaneous activity and rectal temperature relate to effects in humans. Nonetheless, the rather wide dosage range of Δ^9-THC and morphine sulfate which resulted in less-than-additive effects on either spontaneous activity and rectal temperature is encouraging. It is particularly noteworthy that the less-than-additive effects were found at the higher dose range where adverse effects are more likely to be observed. Additional encouragement is provided by recent studies in which intrathecal co-administration of Δ^9-THC and morphine sulfate produces a fivefold increase in the potency of morphine sulfate (Sandra P. Welch, unpublished observations).

In summary, dose–response surface analysis revealed that the antinociceptive effects of the combination of Δ^9-THC and morphine sulfate were additive while their effects on spontaneous activity and rectal temperature were significantly less than additive. This methodology also demonstrated that the nature of a drug interaction could be associated with a selected dose range. The additive antinociceptive effects of Δ^9-THC and morphine sulfate could serve as an additional lead for development of an analgesic combination which produces less adverse effects than those observed with opioid treatment alone.

ACKNOWLEDGMENT

This work was funded in part by NIDA grant # DA-05274.

QUESTIONS AND PROBLEMS

1. Consider the model $y = \beta_0 + \beta_1 x_1 + \beta_2 x_2 + \beta_3 x_1 x_2 + \epsilon$, where x_1 and x_2 represent doses of two compounds of interest. Suppose that β_1 and β_2 are both positive. For a synergistic interaction (i.e., $\beta_3 > 0$), show graphically that the dose–response curve for one compound at a fixed dose of the other is to the left of the dose–response curve under the hypothesis of additivity, and that a contour of constant response is concave upward and falls below the contour associated with additivity (i.e., the line of additivity). Show the reverse is true for decreasing dose–response curves.

2. Verify the form of the simultaneous confidence band on the response $\mathbf{x}\boldsymbol{\beta}$ for the model given in equation (1).

3. The analysis of the spontaneous activity used in the chapter followed normal theory by taking the square root of the count variable. Use a Poisson regression model to verify the less than additive relationship between Δ^9-THC and morphine in regard to spontaneous activity.

4. Use the Cox proportional hazards model to verify the additive relationship between Δ^9-THC and morphine in regard to tail-flick latency. Discuss the effect of the heavy censoring on the analysis.

APPENDIX

About the Diskette

The diskette that accompanies *Case Studies in Biometry* contains all the data used by its authors. The diskette also contains a README file, a menu-driven program that decompresses and installs the data sets, text files that describe the data sets, and sample SAS input programs.

Please note the permissions statements given in the text files accompanying the data sets.

A.1 DISKETTE CONTENTS

Chapters 1, 3, 4, 11, 16, 18, and 21 include two data sets. The rather large data set for Chapter 19 has been divided into seven subsets to allow you handle it more easily. The remaining chapters use only one data set. Please refer to the text files associated with each chapter for more information on variable names and coding conventions.

The diskette installation program will install the following files:

Text Summary Files	Data Files	SAS Program Files
README		
CH1A.TXT	CH1A.DAT	CH1A.SAS
CH1B.TXT	CH1B.DAT	CH1B.SAS
CH2.TXT	CH2.DAT	CH2.SAS
CH3A.TXT	CH3A.DAT	CH3A.SAS
CH3B.TXT	CH3B.DAT	CH3B.SAS
CH4A.TXT	CH4A.DAT	CH4A.SAS
CH4B.TXT	CH4B.DAT	CH4B.SAS
CH5.TXT	CH5.DAT	CH5.SAS
CH6.TXT	CH6.DAT	CH6.SAS
CH7.TXT	CH7.DAT	CH7.SAS
CH8.TXT	CH8.DAT	CH8.SAS

CH9.TXT	CH9.DAT	CH9.SAS
CH10.TXT	CH10.DAT	CH10.SAS
CH11A.TXT	CH11A.DAT	CH11A.SAS
CH11B.TXT	CH11B.DAT	CH11B.SAS
CH12.TXT	CH12.DAT	CH12.SAS
CH13.TXT	CH13.DAT	CH13.SAS
CH14.TXT	CH14.DAT	CH14.SAS
CH15.TXT	CH15.DAT	CH15.SAS
CH16A.TXT	CH16A.DAT	CH16A.SAS
CH16B.TXT	CH16B.DAT	CH16B.SAS
CH17.TXT	CH17.DAT	CH17.SAS
CH18A.TXT	CH18A.DAT	CH18A.SAS
CH18B.TXT	CH18B.DAT	CH18B.SAS
CH19.TXT	CH19A.DAT	CH19.SAS
•	CH19B.DAT	•
•	CH19C.DAT	•
•	CH19D.DAT	•
•	CH19E.DAT	•
•	CH19F.DAT	•
•	CH19G.DAT	•
CH20.TXT	CH20.DAT	CH20.SAS
CH21A.TXT	CH21A.DAT	CH21A.SAS
CH21B.TXT	CH21B.DAT	CH21B.SAS

A.2 HARDWARE AND SOFTWARE REQUIREMENTS

The data sets can be installed on any IBM PC compatible computer with a hard disk drive. You will need approximately 7MB of free disk space on your hard drive. Each data set is provided as printable ASCII text. You can also use SAS to compile the SAS programs that read the data sets into that package once they have been installed. The SAS programs do not include any data analysis functions, only input statements.

A.3 MAKING A BACKUP COPY

Before using the enclosed diskette, make a backup copy of the original. This backup is for personal use and will only be required in case of damage to the original. Any other use of the diskette violates copyright law. Assuming the floppy drive you will be using is drive A, please do the following:

1. First make sure that you have formatted your backup target diskette.
2. Insert the original source diskette in drive A.

3. At the A:> prompt, type DISKCOPY A: A: and press Return. (You will be prompted to place the source diskette in drive A, which you have already done.)

4. Press Return. Wait until you are prompted to place the target diskette in drive A.

5. Remove the original source diskette and replace it with your formatted blank diskette. Press Return and follow the instructions. You may need to alternate between source and target diskettes to complete the backup procedure.

A.4 INSTALLING THE DATA SETS

The default disk drive is drive C, and the default installation directory is CSB. At the end of installation, you will be given the opportunity to review the README file for more information. To install the data sets:

1. Assuming that you use drive A as the floppy drive for your installation, at the A:> prompt type INSTALL. Alternatively, you may type A:INSTALL at the C:> prompt.

2. Follow the instructions displayed by the installation program.

References

Aalen, O. O., Borgan, O., Keiding, N., and Thormann, J. (1980). Interaction between life history events: non-parametric analysis for prospective and retrospective data in the presence of censoring. *Scandinavian Journal of Statistics* **7,** 161–171.

Abbott, R. D. (1985). Logistic regression in survival analysis. *American Journal of Epidemiology* **121,** 465–471.

Aboufirassi, M., and Mariño, M. (1983). Kriging of water levels in the Souss Aquifer, Morocco. *Mathematical Geology* **15,** 537–551.

Agresti, A. (1988). A model for agreement between ratings on an ordinal scale. *Biometrics* **44,** 539–548.

Agresti, A. (1990). *Categorical Data Analysis.* New York: John Wiley & Sons.

Aitken, M., and Clayton, D. G. (1980). The fitting of exponential, Weibull and extreme value distributions to complex censored survival data using GLIM. *Applied Statistics* **29,** 156–163.

Aitkin, M., and Wilson, G. T. (1980). Mixture models, outliers, and the EM algorithm. *Technometrics* **22,** 325–331.

Albert, A., and Anderson, J. A. (1984). On the existence of maximum likelihood estimates in logistic regression models. *Biometrika* **71,** 1–10.

Albert, A., and Harris, E. K. (1987). *Multivariate Interpretation of Clinical Laboratory Data.* New York: Marcel Dekker.

Albert, A., and Lesaffre, E. (1986). Multiple group logistic discrimination. *Computers and Mathematics with Applications* **12,** 209–224.

Alderson, M. R., Lee, P. N., and Wang, R. (1985). Risks of lung cancer, chronic bronchitis, ischaemic heart disease, and stroke in relation to type of cigarette smoked. *Journal of Epidemiology and Community Health* **39,** 286–293.

Alldredge, J. R., and Ratti, J. T. (1986). Comparison of some statistical techniques for analysis of resource selection. *Journal of Wildlife Management* **50,** 157–165.

Alldredge, J. R., and Ratti, J. T. (1992). Further comparison of some statistical techniques for analysis of resource selection. *Journal of Wildlife Management* **56,** 1–9.

Allison, P. D. (1982). Discrete time methods for the analysis of event histories. In *Sociological Methodology*, S. Leinhart (ed.), San Francisco: Jossey-Bass, pp. 61–98.

Allison, P. D. (1984). *Event History Analysis*, Sage University Paper Series on Quantitative Applications in the Social Sciences 07-046. Beverly Hills, Calif.: Sage Publications.

Andelman, J. B. (1985). Human exposures to volatile halogenated organic chemicals in indoor and outdoor air. *Environmental Health Perspectives* **62**, 313–318.

Andersen, P. K., and Gill, R. D. (1982). Cox's regression model for counting processes: a large sample study. *Annals of Statistics* **10**, 1100–1120.

Anderson, T. W. (1958). *An Introduction to Multivariate Statistical Analysis*. New York: John Wiley & Sons.

Anderson, J. A. (1972). Separate sample logistic discrimination. *Biometrika* **59**, 19–35.

Anderson, J. A. (1984). Regression and ordered categorical variables. *Journal of the Royal Statistical Society Series B* **46**, 1–30.

Armitage, P. (1975). *Statistical Methods in Medical Research*. Oxford: Blackwell.

Armitage, P. K., McPherson, D. K., and Rowe, B. C. (1969). Repeated significance tests on accumulating data. *Journal of the Royal Statistical Society Series A* **132**, 235–244.

Ashford, J. R., and Smith, C. S. (1964). General models for quantal response to the joint action of a mixture of drugs. *Biometrika* **51**, 413–428.

Atkinson, E. N., Bartoszynski, R., Brown, B. W., and Thompson, J. R. (1983). On estimating the growth function of tumors. *Mathematical Biosciences* **67**, 145–166.

Avery, R. A. (1982). Field studies of body temperatures and thermoregulation. In *Biology of the Reptilia*, Vol. 13, C. Gans and F. H. Pough (eds.), pp. 93–165. New York: Academic Press.

Azarovitz, T. R. (1991). *A Brief Historical Review of the Woods Hole Laboratory Trawl Time Series*. Woods Hole, Mass.: National Marine Fisheries Service.

Bailer, A. J., and Oris, J. T. (1993). Modeling reproductive toxicity in Ceriodaphnia tests. *Environmental Toxicology and Chemistry* **12**, 787–791.

Barber, B. J., and Crawford, E. C., Jr. (1977). A stochastic dual-limit hypothesis for behavioural thermoregulation in lizards. *Physiological Zoology* **50**, 53–60.

Bartholomew, G. A. (1982). Body temperature and energy metabolism. In *Animal Physiology: Principles and Adaptations*, 4th ed., M. S. Gordon et al. (eds.), pp. 333–406. New York: Macmillan.

Bartholomew, D. J. (1987). *Latent Variable Models and Factor Analysis*. New York: Oxford University Press.

Bartuska, A. M., and Joyner, K. C. (1987). Status report on the Southern Commercial Forest Research Cooperative. In *Proceedings of the 80th Annual Meeting of the Air Pollution Control Association*, Paper 87-34.3. New York: Air Pollution Control Association.

Becker, M. P. (1989). Using association models to analyse agreement data: two examples. *Statistics in Medicine* **8**, 1199–1207.

Becker, M. P. (1989). Square contingency tables having ordered categories and GLIM. *GLIM Newsletter* **19**, 22–31.

Becker, M. P. (1990). Quasisymmetric models for the analysis of square contingency tables. *Journal of the Royal Statistical Society Series B* **52**, 369–378.

Becker, M. P., and Agresti, A. (1992). Log-linear modelling of pairwise interobserver agreement on a categorical scale. *Statistics in Medicine* **11**, 101–114.

Belsley, D. A., Kuh, E., and Welsch, R. E. (1980). *Regression Diagnostics: Identifying Influential Data and Sources of Collinearity.* New York: John Wiley & Sons.

Bennett, A. F. (1987). Interindividual variability: an underutilized resource. In *New Directions in Ecological Physiology*, M. E. Feder, A. F. Bennett, W. W. Burggren, and R. B. Huey (eds.), pp. 147–165. Cambridge: Cambridge University Press.

Berenbaum, M. C. (1981). Criteria for analyzing interactions between biological active agents. *Advances in Cancer Research* **35**, 269–333.

Berenbaum, M. C. (1985). The expected effect of a combination of agents: the general solution. *Journal of Theoretical Biology* **114**, 413–431.

Berkson, J. (1949). Minimum chi-square and maximum likelihood solution in terms of a linear transform, with particular reference to bio-assay. *Journal of the American Statistical Association* **50**, 273–278.

Berkson, J. (1951). Relative precision of minimum chi-square and maximum likelihood estimates of regression coefficients. In *Proceedings of the 2nd Berkeley Symposium on Mathematical Statistics and Probability*, pp. 471–479. Berkeley, Calif.: University of California Press.

Berkson, J. (1980). Minimum chi-square, not maximum likelihood! (with discussion). *The Annals of Statistics* **8**, 457–479.

Berlin, N. I., Buncher, C. R., Fontana, R. S., Frost, J. K., and Melamed, M. R. (1984). The National Cancer Institute Cooperative Early Lung Cancer Detection Program: results of the initial screen (prevalence): early lung cancer detection: introduction. *American Review of Respiratory Diseases* **130**, 545–549.

Berman, E., Heller, G., Santorsa, J., McKenzie, S., Gee, T., Kempin, S., Gulati, S., Andreeff, M., Kolitz, J., Gabrilove, J., Reich, L., Mayer, K., Keefe, D., Trainor, K., Schluger, A., Penenberg, D., Raymond, V., O'Reilly, R., Jhanwar, S., Young, C., and Clarkson, B. (1991). Results of a randomized trial comparing idarubicin and cytosine arabinoside with daunorubicin and cytosine aroabinoside in adult patients with newly diagnosed acute myelogenous leukemia. *Blood* **77**, 1666–1674.

Besag, J., and Diggle, P. J. (1977). Simple Monte Carlo tests for spatial pattern. *Applied Statistics* **26**, 327–333.

Besag, J., and Newell, J. (1991). The detection of clusters in rare diseases. *Journal of the Royal Statistical Society Series A* **154**, 143–155.

Bickel, P. J., and Doksum, K. A. (1977). *Mathematical Statistics.* Oakland, Calif.: Holden-Day.

Binder, D. (1981). On the variances of asymptotically normal estimators for complex surveys. *Survey Methodology* **7**, 157–170.

Bliss, C. I. (1967). *Statistics in Biology.* New York: McGraw-Hill.

Bloom, B. S., Hauck, W. W., Peterson, O. L., Nickerson, R. J., and Colton, T. (1978). Surgeons in the United States. *Archives of Surgery* **113**, 188–193.

Boring, C. C., Squires, T. S., and Tong, T. (1992). Cancer statistics, 1992. *Ca: A Cancer Journal for Clinicians* **42**, 19–38.

Boutton, T. W., and Flagler, R. B. (1990). Growth and water-use efficiency of shortleaf pine as affected by ozone and acid rain. In *Proceedings of the 83rd Annual Meet-*

ing and Exhibition of Air and Waste Management Association, Paper 90-187.7. Pittsburgh, Pa.: Air and Waste Management Association.

Bowe, C. A. (1984). Spatial relations in Animal learning and behavior. *Psychological Record* **34**, 181–209.

Bowker, R. G. (1984). Precision of thermoregulation of some African lizards. *Physiological Zoology* **57**, 401–412.

Box, G. E. P., and Cox, D. R. (1964). An analysis of transformations. *Journal of the Royal Statistical Society Series B* **26**, 211–243.

Box, G. E. P., and Jenkins, G. M. (1976). *Time Series Analysis: Forecasting and Control*, rev. ed. Oakland, Calif.: Holden-Day.

Box, G. E. P., and Tiao, G. C. (1975). Intervention analysis with applications to economic and environmental problems. *Journal of the American Statistical Association* **70**, 70–79.

Box, G. E. P., Hunter, W. G., and Hunter, J. S. (1978). *Statistics for Experimenters: An Introduction to Design, Data Analysis, and Model Building*. New York: John Wiley & Sons.

Bradu, D., and Mundlak, Y. (1970). Estimation in lognormal linear models. *Journal of the American Statistical Association* **65**, 198–211.

Breslow, N. E. (1974). Covariance analysis of censored survival data. *Biometrics* **30**, 89–99.

Breslow, N. E. (1984). Extra-Poisson variation in log-linear models. *Applied Statistics* **33**, 38–44.

Breslow, N. E., and Clayton, D. G. (1993). Approximate Inference in Generalized Linear Mixed Models. *Journal of the American Statistical Association* **88**, 9–25.

Breslow, N. E., and Day, N. E. (1980). *Statistical Methods in Cancer Research*, vol. 1, *The Analysis of Case-Control Studies*, Scientific Publication 32. Lyon, France: International Agency for Research on Cancer (WHO).

Breslow, N. E., Lubin, J. H., Marek, P., and Langholz, B. (1983). Multiplicative models and cohort analysis. *Journal of the American Statistical Association* **78**, 1–12.

Brett, G. Z. (1969). Earlier diagnosis and survival in lung cancer study. *British Medical Journal* **4**, 260–262.

Bromenshenk, J., Carlson, S., Simpson, J., and Thomas J. (1985). Pollution monitoring of Puget Sound with honeybees. *Science* **227**, 632–634.

Brookmeyer, R., Day, N. E., and Moss, S. (1986). Case-control studies for estimation of the natural history of preclinical disease from screening data. *Statistics in Medicine* **5**, 127–138.

Brown, C. C., and Chu, K. C. (1987). Use of multistage models to infer stage affected by carcinogenic exposure: example of lung cancer and cigarette smoking. *Journal of Chronic Diseases* **40**, 171S–179S.

Brown, H. S., Bishop, D. R., and Rowan, C. A. (1984). The role of skin absorption as a route of exposure for volatile organic compounds (VOCs) in drinking water. *American Journal of Public Health* **74**, 479–484.

Brownlee, K. A. (1965). *Statistical Theory and Methodology in Science and Engineering*, 2nd ed. New York: John Wiley & Sons.

Bull, S. B., and Pederson, L. L. (1988). Variances for polychotomous logistic regression using complex survey data. *Proceedings of the 1987 Survey Research Methods Section, American Statistical Association*, pp. 507–512.

Burden, R. L., Faires, J. D., and Reynolds, A. C. (1978). *Numerical Analysis.* Boston: Prindle, Weber & Schmidt.

Cain, K. C., and Lange, N. T. (1984). Approximate case influence for the proportional hazards regression model with censored data. *Biometrics* **40**, 493–499.

Carpenter, S. R. (1990). Large-scale perturbations: opportunities for innovation. *Ecology* **71**, 2038–2043.

Carroll, R. J., and Ruppert, D. (1988). *Transformations and Weighting in Regression.* London: Chapman & Hall.

Carroll, R. J., and Spiegelman, C. H. (1992). Diagnostics for nonlinearity and heteroscedasticity in errors-in-variables regression. *Technometrics* **34**, 186–196.

Carroll, R. J., Eltinge, J. L., and Ruppert, D. (1993). Robust linear regression in replicated measurement error models. *Statistics and Probability Letters* **16**, 169–176.

Carter, W. H., Jr., Chinchilli, V. M., Wilson, J. D., Campbell, E. D., Kessler, F. K., and Carchman, R. A. (1986). An asymptotic confidence region for the ED100p from the logistic response surface for a combination of agents. *The American Statistician* **40**, 124–128.

Carter, W. H., Jr., Gennings, C., Staniswalis, J. G., Campbell, E. D., and White, K. L., Jr. (1988). A statistical approach to the construction and analysis of isobolograms. *Journal of the American College of Toxicology* **7**, 963–973.

Casella, G., and Berger, R. L. (1990). *Statistical Inference.* Pacific Grove, Calif.: Wadsworth and Brooks/Cole.

Chambers, W. J., Puig-Antich, J., Hirsch, M., Paez, P., Ambrosini, P. J., Tabrizi, M. A., and Davies, M. (1985). The assessment of affective disorders in children and adolescents by semistructured interview: test–retest reliability of the schedule for affective disorders and schizophrenia for school-age children, present episode version. *Archives of General Psychiatry* **42**, 696–702.

Chambless, L. E., and Boyle, K. E. (1985). Maximum likelihood methods for complex sample data: logistic regression and discrete proportional hazards models. *Communications in Statistics* **14**, 1377–1392.

Chang, M. N. (1989). Confidence intervals for a normal mean following a group sequential test. *Biometrics* **45**, 247–254.

Chappelka, A. H., Lockaby, B. G., Mitchell, R. J., Medahl, R. S., Kush, J. S., and Jordan, D. N. (1990). Growth and physiological responses of loblolly pine exposed to ozone and simulated acidic rain in the field. In *Proceedings of the 83rd Annual Meeting and Exhibition of Air and Waste Management Association*, Paper 90-187.5. Pittsburgh, Pa.: Air and Waste Management Association.

Chatfield, C. (1979). Inverse autocorrelations. *Journal of the Royal Statistical Society Series A* **142**, 363–377.

Chatfield, C. (1980). *The Analysis of Time Series: An introduction*, 2nd ed. London: Chapman & Hall.

Clayton, D. G. (1988a). The analysis of event history data: a review of progress and the outstanding problems. *Statistics in Medicine* **7**, 819–841.

Clayton, D. G. (1988b). *Simulation in Hierarchical Models*. Technical report. Leicester, U.K.: University of Leicester.

Clayton, D. G., and Cuzick, J. (1985). The EM algorithm for Cox's regression model using GLIM. *Applied Statistics* **34**, 148–156.

Cleveland, W. S. (1979). Robust locally weighted regression and smoothing scatterplots. *Journal of the American Statistical Association* **74**, 829–836.

Cochran, W. G. (1977). *Sampling Techniques*, 3rd ed. New York: John Wiley & Sons.

Cochrane, D., and Orcutt, G. H. (1949). Application of least-squares regression to relationships containing autocorrelated error terms. *Journal of the American Statistical Association* **71**, 961–967.

Cohen, J. (1960). A coefficient of agreement for nominal tables. *Educational and Psychological Measurement* **20**, 37–46.

Cohen, J. (1968). Weighted kappa: nominal scale agreement with provision for scaled disagreement or partial credit. *Psychological Bulletin* **70**, 378–382.

Collaborative Ocular Melanoma Study (1989). *COMS Manual of Procedures*, NTIS Accession PB90-115536. Springfield, Va.: National Technical Information Service.

Conger, A. J. (1980). Integration and generalization of kappa for multiple raters. *Psychological Bulletin* **88**, 322–328.

Conover, W. (1971). *Practical Nonparametric Statistics*. New York: John Wiley & Sons.

Cook, R. D., and Weisberg, S. (1982). *Residuals and Influence in Regression*. London: Chapman & Hall.

Cook-Mozaffari, P. J., Darby, S. C., Doll, R., Forman, D., Hermon, C., Pike, M. C., and Vincent, T. (1989). Geographical variation in mortality from leukaemia and other cancers in England and Wales in relation to proximity to nuclear installations, 1969–78. *British Journal of Cancer* **59**, 476–485.

Coppleson, L. W., and Brown, B. (1975). Observations on a model of the biology of carcinoma of the cervix: a poor fit between observation and theory. *American Journal of Obstetrics and Gynecology* **122**, 127–136.

Costlow, R. D., Hirsekorn, J. M., Stiratelli, R. G., O'Hara, G. P., Black, D. L., Kane, W. W., Burke, S. S., Smith, J. M., and Hayes, A. W. (1983). The effects on rat pups when nitrofen (4-(2,4-dichlorophenoxy)nitrobenzene) was applied dermally to the dam during organogenesis. *Toxicology* **28**, 37–50.

Cothern, C. R. (1988). Uncertainties in quantitative risk assessment—two examples: trichloroethylene and radon in drinking water. In *Risk Assessment and Risk Management of Industrial and Environmental Chemicals*, C. R. Cothern, M. A. Mehlman, and W. L. Marcus, (eds.), pp. 159–180. Princeton, N.J.: Princeton Scientific Publishing Co.

Cox, B. G., and Cohen, S. B. (1985). *Methodological Issues for Health Care Surveys*. New York: Marcel Dekker.

Cox, D. R. (1966). Some procedures connected with the logistic qualitative response curve. In *Research Papers in Statistics: Festschrift for Jerzy Neyman* (F. N. David, ed.). London: John Wiley & Sons.

Cox, D. R. (1972). Regression models and life tables. *Journal of the Royal Statistical Society Series B* **34**, 187–220.

Cox, D. R., and Hinkley, D. V. (1974). *Theoretical Statistics.* London: Chapman & Hall.

Cox, D. R., and Miller, H. D. (1965). *The Theory of Stochastic Processes.* London: Chapman & Hall.

Cox, D. R., and Oakes, D. (1990). *Analysis of Survival Data.* London: Chapman & Hall.

Cox, D. R., and Snell, E. J. (1968). A general definition of residuals. *Journal of the Royal Statistical Society Series B* **30,** 248–275.

Cox, D. R., and Snell, E. J. (1989). *Analysis of Binary Data,* 2nd ed. New York: Chapman & Hall.

Cressie, N. (1991). *Statistics for Spatial Data.* New York: John Wiley & Sons.

Cryder, C. M., Corgan, J. N., Urquhart, N. S., and Clason, D. (1991). Isozyme analysis of progeny derived from (*Allium fistulosum* × *Allium cepa*) × *Allium cepa. Theoretical and Applied Genetics* **82,** 337–345.

Curran, P. (1988). The semivariogram in remote sensing: an introduction. *Remote Sensing of Environment* **24,** 493–507.

Cuzick, J. (1984). A review of semi-parametric models for life histories. *I.M.A. Journal of Mathematics Applied in Medicine and Biology* **1,** 323–332.

D'Agostino, R. B., Lee, M.-L., Belanger, A. J., Cupples, L. A., Anderson, K., and Kannel, W. B. (1990). Relation of pooled logistic regression to time dependent Cox regression analysis: the Framingham heart study. *Statistics in Medicine* **9,** 1501–1515.

Darroch, J. N., and McCloud, P. I. (1986). Category distinguishability and observed agreement. *Australian Journal of Statistics* **28,** 371–388.

Davies, M., and Fleiss, J. L. (1982). Measuring agreement for multinomial data. *Biometrics* **38,** 1047–1051.

Day, N. E., and Moss, S. (1986). Screening for squamous cervical cancer: duration of low risk after negative results of cervical cytology and its implication for screening policies. *British Medical Journal* **293,** 659–664.

Day, N. E., and Walter, S. D. (1984). Simplified models of screening for chronic disease: estimation procedures for mass screening programmes. *Biometrics* **40,** 1–14.

Dean, T. J., and Johnson, J. D. (1990). Proportional-plus-integral control of experimental ozone concentrations in a large open-top chamber. *Atmospheric Environment* **25,** 1123–1126.

Dean, C., and Lawless, J. F. (1989). Tests for detecting overdispersion in Poisson regression models. *Journal of the American Statistical Association* **84,** 467–472.

Dellaportas, P., and Smith, A. F. M. (1993). Bayesian inference for generalized linear and proportional hazards models via Gibbs sampling. *Applied Statistics* **42,** 443–460.

DeMets, D. L. (1984). Stopping guidelines versus stopping rules: a practitioners point of view. *Communications in Statistics: Theory and Methods* **13,** 2395–2417.

DeMets, D. L., and Ware, J. H. (1980). Group sequential methods in clinical trials with a one-sided hypothesis. *Biometrika* **67,** 651–660.

Deming, W. E. (1977). An essay on screening, or two-phase sampling, applied to surveys of a community. *International Statistical Review* **45,** 29–37.

Dewey, W. L., Harris, L. S., Howes, J. F., and Nuite, J. A. (1970). The effect of various neurohumoral modulators on the activity of morphine and the narcotic antagonists in the tailflick and phenylquinone test. *Journal of Pharmacology and Experimental Therapeutics* **175**, 435–442.

Diaconis, P., and Mosteller, F. (1989). Methods of studying coincidences. *Journal of the American Statistical Society* **84**, 853–861.

Diagnostic and Statistical Manual of Mental Disorders, 3rd ed. (1980). Washington, D.C.: American Psychiatric Association.

Diggle, P. J. (1990). A point process modeling approach to raised incidence of a rare phenomenon in the vicinity of a prespecified point. *Journal of the Royal Statistical Society Series A* **153**, 349–362.

Diggle, P. J., Lange, N., and Beneš, F. M. (1991). Analysis of variance for replicated spatial point patterns in clinical neuroanatomy. *Journal of the American Statistical Association* **86**, 618–625.

Dill, C. D. (1972). Reptilian core temperatures: variation within individuals. *Copeia* **1972**, 577–579.

Dockery, D. W., and Spengler, J. D. (1981). Personal exposures to respirable particulates and sulfates. *Journal of the Air Pollution Control Association* **31**, 153–159.

Doll, R. (1989). The epidemiology of childhood leukaemia. *Journal of the Royal Statistical Society Series A* **152**, 341–351.

Doll, R., Evans, H. J., and Darby, S. C. (1994). Paternal exposure not to blame. *Nature* **367**, 678–680.

Draper, N. R., and Smith, H. (1981). *Applied Regression Analysis*, 2nd ed. New York: John Wiley & Sons.

Draper, W. M., and Casida, J. E. (1983). Diphenyl ether herbicides and related compounds: structure–activity relationships as bacterial mutagens. *Journal of Agricultural and Food Chemistry* **31**, 1201–1207.

Drut, M. S. (1992). Habitat use and selection by sage grouse broods in southeastern Oregon. M.S. thesis. Department of Fisheries and Wildlife, Oregon State University, Corvallis, Oreg.

Duan, N. (1982). Model for human exposure to air pollution. *Environment International* **8**, 305–309.

Dubin, N., and Pasternack, B. S. (1986). Risk assessment for case-control subgroups by polychotomous logistic regression. *American Journal of Epidemiology* **123**, 1101–1117.

Duncan, A. J. (1974). *Quality Control and Industrial Statistics*, 4th ed. Homewood, Ill.: Richard D. Irwin.

Dyer, A. R., Stamler, J., Paul, O., Lepper, M., Shekelle, R. B., McKean, H., and Garside, D. (1980). Alcohol consumption and 17-year mortality in the Chicago Western Electric Company Study. *Preventive Medicine* **9**, 78–90.

Eckert, R. E. (1988). *Animal Physiology: Mechanisms and Adaptations*, 3rd ed. New York: W. H. Freeman.

Eddy, D. M. (1989). Screening for lung cancer. *Annals of Internal Medicine* **111**, 232–237.

Efron, B. (1975). The efficiency of logistic regression compared to normal theory discriminant analysis. *Journal of the American Statistical Association* **70**, 892–898.

Efron, B. (1977). The efficiency of Cox's likelihood function for censored data. *Journal of the American Statistical Association* **72**, 557–565.

Efron, B. (1982). *The Jackknife, the Bootstrap, and Other Resampling Plans.* Philadelphia: Society for Industrial and Applied Mathematics.

Efron, B. (1988). Logistic regression, survival analysis and the Kaplan–Meier curve, *Journal of the American Statistical Association* **83**, 414–425.

Elandt-Johnson, R. C., and Johnson, N. L. (1980). *Survival Models and Data Analysis.* New York: John Wiley & Sons.

Emerson, S. S. (1993). Computation of the uniform minimum variance unbiased estimator of a normal mean following a group sequential trial. *Computers and Biomedical Research* **26**, 68–73.

Emerson, S. S., and Fleming, T. R. (1989). Symmetric group sequential designs. *Biometrics* **45**, 905–923.

Emerson, S. S., and Fleming, T. R. (1990a). Interim analyses in clinical trials. *Oncology* **4**, 126–133.

Emerson, S. S., and Fleming, T. R. (1990b). Parameter estimation following group sequential hypothesis testing. *Biometrika* **77**, 875–892.

Evans, D. M. D., Hudson, E. A., Brown, C. L., Boddington, M. M., Hughes, H. E., MacKenzie, E. F. D., and Marshall, T. (1986). Terminology in gynecological cytopathology: report of the British society for clinical cytology. *Journal of Clinical Pathology* **39**, 933–944.

Ewings, P. D., Bowie, C., Phillips, M. J., and Johnson, S. A. N. (1989). Incidence of leukaemia in young people in the vicinity of Hinkley Point nuclear power station, 1959–86. *British Medical Journal* **299**, 289–293.

Eynon, B., and Switzer, P. (1983). The variability of rainfall acidity. *The Canadian Journal of Statistics* **11**, 11–24.

Fienberg, S. E., and Kaye, D. H. (1991). Legal and statistical aspects of some mysterious clusters. *Journal of the Royal Statistical Society Series A* **154**, 143–155.

Finerty, J. P. (1980). *The Population Ecology of Cycles in Small Mammals.* New Haven, Conn.: Yale University Press.

Finney, D. (1941). On the distribution of a variate whose logarithm is normally distributed. *Supplement to the Journal of the Royal Statistical Society* **7**, 155–161.

Fisher, R. A. (1935). *The Design of Experiments.* Edinburgh: Oliver & Boyd.

Fisher, R. A. (1958). *Statistical Methods for Research Workers*, 13th ed. New York: Hafner Press.

Fisher, R. A., and Yates, F. (1963). *Statistical Tables for Biological, Agricultural and Medical Research*, 3rd ed. New York: Hafner Press.

Flehinger, B. J., Kimmel, M., and Melamed, M. R. (1988). Natural history of adenocarcinoma–large cell carcinoma of lung: conclusions from screening programs in New York and Baltimore. *Journal of the National Cancer Institute* **80**, 337–344.

Flehinger, B. J., Kimmel, M., and Melamed, M. R. (1992). The effect of surgical treatment on survival from lung cancer: implications for screening. *Chest* **101**, 1013–1018.

Flehinger, B. J., Melamed, M. R., Zaman, M. B., Heelan, R. J., Perchick, W. B., and

Martini, N. (1984). Early lung cancer detection: results of the initial (prevalence) radiologic and cytologic screening in the Memorial Sloan-Kettering study. *American Review of Respiratory Diseases* **130,** 555–560.

Flehinger, B. J., and Kimmel, M. (1987). The natural history of lung cancer in a periodically screened population. *Biometrics* **43,** 44–53.

Flehinger, B. J., Kimmel, M., Polyak, T., and Melamed, M. R. (1993). Screening for lung cancer: The Mayo Lung Project revisited. *Cancer* **72,** 1573–1580.

Fleiss, J. L. (1986). *The Design and Analysis of Clinical Experiments.* New York: John Wiley & Sons.

Fleming, T. R., and Harrington, D. P. (1991). *Counting Processes and Survival Analysis.* New York: John Wiley & Sons.

Fontana, R. S., Sanderson, D. R., Taylor, W. F., Woolner, L. B., Miller, W. E., Muhm, J. R., and Uhlenhopp, M. A. (1984). Early lung cancer detection: results of the initial (prevalence) radiologic and cytologic screening in the Mayo Clinic study. *American Review of Respiratory Diseases* **130,** 561–565.

Fontana, R. S., Sanderson, D. R., Woolner, L. B., Taylor, W. F., Miller, W. E., and Muhm, J. R. (1986). Lung cancer screening: the Mayo program. *Journal of Occupational Medicine* **28,** 746–750.

Foster, R. B. (1985). Environmental legislation. In *Fundamentals of Aquatic Toxicology*, G. M. Rand and S. R. Petrocelli (eds.), pp. 587–600. Washington, D.C.: Hemisphere Publishing Corporation.

Francis, B. M. (1989). Relative developmental toxicities on nine diphenyl ethers related to nitrofen. *Environmental Toxicology and Chemistry* **8,** 681–688.

Fraser, T. R. (1872). The antagonism between the actions of active substances. *British Medical Journal* **2,** 485–487.

Frost, J. K., Ball, W. C., Levin, M. L., Tockman, M. S., Baker, R. R., Carter, D., et al. (1984). Early lung cancer detection: results of the initial (prevalence) radiologic and cytologic screening in the Johns Hopkins Study. *American Review of Respiratory Diseases* **130,** 549–554.

Fuller, W. A. (1987). *Measurement Error Models.* New York: John Wiley & Sons.

Garber, A. M., and MaCurdy, T. (1989). *Predicting Nursing Home Utilization Among the High-Risk Elderly*, Working Paper Series 2843. Cambridge, Mass.: National Bureau of Economic Research, pp. 1–44.

Gardner, M. J. (1989). Review of reported incidence of childhood cancer rates in the vicinity of nuclear installations in the UK. *Journal of the Royal Statistical Society Series A* **152,** 307–325.

Garfinkel, L., and Stellman, S. D. (1988). Smoking and lung cancer in women: findings in a prospective study. *Cancer Research* **48,** 6951–6955.

Garland, T., Jr., and Adolph, S. C. (1991). Physiological differentiation of vertebrate populations. *Annual Review of Ecology and Systematics* **22,** 193–228.

Garrison, C. Z., Schluchter, M. D., Schoenback, V. J., and Kaplan, B. K. (1989). Epidemiology of depressive symptoms in young adolescents. *Journal of the American Academy of Child and Adolescent Psychiatry* **28,** 343–351.

Garrison, C. Z., Jackson, K. L., Addy, C. L., McKeown, R. E., and Waller, J. L. (1991).

Suicidal behaviors in young adolescents. *American Journal of Epidemiology* **133**, 1005–1014.

Garrison, C. Z., Addy, C. L., Jackson, K. L., McKewon, R. E., and Waller, J. L. (1992). Major depressive disorder and dysthymia in young adolescents. *American Journal of Epidemiology* **135**, 792–802.

Gelfand, A. E., and Smith, A. F. M. (1990). Sampling-based approaches to calculating marginal densities. *Journal of the American Statistical Association* **85**, 398–409.

Gelfand, A. E., Hills, S. E., Racine-Poon, A., and Smith, A. F. M. (1990). Illustration of Bayesian inference in normal data models using Gibbs sampling. *Journal of the American Statistical Association* **85**, 972–985.

Gelman, A., and Rubin, D. R. (1992). A single series from the Gibbs sampler provides a false sense of security. In *Bayesian Statistics*, vol. 4, J. M. Bernardo, J. Berger, A. P. Dawid, and A. F. M. Smith (eds.), pp. 627–633. Oxford: Oxford University Press.

Geman, S., and Geman, D. (1984). Stochastic relaxation, Gibbs distributions, and the Bayesian restoration of images. *IEEE Transactions on Pattern Analysis and Machine Intelligence* **6**, 721–741.

Gennings, C., Carter, W. H., Jr., Campbell, E. D., Staniswalis, J. G., Martin, T. J., Martin, B. R., and White, K. L., Jr. (1990). Isobolographic characterization of drug interactions incorporating biological variability. *Journal of Pharmacology and Experimental Therapeutics* **252**, 208–217.

Giesbrecht, F. G. (1983). An efficient procedure for computing MINQUE of variance components and generalized least squares estimates of fixed effects. *Communications in Statistics: Theory and Methods* **12**, 2169–2177.

Gilbert, E. W. (1958). Pioneer maps of health and disease in England. *Geographical Journal* **124**, 172–183.

Gilbert, R., and Simpson, J. (1985). Kriging for estimating spatial patterns of contaminants: potential and problems. *Environmental Monitoring and Assessment* **5**, 113–135.

Gilks, W. R., and Wild, P. (1992). Adaptive rejection sampling for Gibbs sampling. *Applied Statistics* **41**, 337–348.

Gilks, W. R., Clayton, D. G., Spiegelhalter, D. J., Best, N. G., McNeil, A. J., Sharples, L. D., and Kirby, A. J. (1993). Modelling complexity: applications of Gibbs sampling in medicine. *Journal of the Royal Statistical Society Series B* **55**, 39–52.

Ginsberg, C. K. (1991). Exfoliative cytological screening: the Papanicolaou test. *Journal of Obstetric, Gynecologic, and Neonatal Nursing* **20**, 39–46.

Goggans, R. (1986). Habitat use by flammulated owls in northeastern Oregon. M.S. Thesis. Department of Fisheries and Wildlife. Oregon State University, Corvallis, Oreg.

Goodman, L. A. (1979). Simple models for the analysis of assiciation in cross-classifications having ordered categories. *Journal of the American Statistical Association* **74**, 537–552.

Goodman, L. A. (1985). The analysis of cross-classified data having ordered and/or unordered categories: association models, correlation models, and asymmetry models for contingency tables with or without missing entries. *Annals of Statistics* **13**, 10–69.

Gori, D. F. (1989). Floral color change in *Lupinus argenteus* (Fabaceae): why should plants advertise the location of unrewarding flowers to pollinators? *Evolution* **43,** 870–881.

Graham, J. (1991). Longitudinal analysis for binary and count data. M.Sc. thesis. Department of Statistics, University of British Columbia, Vancouver, British Columbia, Canada.

Graybill, F. A. (1976). *Theory and Application of the General Linear Model.* Pacific Grove, Calif.: Wadsworth.

Greenhouse, S. W., and Geisser, S. (1959). On methods in the analysis of profile data. *Psychometrika* **24,** 95–112.

Haberman, S. J. (1974). Log-linear models for frequency tables with ordered classifications. *Biometrics* **30,** 589–600.

Halliday, R. G., and Koeller, P. A. (1981). A history of Canadian groundfish trawling surveys and data usage in ICNAF Divisions 4TVWX, in *Bottom Trawl Surveys,* Canadian Special Publication of Fisheries and Aquatic Science 58, W. G. Doubleday and D. Rivard (eds.), pp. 27–42.

Halpern, M. T., Gillespie, B. W., and Warner, K. E. (1993). Patterns of absolute risk of lung cancer mortality in former smokers. *Journal of the National Cancer Institute* **85,** 457–464.

Hartley, D., and Kidd, H. (eds.) (1987). *The Agrochemicals Handbook,* 2nd ed. Nottingham, U.K.: The Royal Society of Chemistry Information Services.

Hasabelnaby, N. A., and Fuller, W. A. (1991). Measurement error models with unequal error variances. In *Proceedings of the International Workshop on Statistical Modelling and Latent Variables,* K. Haagen, D. Bartholomew, and M. Deistler, (eds.). Amsterdam: North-Holland/Elsevier.

Hastie, T., and Tibshirani, R. (1990a). Exploring the nature of covariate effects in the proportional hazards model. *Biometrics* **46,** 1005–1016.

Hastie, T., and Tibshirani, R. (1990b). *Generalized Additive Models.* London: Chapman & Hall.

Hastings, W. K. (1970). Monte Carlo sampling methods using Markov chains and their applications. *Biometrika* **57,** 97–109.

Heck, W. W., Heagle, A. S., Miller, J. E., and Rawlings, J. O. (1991). A national program (NCLAN) to assess the impact of ozone on agricultural resources. In *Tropospheric Ozone and the Environment; Papers from an International Conference,* Los Angeles, R. L. Berglund, D. R Lawson, and D. J. McKee (eds.), pp. 225–254, Transaction Series 19. Pittsburgh, Pa.: Air and Waste Management Association.

Heisey, D. M. (1985). Analyzing selection experiments with log-linear models. *Ecology* **66,** 1744–1748.

Higgins, I. T., and Wynder, E. L. (1988). Reduction in risk of lung cancer among ex-smokers with particular reference to histologic type. *Cancer* **62,** 2397–2401.

Hoaglin, D. C., and Welsch, R. E. (1978). The hat matrix in regression and ANOVA. *American Statistician* **32,** 17–22 (Corr. **32,** 146).

Hosmer, D. W., Jr. (1973). A comparison of iterative maximum likelihood estimates of the parameters of a mixture of two normal distributions under three different types of sample. *Biometrics* **29,** 761–770.

Hosmer, D. W., Jr., and Lemeshow, S. (1980). Goodness-of-fit tests for the multiple logistic regression model. *Communications in Statistics: Theory and Methods* **10**, 1043–1069.

Hosmer, D. W., and Lemeshow, S. (1989). *Applied Logistic Regression*. New York: John Wiley & Sons.

Hosmer, D. W., Lemeshow, S., and Klar, J. (1988). Goodness-of-fit testing for multiple logistic regression analysis when the estimated probabilities are small. *Biometrical Journal* **30**, 911–924.

Hosmer, D. W., Taber, S., and Lemeshow, S. (1991). The importance of assessing the fit of logistic regression models: a case study. *American Journal of Public Health* **81**, 1630–1635.

Huey, R. (1982). Temperature, physiology and the ecology of reptiles. In *Biology of the Reptilia*, vol. 13, C. Gans and F. H. Pough (eds.), pp. 25–91. New York: Academic Press.

Huynh, H., and Feldt, L. S. (1970). Conditions under which mean square ratios in repeated measurements designs have exact F-distributions. *Journal of the American Statistical Association* **65**, 1582–1589.

Ikeda, S., Yanai, N., and Ishikawa, S. (1968). Flexible bronchofiberscope. *Keio Journal of Medicine* **17**, 16–18.

Ingram, D. D., and Kleinman, J. C. (1989). Empirical comparisons of proportional hazards and logistic regression models. *Statistics in Medicine* **8**, 525–538.

Isaaks, E., and Srivastava, R. (1989). *An Introduction to Applied Geostatistics*. New York: Oxford University Press.

Jassby, A. D., and Powell, T. M. (1990). Detecting changes in ecological time series. *Ecology* **71**, 2044–2052.

Jennings, D. E. (1986). Judging inference adequacy in logistic regression. *Journal of the American Statistical Association* **81**, 471–476.

Jennison, C., and Turnbull, B. W. (1984). Repeated confidence intervals for group sequential trials. *Controlled Clinical Trials* **5**, 33–45.

Jennison, C., and Turnbull, B. W. (1989). Interim analyses: the repeated confidence interval approach (with discussion). *Journal of the Royal Statistical Society Series B* **51**, 305–361.

Johnson, D. H. (1980). The comparison of usage and availability measurements for evaluating resource preference. *Ecology* **61**, 65–71.

Jones, R. H. (1980). Maximum likelihood fitting of ARMA models to time series with missing observations. *Technometrics* **22**, 389–395.

Kahn, H. A., and Sempos, C. T. (1989). *Statistical Methods in Epidemiology*. New York: Oxford University Press.

Kalbfleisch, J. B., and Lawless, J. F. (1985). The analysis of panel data under a Markov assumption. *Journal of the American Statistical Association* **80**, 863–871.

Kalbfleisch, J. D., and Prentice, R. L. (1980). *The Statistical Analysis of Failure Time Data*. New York: John Wiley & Sons.

Kaldor, J., and Clayton, D. G. (1985). Latent class analysis in chronic disease epidemiology. *Statistics in Medicine* **4**, 327–336.

Kaplan, E. L., and Meier, P. (1958). Nonparametric estimation from incomplete observations. *Journal of the American Statistical Association* **53**, 457–481.

Karasov, W. H. (1992). Daily energy expenditure and the cost of activity in mammals. *American Zoologist* **32**, 238–248.

Katz, R. H. (1981). On some criteria for estimating the order of a Markov chain. *Technometrics* **23**, 243–249.

Katz, S., and Akpom, C. A. (1976). Index of ADL. *Medical Care* **14**, 116–118.

Kemmerlin, W. R. (1986). Efficiency in two stage sampling for a normal mixture. Master's thesis, University of South Carolina, Columbia, S.C.

Kemmerlin, W. R., and Jackson, K. L. (1987). Maximum likelihood estimation and simulation for one and two stage sampling of normal mixtures using SAS software. *SUGI Proceedings* **12**, 1137–1140.

Kimbrough, R. D., Gaines, T. B., and Linder, R. E. (1974). 2,4-Dichlorophenyl-*p*-nitrophenyl ether: effects on lung maturation of rat fetus. *Archives of Environmental Health* **28**, 316–320.

Kimbrough, R. D., Mitchell, F. L., and Houk, V. N. (1985). Trichloroethylene: an update. *Journal of Toxicology and Environmental Health* **15**, 369–383.

Kimmel, M., and Flehinger, B. J. (1991). Nonparametric estimation of the size–metastasis relationship in solid cancers. *Biometrics* **47**, 987–1004.

Kingsolver, J. G., and Watt, W. B. (1983). Thermoregulatory strategies in *Colias* butterflies: thermal stress and the limits to adaptation in temporally varying environments. *The American Naturalist* **121**, 32–55.

Kirby, A. J., Spiegelhalter, D. J., Day, N. E., Fenton, L., and McGregor, E. J. (1992). Conservative treatment of mild/moderate dyskaryosis: long term outcome. *Lancet* **339**, 828–831.

Knox, E. G. (1988). Evaluation of a proposed breast cancer screening programme. *British Medical Journal* **297**, 650–654.

Koenig, J. Q., Covert, D. S., Marshall, S. G., van Belle, G., and Peirson, W. E. (1987). The effects of ozone and nitrogen dioxide on pulmonary function in healthy and in asthmatic adolescents. *American Review of Respiratory Diseases* **136**, 1152–1157.

Korn, E. L., and Graubard, B. I. (1991). Epidemiologic studies utilizing surveys: accounting for the sampling design. *American Journal of Public Health* **81**, 1166–1173.

Korn, L. R., Hosmer, D. W., and Lemeshow, S. (1986). The performance of a goodness-of-fit test for logistic regression with discrete covariates. *Biometrical Journal* **28**, 697–708.

Koutrakis, P., Wolfson, J. M., Bunyaviroch, A., Froehlich, S. E., Kirano, K., and Mulik, J. D. (1993). Measurement of ambient ozone using a nitrite-coated filter. *Analytical Chemistry* **65**, 209–214.

Kress, L. W., and Allen, H. L. (1991). Impact of ozone and acidic precipitation on the growth of loblolly pine seedlings. In *Proceedings of the 84th Annual Meeting and Exhibition of Air and Waste Management Association*, Vancouver, British Columbia, Canada, Paper 91-142.9. Pittsburgh, Pa.: Air and Waste Management Association.

Kress, L. W., Allen, H. L., Mudano, J. E., and Heck, W. W. (1988). Response of loblolly pine to acidic precipitation and ozone. In *Proceedings of the 81st Annual Meeting of the Air Pollution Control Association*, Dallas, Paper 88-70.5. Pittsburgh, Pa.: Air Pollution Control Association.

Krige, D., and Magri, E. (1982). Geostatistical case studies of the advantages of lognormal–de Wijsian kriging with mean for a base metal mine and a gold mine. *Mathematical Geology* **14**, 547–555.

Kulle, T. J., Sauder, L. R., Hebel, J. R., and Chatham, M. D. (1985). Ozone response relationships in healthy nonsmokers. *American Review of Respiratory Diseases* **132**, 36–41.

Kuo, L., and Yiannoutsos, C. (1991). *Emiprical Bayes Risk Evaluation with Type II Censored Data*. Monterey, Calif.: United States Navy, Naval Postgraduate School.

Kupper, L. L., Janis, J. M., Karmous, A., and Greenberg, B. G. (1985). Statistical age–period–cohort analysis: a review and critique. *Journal of Chronic Diseases* **38**, 811–830.

Lagakos, S. W., Wessen, B. J., and Zelen, M. (1986). An analysis of contaminated water and health effects in Woburn, Massachusetts (with discussion). *Journal of the American Statistical Society* **81**, 583–614.

Laird, N., and Olivier, D. (1981). Covariance analysis of censored survival data using log-linear analysis techniques. *Journal of the American Statistical Association* **76**, 231–240.

Lan, K. K. G., and DeMets, D. L. (1983). Discrete sequential boundaries for clinical trials. *Biometrika* **70**, 659–663.

Lancaster, T. (1990). *The Economic Analysis of Transition Data*. New York: Cambridge University Press.

Landis, J. R., and Koch, G. G. (1977). The measurement of observed agreement for categorical data. *Biometrics* **33**, 159–174.

Landwehr, J. M., Pregibon, D., and Shoemaker, A. C. (1984). Graphical methods for assessing logistic regression models. *Journal of the American Statistical Association* **79**, 61–71.

Lange, N. (1992). Graphs and stochastic relaxation for hierarchical Bayes models. *Statistics in Medicine* **11**, 2001–2016.

Lange, N., Carlin, B. P., and Gelfand, A. E. (1992). Hierarchical Bayes models for the progression of HIV infection using longitudinal CD4 T-cell numbers (with discussion). *Journal of the American Statistical Association* **87**, 615–626.

Lawless, J. F. (1982). *Statistical Models and Methods for Lifetime Data*. New York: John Wiley & Sons.

Lawless, J. F., and Singhal, K. (1978). Efficient screening of non-normal regression models. *Biometrics* **34**, 318–328.

Lawson, A. (1993). On the analysis of mortality events associated with a prespecified fixed point. *Journal of the Royal Statistical Society Series A* **156**, 363–377.

Lee, H.-H., Lu, P.-Y., Metcalf, R. L., and Hsu, E.-L. (1976). The environmental fate of three dichlorophenyl nitrophenyl ether herbicides in a rice paddy model ecosystem. *Journal of Environmental Quality* **5**, 482–486.

Lesaffre, E., and Albert, A. (1989a). Partial separation in logistic discrimination. *Journal of the Royal Statistical Society Series B* **51**, 109–116.

Lesaffre, E., and Albert, A. (1989b). Multiple-group logistic regression diagnostics. *Applied Statistics* **38**, 425–440.

Lesser, V. M., Rawlings, J. O., Spruill, S. E., and Somerville, M. C. (1990). Ozone effects on agricultural crops: statistical methodologies and estimated dose-response relationships. *Crop Science* **30**, 148–155.

Levison, M. E., and Haddon, W. (1965). The area adjusted map: an epidemiologic device. *Public Health Reports* **80**, 55–59.

Lewis, P. A. W., and Orav, E. J. (1989). *Simulation Methodology for Statisticians, Operations Analysts, and Engineers*, Vol. 1. Belmont, Calif.: Wadsworth.

Liang, K. Y., and Zeger, S. L. (1986). Longitudinal data analysis using generalized linear models. *Biometrika* **73**, 13–22.

Light, R. J. (1971). Measures of response agreement for qualitative data: some generalizations and alternatives. *Psychological Bulletin* **5**, 365–377.

Limam, M. M. T., and Thomas, D. R. (1988). Simultaneous tolerance intervals for the linear regression model. *Journal of the American Statistical Association* **83**, 801–804.

Lin, L. I. K. (1989). A concordance correlation coefficient to evaluate reproducibility. *Biometrics* **45**, 255–268.

Lippmann, M. (1989). Health effects of ozone: a critical review. *Journal of the Air Pollution Control Association* **39**, 672–695.

Liu, K., Cougthlin, T., and McBridmam, T. (1991). Predicting nursing-home admission and length of stay: a duration analysis. *Medical Care* **29**, 1–18.

Liu, L.-J. S., Koutrakis, P., Suh, H. H., Mulik, J. D., and Burton, R. M. (1993). Use of personal measurements for ozone exposure assessment: a pilot study. *Environmental Health Perspectives* **101**, 318–324.

Ljung, G. M., and Box, G. E. P. (1978). On a measure of a lack of fit in time series models. *Biometrika* **65**, 297–303.

Loewe, S. (1957). Antagonisms and antagonists. *Pharmacology Review* **9**, 237–242.

Lubin, J. H., Blot, W. J., Berrino, F., Flamant, R., Gillis, C. R., Kunze, M., Schmahl, D., and Visco, G. (1984). Modifying risk of developing lung cancer by changing habits of cigarette smoking. *British Medical Journal* **288**, 1953–1956.

Lunney, D., Barker, J., Priddel, D., and O'Connell, M. (1988). Roost selection by Gould's long-eared bat, *Nyctophilus gouldi* Tomes (Chiroptera: Vespertilionidae), in logged forest on the south coast of New South Wales. *Australian Wildlife Research* **15**, 375–384.

MacKay, R. S. (1964). Galapagos tortoise and marine iguana deep body temperatures measured by radiotelemetry. *Nature* **204**, 355–358.

Mackintosh, N. J. (1983). *Conditioning and Associative Learning*. Oxford: Clarendon Press.

Maclure, M., and Willett, W. C. (1987). Reviews and commentary: misinterpretation and misuse of the kappa statistic. *American Journal of Epidemiology* **126**, 161–169.

Mandelli, F., Petti, M. C., Ardia, A., Di Pietro, N., Di Raimondo, F., Ganzina, F., Falconi, E., Geraci, E., Ladogana, S., Latagliata, R., Malleo, C., Nobile, F., Petti, N., Rotoli, B., Specchi, G., Tabilio, A., and Resegotti, L. (1991). A randomized clinical trial comparing idarubicin and cytarabine to daunorubicin and cytarabine in the treatment of acute nonlymphoid leukemia. *European Journal of Cancer* **27**, 750–755.

Mantel, N. (1966). Models for complex contingency tables and polychotomous dosage response curves. *Biometrics* **22**, 83–95.

Mantel, N. (1973). Synthetic retrospective studies and related topics. *Biometrics* **29**, 479–486.

Marcum, C. L., and Loftsgaarden, D. O. (1980). A nonmapping technique for studying habitat preferences. *Journal of Wildlife Management* **44**, 963–968.

Marshall, R. J. (1991). A review of methods for the statistical analysis of spatial patterns of disease. *Journal of the Royal Statistical Society Series A* **154**, 421–441.

Marshall, R. J., and Chisolm, E. M. (1985). Hypothesis testing in the polychotomous logistic model with an application to detecting gastrointestinal cancer. *Statistics in Medicine* **4**, 337–344.

Mather, D., and Silver, C. A. (1980). Statistical problems in studies of temperature preference of fishes. *Canadian Journal of Fisheries and Aquatic Science* **37**, 733–737.

Matheron, G. (1963). Principles of geostatistics. *Economic Geology* **58**, 1246–1266.

McCullagh, P., and Nelder, J. A. (1989). *Generalized Linear Models*, 2nd ed. London: Chapman & Hall.

McDonnell, W. F., Horstman, D. H., Hazucha, M. J., Seal, E., Jr., Haak, E. D., Salaam, S. A., and House, D. E. (1983). Pulmonary effects of ozone exposure during exercise: dose-response characteristics. *Journal of Applied Physiology* **54**, 1345–1397.

McKone, T. E. (1987). Human exposure to volatile organic compounds in household tap water: the indoor inhalation pathway. *Environmental Science and Technology* **21**, 1194–1201.

McKone, T. E., and Bogen, K. T. (1991). Predicting the uncertainties in risk assessment: a California groundwater case study. *Environmental Science and Technology* **25**, 1674–1681.

McKone, T. E., and Bogen, K. T. (1992). Uncertainties in health risk assessment: an integrated case study based on tetrachloroethylene in California groundwater. *Regulatory Toxicology and Pharmacology* **15**, 86–103.

Melamed, M. R., Flehinger, B., Miller, D., Osborne, R., Zaman, J., McGinnis, C., and Martini, N. (1977). Preliminary report of the lung cancer detection program in New York. *Cancer* **39**, 369–382.

Melamed, M. R., Flehinger, B. J., Zaman, M. B., Heelan, R. T., Hallerman, R. T., and Martini, N. (1981). Detection of true pathologic Stage I lung cancer in a screening program and the effect on survival. *Cancer* **47**, March 1 Supplement, 1182–1187.

Melamed, M. R., Flehinger, B. J., Zaman, M. B., Heelan, R. T., Perchick, W. A., and Martini, N. (1984). Screening for early lung cancer: results of the Memorial Sloan-Kettering study in New York. *Chest* **86**, 44–53.

Melamed, M. R., Flehinger, B. J., and Fontana, R. S. (1990). Should asymptomatic cigarette smokers have annual chest x-rays after age 55 years? In *Debates in Medicine*, Vol. 3, G. Gitnick, H. V. Barnes, T. P. Duffy, R. P. Lewis, and R. H. Winterbauer (eds.). Chicago: Year Book Medical Publishers.

Metropolis, N., Rosenbluth, A. W., Rosenbluth, M. N., Teller, A. H., and Teller, E.

(1953). Equation of state calculations by fast computing machines. *The Journal of Chemical Physics* **21,** 1087–1092.

Miller, R. G. (1981). *Simultaneous Statistical Inference,* 2nd ed. New York: Springer-Verlag.

Miller, R. G., Efron, B., Brown, B. W., and Moses, L. E. (1980). *Biostatistics Casebook.* New York: John Wiley & Sons.

Morel, J. G. (1989). Logistic regression under complex survey designs. *Survey Methodology* **15,** 203–233.

Morrison, A. S. (1985). *Screening in Chronic Diseases.* New York: Oxford University Press.

Morrison, D. F. (1976). *Multivariate Statistical Methods.* New York: McGraw-Hill.

Mosteller, F., and Tukey, J. W. (1977). *Data Analysis and Regression.* Reading, Mass.: Addison-Wesley.

Mount, D. I. (1977). Present approaches to toxicity testing: a perspective. In *Aquatic Toxicology and Hazard Evaluation,* ASTM STP 624, F. L. Mayer and J. L. Hamelink (eds.), pp. 5–14. Philadelphia: American Society for Testing and Materials.

Mount, D. I., and Brungs, W. A. (1967). A simplified dosing apparatus for fish toxicology studies. *Water Resources* **1,** 21–29.

Myers, R. H. (1990). *Classical and Modern Regression with Applications,* 2nd ed. Boston, PWS-Kent.

Naiman, R. J., Melillo, J. M., and Hobbie, J. E. (1986). Ecosystem alteration of boreal forest streams by beaver (*Castor canadensis*). *Ecology* **67,** 1254–1269.

Nash, F. A., Morgan, J. M., and Tompkins, J. G. (1986). South London lung cancer study. *British Medical Journal* **2,** 715–721.

Neilson, J. D., and Bowering, W. R. (1989). Minimum size regulations and the implications for yield and value in the Canadian Atlantic halibut (*Hippoglossus hippoglossus*) fishery. *Canadian Journal of Fisheries and Aquatic Sciences* **46,** 1899–1903.

Neilson, J. D., Waiwood, K. G., and Smith, S. J. (1989). Survival of Atlantic halibut (*Hippoglossus hippoglossus*) caught by longline and otter trawl gear. *Canadian Journal of Fisheries and Aquatic Sciences* **46,** 887–897.

Neter, J., Wasserman, W., and Kutner, M. H. (1989). *Applied Linear Regression Models,* 2nd ed. Homewood, Ill.: Richard D. Irwin.

Neter, J., Wasserman, W., and Kutner, M. H. (1990). *Applied Linear Statistical Models,* 3rd ed. Homewood, Ill.: Richard D. Irwin.

Neu, C. W., Byers, C. R., and Peek, J. M. (1974). A technique for analysis of utilization–availability data. *Journal of Wildlife Management* **38,** 541–545.

New York State Department of Environmental Conservation (1987). *Inactive Hazardous Waste Disposal Sites in New York State,* Vol. 7. Albany, N.Y.: New York State.

Neyman, J. (1938). Contributions to the theory of sampling human populations. *Journal of the American Statistical Association* **33,** 101–116.

Neyman, J. (1949). Contribution to the theory of the chi-square test. In *Proceedings of the Berkeley Symposium on Mathematical Statistics and Probability,* pp. 239–273. Berkeley, Calif.: University of California Press.

Norberg-King, T. J. (1988). *An Interpolation Estimate for Chronic Toxicity: The ICp Approach.* National Effluent Toxicity Assessment Center Technical Report 05-88.

Duluth, Minn.: U.S. Environmental Protection Agency, Environmental Research Laboratory–Duluth.

Noyes, R., Jr., Brunk, S. F., Avery, D. H., and Canter, A. (1975). The analgesic properties of Δ^9-tetrahydrocannabinol and codeine. *Clinical Pharmacology and Therapeutics* **18,** 84–89.

O'Brien, P. C., and Fleming, T. R. (1979). A multiple testing procedure for clinical trials. *Biometrics* **35,** 549–565.

Ockene, J. K., Kuller, L. H., Svendsen, K. H., and Meilahn, E. (1990). The relationship of smoking cessation to coronary heart disease and lung cancer in the Multiple Risk Factor Intervention Trial (MRFIT). *American Journal of Public Health* **80,** 954–958.

O'Connell, D. L., and Dobson, A. J. (1984). General observer-agreement measures on individual subjects and groups of subjects. *Biometrics* **40,** 973–983.

Olson, D., Bell, R., and Portner, J. (1982). *FACES II.* St. Paul, Minn.: University of Minnesota.

Openshaw, S., Craft, A. W., Charlton, M., and Birch, J. M. (1988). Investigation of leukemia clusters by use of a geographical analysis machine. *Lancet,* 272–273.

Oris, J. T., and Bailer, A. J. (1993). Statistical analysis of the Ceriodaphnia toxicity test: sample size determination for reproductive effects. *Environmental Toxicology and Chemistry* **12,** 85–90.

Oris, J. T., Winner, R. W., and Moore, M. V. (1991). A four-day Ceriodaphnia survival and reproduction toxicity test. *Environmental Toxicology and Chemistry* **10,** 217–224.

O'Rourke, D., and Blair, J. (1983). Improving random respondent selection in telephone surveys. *Journal of Marketing Research* **20,** 428–432.

Osborne, C. (1992). Statistical calibration: a review. *International Statistical Review* **60.**

Paul, C. (1988). The New Zealand cervical cancer study: could it happen again? *British Medial Journal* **297,** 533–539.

Paynter, V. A., Reardon, J. C., and Shelburne, V. B. (1991). Carbohydrate changes in shortleaf pine (*Pinus echinata*) needles exposed to acid rain and ozone. *Canadian Journal of Forest Research* **21,** 666–671.

Pederson, L. L., Bull, S. B., Ashley, M. J., and Lefcoe, N. M. (1987). A population survey in Ontario regarding restrictive measures on smoking: relationship of smoking status to knowledge, attitudes and predicted behaviour. *International Journal of Epidemiology* **16,** 383–391.

Pederson, L. L., Bull, S. B., Ashley, M. J., and Lefcoe, N. M. (1989). A population survey on legislative measures to restrict smoking in Ontario. 3. Variables related to attitudes of smokers and nonsmokers. *American Journal of Preventive Medicine* **5,** 313–322.

Pederson, L. L., Wanklin, J. M., Bull, S. B., and Ashley, M. J. (1991). A conceptual framework for the roles of legislation and education in reducing exposure to environmental tobacco smoke. *American Journal of Health Promotion* **6,** 105–111.

Pederson, L. L., Bull, S. B., Ashley, M. J., Garcia, J. M., and Lefcoe, N. M. (1993). Evaluation of the workplace smoking by-law in the City of Toronto. *American Journal of Public Health* **83,** 1342–1345.

Peffley, E. B., Corgan, J. N., Horak, K. E., and Tanksley, S. D. (1985). Electrophoretic analysis of Allium alien addition lines. *Theoretical and Applied Genetics* **71**, 176–184.

Pennington, M. (1983). Efficient estimates of abundance for fish and plankton surveys. *Biometrics* **39**, 281–286.

Pereira, J. M. C., and Itami, R. M. (1991). GIS-based habitat modeling using logistic multiple regression: a study of the Mt. Graham red squirrel. *Photogrammetric Engineering and Remote Sensing* **57**, 1475–1486.

Peterson, C. R. (1987). Daily variation in the body temperatures of free-ranging garter snakes. *Ecology* **68**, 160–169.

Pocock, S. J. (1977). Group sequential methods in the design and analysis of clinical trials. *Biometrika* **64**, 191–199.

Pocock, S. J. (1983). *Clinical Trials: A Practical Approach.* New York: John Wiley & Sons.

Pocock, S. J., Geller, N. L., and Tsiatis, A. A. (1987). The analysis of multiple endpoints in clinical trials. *Biometrics* **43**, 487–498.

Poole, S., and Stephenson, J. E. (1977). Core temperature: some short-comings of rectal temperature measurements. *Physiology and Behaviour* **18**, 203–205.

Posner, K. L., Sampson, P. D., Caplan, R. A., Ward, R. J., and Cheney, F. W. (1990). Measuring interrater reliability among multiple raters: an example of methods for nominal data. *Statistics in Medicine* **9**, 1103–1115.

Pregibon, D. (1981). Logistic regression diagnostics. *Annals of Statistics* **9**, 705–724.

Prentice, R. L., and Pyke, R. (1979). Logistic disease incidence models and case-control studies. *Biometrika* **66**, 403–411.

Press, S. J. (1972). *Applied Multivariate Analysis.* New York: Holt, Rinehart and Winston.

Press, S. J., and Wilson, S. (1978). Choosing between logistic regression and discriminant analysis. *Journal of the American Statistical Association* **73**, 699–705.

Prichard, M. N., and Shipman, C., Jr. (1990). Mini review: a three-dimensional model to analyze drug–drug interactions. *Antiviral Research*, **14**, 181–205.

Prorok, P. C. (1976a). The theory of periodic screening. I. Lead time and proportion detected. *Advances in Applied Probability* **8**, 127–143.

Prorok, P. C. (1976b). The theory of periodic screening. II. Doubly bounded recurrence times and mean lead time and detection probability estimation. *Advances in Applied Probability* **8**, 460–476.

Radloff, L. S. (1977). The CES-D scale: a self-report depression scale for research in the general population. *Applied Psychological Measurement* **1**, 385–401.

Raftery, A., and Lewis, S. (1991). How many iterations in the Gibbs sampler? In *Bayesian Statistics*, Vol. 4, J. M. Bernardo, J. Berger, A. P. Dawid, and A. F. M. Smith (eds.). Oxford: Oxford University Press.

Rao, C. R. (1973). *Linear Statistical Inference and Its Application*, 2nd ed. New York: John Wiley & Sons.

Rao, J. N. K., Kumar, S., and Roberts, G. (1989). Analysis of sample survey data involving categorical response variables: methods and software. *Survey Methodology* **15**, 161–186.

Rawlings, J. O. (1988). *Applied Regression Analysis: A Research Tool.* Pacific Grove, Calif.: Wadsworth and Brooks/Cole.

Rawlings, J. O., and Cure, W. W. (1985). The Weibull function as a dose-response model to describe ozone effects on crop yield. *Crop Science* **25,** 807–814.

Raynor, W. J., Shekelle, R. B., Rossof, A. H., Maliza, C., and Paul, O. (1981). High blood pressure and 17-year cancer mortality in the Western Electric Health Study. *American Journal of Epidemiology* **13,** 371–377.

Reid, N., and Crepeau, H. (1985). Influence functions for proportional hazards regression. *Biometrika* **72,** 1–9.

Reynolds, T. D., and Laundré, J. W. (1990). Time intervals for estimating pronghorn and coyote home ranges and daily movements. *Journal of Wildlife Management* **54,** 316–322.

Ripley, B. D. (1977). Modelling spatial patterns. *Journal of the Royal Statistical Society Series B* **39,** 172–212.

Ripley, B. D. (1981). *Spatial Statistics.* New York: John Wiley & Sons.

Ripley, B. D. (1987). *Stochastic Simulation.* New York: John Wiley & Sons.

Ripple, W. J., Johnson, D. H., Hershey, K. T., and Meslow, E. C. (1991). Old-growth and mature forests near spotted owl nests in western Oregon. *Journal of Wildlife Management* **55,** 316–318.

Roberts, G., Rao, J. N. K., and Kumar, S. (1987). Logistic regression analysis of sample survey data. *Biometrika* **74,** 1–12.

Robertson, G. (1987). Geostatistics in ecology: interpolating with known variance. *Ecology* **68,** 744–748.

Rosner, G. L., and Tsiatis, A. A. (1988). Exact confidence intervals following a group sequential trial: a comparison of methods. *Biometrika* **75,** 723–729.

Samarov, A., and Taqqu, M. S. (1988). On the efficiency of the sample mean in long-memory noise. *Journal of Time Series Analysis* **9,** 191–200.

Santner, T. J., and Duffy, D. E. (1986). A note on Albert and Anderson's conditions for the existence of maximum likelihood estimates in logistic regression models. *Biometrika* **73,** 755–758.

Schoenfeld, D. (1982). Partial residuals for the proportional hazards regression model. *Biometrika* **69,** 239–241.

Schulman, J., Selvin, S., and Merrill, D. W. (1988). Density equalized map projections: a method for analysing clustering around a fixed point. *Statistics in Medicine* **7,** 491–505.

Schwartz, J. L. (1987). *Review and Evaluation of Smoking Cessation Methods: The United States and Canada, 1978–1985,* NIH Publication 87-2940. Washington, D.C.: U.S. Department of Health and Human Services.

Scott, A. J., and Wild, C. J. (1986). Fitting logistic models under case-control or choice based sampling. *Journal of Royal Statistical Society Series B* **48,** 170–182.

Seigel, D. G., and Greenhouse, S. W. (1973). Multiple relative risk functions in case-control studies. *American Journal of Epidemiology* **97,** 324–331.

Shaffer, D., Gould, M. S., Brasic, J., Ambrosini, P., Fisher, P., and Bird, H. (1983). A children's global assessment scale (CGAS). *Archives of General Psychiatry* **40,** 1228–1231.

Shapiro, S. S., and Wilk, M. (1965). An analysis of variance test for normality (complete samples). *Biometrika* **52**, 591–611.

Shillington, E. R. (1978). A chi-square goodness-of-fit test for logistic data, presented at *Joint Statistical Meetings*, San Diego, Calif.

Shrout, P. E., and Newman, S. C. (1989). Design of two-phase prevalence surveys of rare disorders. *Biometrics* **45**, 549–555.

Sievert, L. M. (1989). Postprandial temperature selection in *Crotophytus collaris*. *Copeia* **1989**, 987–993.

Silverman, B. W. (1986). *Density Estimation for Statistics and Data Analysis.* London: Chapman & Hall.

Slud, E. V., and Wei, L. J. (1982). Two-sample repeated significance tests based on the modified wilcoxon statistic. *Journal of the American Statistical Association* **77**, 855–861.

Smith, A. F. M. (1992). Bayesian computational methods. *Philosophical Transactions of the Royal Society of London A* **337**, 369–386.

Smith, A. F. M., and Roberts, G. O. (1993). Bayesian computation via the Gibbs sampler and related Monte Carlo methods. *Journal of the Royal Statistical Society Series B* **55**, 3–23.

Smith, P. L. (1979). Splines as a useful and convenient statistical tool. *The American Statistician* **33**, 57–62.

Starks, T., Behrens, N., and Fang, J. (1982). The combination of sampling and kriging in the regional estimation of coal resources. *Mathematical Geology* **14**, 87–106.

Steel, R. G. D., and Torrie, J. H. (1980). *Principles and Procedures of Statistics*, 2nd ed. New York: McGraw-Hill.

Stein, G. Z. (1988). Modelling counts in biological populations. *Mathematical Scientist* **13**, 56–65.

Stellman, S. D., Bofetta, P., and Garfinkel, L. (1988). Smoking habits of 800,000 American men and women in relation to their occupations. *American Journal of Industrial Medicine* **13**, 43–58.

Stellman, S. D., and Garfinkel, L. (1989). Proportions of cancer deaths attributable to cigarette smoking in women. *Women and Health* **15**, 19–28.

Stone, R. A. (1988). Investigations of excess environmental risks around putative sources: statistical problems and a proposed test. *Statistics in Medicine* **7**, 649–660.

Tanner, M. A., and Young, M. A. (1985). Modeling agreement among raters. *Journal of the American Statistical Association* **80**, 175–180.

Tenenbein, A. (1970). A double sampling scheme for estimating from binomial data with misclassifications. *Journal of the American Statistical Association* **65**, 1350–1361.

Therneau, T. M., Grambsch, P. M., and Fleming, T. R. (1990). Martingale-based residuals for survival models, *Biometrika* **77**, 147–160.

Thomas, D. L., and Taylor, E. J. (1990). Study designs and tests for comparing resource use and availability. *Journal of Wildlife Management* **54**, 322–330.

Tregust, D. F., Folk, G. E., Jr., Randall, W., and Folk, M. A. (1979). The circadian rhythm of body temperature of unrestrained opossums, *Didelphis virginiana. Journal of Thermal Biology* **4**, 251–255.

Tsay, R. (1984). Regression models with time-series error. *Journal of the American Statistical Association* **79**, 118–124.

Tsiatis, A. A. (1980). A note on a goodness-of-fit test for the logistic regression model. *Biometrika* **67**, 250–251.

Tsiatis, A. A., Rosner, G. L., and Mehta, C. R. (1984). Exact confidence intervals following a group sequential test. *Biometrics* **40**, 797–803.

Tufte, E. R. (1983). *The Visual Display of Quantitative Information.* Cheshire, Conn.: Graphics Press.

Tummon, I. S., Ali, A., Pepping, M. E., Radwanska, E., Binor, Z., and Dmowksi, W. P. (1988). Bone mineral density in women with endometriosis before and during ovarian suppression with gonadotropin-releasing hormone agonists or Danazol. *Fertility and Sterility* **49**, 792–796.

Turchin, P. (1990). Rarity of density dependence or population regulation with lags? *Nature* **344**, 660–663.

Turchin, P., and Taylor, A. D. (1992). Complex dynamics in ecological time series. *Ecology* **73**, 289–305.

Turnbull, B. W., Iwano, E. J., Burnett, W. S., Howe, H. L., and Clark, L. C. (1990). Monitoring for clustering of disease: application to leukemia incidence in upstate New York. *American Journal of Epidemiology* **132**, supplement, S136–S143.

Update, January (1992). The American Cancer Society guidelines for the cancer-related checkup. *Ca: A Cancer Journal for Clinicians* **42**, 44–45.

U.S. Department of Health and Human Services (1989a). *Trends in Public Beliefs, Attitudes, and Opinions in Smoking. A Report of the Surgeon General*, DHHS Publication 89(8411). Washington, D.C.: U.S. Government Printing Office.

U.S. Department of Health and Human Services (1989b). *Reducing the Health Consequences of Smoking: 25 Years of Progress. A Report of the Surgeon General.* U.S. Department of Health and Human Services, Public Health Service, Centers for Disease Control, Center for Chronic Disease Prevention and Health Promotion, Office on Smoking and Health, DHHS Publication (CDC) 89-8411. Washington, D.C.: U.S. Government Printing Office.

U.S. Department of Health and Human Services (1990). *The Health Benefits of Smoking Cessation.* U.S. Department of Health and Human Services, Public Health Service, Centers for Disease Control, Center for Chronic Disease Prevention and Health Promotion, Office on Smoking and Health, DHHS Publication (CDC) 90-8416. Washington, D.C.: U.S. Government Printing Office.

U.S. Department of Health and Human Services (1991). *Sixth Annual Report on Carcinogens: Summary 1991.* Rockville, Md.: Technical Resources.

U.S. Environmental Protection Agency (USEPA) (1990). *Technical Support Document for Water Quality-Based Toxics Control*, 2nd ed., EPA/505/2-90/001. Washington, D.C.: U.S. EPA, Office of Water.

Vogler, W. R., Velez-Garcia, E., Weiner, R. S., Flaum, M. A., Bartolucci, A. A., Omura, G. A., Gerber, M. C., and Banks, P. L. C. (1992). A phase III trial comparing idarubicin and daunorubicin in combination with cytarabine in acute myelogenous leukemia: a Southeastern Cancer Study Group study. *Journal of Clinical Oncology* **10**, 1103–1111.

Waiwood, K. G. (1988). A transportable seawater holding facility for research vessels. *Aquaculture Engineering* **7**, 127–138.

Wakefield, J. C., Gelfand, A. E., and Smith, A. F. M. (1991). Efficient generation of random variates via the ratio-of-uniforms method. *Statistical Computing* **1**, 129–133.

Wakeford, R. (1990). Some problems in the interpretation of childhood leukemia clusters. In *Spatial Epidemiology* R. W. Thomas (ed.). London: Pion.

Wakeford, R., Binks, K., and Wilkie, D. (1989). Childhood leukemia and nuclear installations. *Journal of the Royal Statistical Society Series A* **152**, 61–86.

Wald, A. (1943). Tests of statistical hypotheses concerning several parameters when the number of observations is large. *Transactions of the American Mathematical Society* **54**, 426–482.

Wald, A. (1947). *Sequential Analysis.* New York: John Wiley & Sons.

Waller, L. A., Turnbull, B. W., Clark, L. C., and Nasca, P. (1992). Chronic disease surveillance and testing of clustering of disease and exposure: application to leukemia incidence and TCE-contaminated dumpsites in upstate New York. *Environmetrics* **3**, 281–300.

Walter, S. D., and Day, N. E. (1983). Estimation of the duration of a pre-clinical disease state using screening data. *American Journal of Epidemiology* **118**, 865–886.

Wang, S. K., and Tsiatis, A. A. (1987). Approximately optimal one-parameter boundaries for group sequential trials. *Biometrics* **43**, 193–199.

Ware, J. H. (1985). Linear models for the analysis of longitudinal studies. *American Statistician* **39**, 95–101.

Weber, C. I., Peltier, W. H., Norberg-King, T. J., Horning, W. B., Kessler, F. A., Menkedick, J. R., Neiheisel, T. W., Lewis, P. A., Klemm, D., Pickering, Q. H., Robinson, E. L., Lazorchak, J. M., Wymer, L. J., and Freyberg, R. W. (1989). *Short-Term Methods for Estimating the Chronic Toxicity of Effluents and Receiving Waters to Freshwater Organisms*, 2nd ed. Cincinnati, Ohio: U.S. Environmental Protection Agency.

Webster, R. (1984). Elucidation and characterization of spatial variation in soil using regionalized variable theory. In *Geostatistics for Natural Resources Characterization*, Part 2, G. Verly et al. (eds.). Boston: D. Reidel.

Wedderburn, R. W. M. (1974). Quasi-likelihood functions, generalized linear models, and the Gauss-Newton method. *Biometrika* **61**, 439–447.

Weiss, W., Boucot, K. R., and Seidman, H. (1982). The Philadelphia pulmonary research project. *Clinical Chest Medicine* **3**, 243–256.

Wessinger, W. D. (1986). Approaches to the study of drug interactions in behavioral pharmacology. *Neuroscience and Biobehavioral Review* **10**, 103–113.

West Publishing (1991). *Selected Environmental Law Statutes*, 1991–92 educ. ed. St. Paul, Minn.: West Publishing Company.

Wheldon, T. E. (1989). The assessment of risk of radiation-induced childhood leukaemia in the vicinity of nuclear installations. *Journal of the Royal Statistical Society Series A* **152**, 327–339.

White, H. (1980). Consistent covariance matrix estimator and a direct test for heteroscedasticity. *Econometrics* **48**, 817–838.

White, G. C., and Garrott, R. A. (1990). *Analysis of Wildlife Radio-Tracking Data.* San Diego, Calif.: Academic Press.

Whitehead, J. (1980). Fitting Cox's regression model to survival data using GLIM. *Applied Statistics* **29,** 268–275.

Whitehead, J. (1983). *The Design and Analysis of Sequential Clinical Trials.* Chichester, U.K.: Ellis Horwood.

Whitehead, J. (1986a). On the bias of maximum likelihood estimation following a sequential test. *Biometrika* **73,** 573–581.

Whitehead, J. (1986b). Supplementary analysis at the conclusion of a sequential clinical trial. *Biometrics* **42,** 461–471.

Whitehead, J., and Facey, K. M. (1992). *Analysis After a Clinical Trial: A Comparison of Orderings of the Sample Space.* Technical report. Reading, U.K.: University of Reading, Department of Applied Statistics.

Whitehead, J., and Marek, P. (1985). A Fortran program for the design and analysis of sequential clinical trials. *Computers and Biomedical Research* **18,** 176–183.

Whitehouse, R. W., Adams, J. E., Bancroft, K., Vaughan-Williams, C. A., and Elstein, M. (1990). The effects of nafarelin and danazol on vertebral trabecular bone mass in patients with endometriosis. *Clinical Endocrinology* **33,** 365–373.

Whittaker, J. (1990). *Graphical Models in Applied Mathematical Multivariate Statistics.* New York: John Wiley & Sons.

Whittemore, A. S. (1985). Analyzing cohort mortality data. *The American Statistician* **39,** 437–441.

Whittemore, A. (1988). Effect of cigarette smoking in epidemiological studies of lung cancer. *Statistics in Medicine* **7,** 223–238.

Whittemore, A. S., Friend, N., Brown, B. W., and Holly, E. A. (1987). A test to detect clusters of disease. *Biometrika* **74,** 631–635.

Wiernik, P. H., Banks, P. L. C., Chase, D. C., Arlin, Z. A., Periman, P. O., Todd, M. B., Ritch, P. S., Enck, R. E., and Weitberg, A. B. (1992). Cytarabine plus idarubicin or daunorubicin as induction and consolidation therapy for previously untreated adult patients with acute myeloid leukemia. *Blood* **79,** 313–319.

Wijesinha, A., Begg, C. B., Funkenstein, H. H., and McNeil, B. J. (1983). Methodology for the differential diagnosis of a complex data-set. *Medical Decision Making* **3,** 133–154.

Wilson, W. W., Jr., and Fontaine, G. A. (1978). Gypsy moth egg mass sampling with fixed and variable radius plots. *U.S. Department of Agriculture Handbook 523.* Washington, D.C.: U.S. Government Printing Office.

Yamaguchi, K. (1991). *Event History Analysis.* Beverly Hills, Calif.: Sage Publications.

Yang, M. C. K., and Carter, R. L. (1983). One-way analysis of variance with time-series data. *Biometrics* **39,** 747–751.

Zeger, S. L., and Liang, K. Y. (1986). Longitudinal data analysis for discrete and continuous outcomes. *Biometrics* **42,** 121–130.

Zeger, S. L., Liang, K. Y., and Self, S. G. (1985). The analysis of binary longitudinal data with time-independent covariates, *Biometrika* **72,** 31–78.

Zelen, M., and Feinleib, M. (1969). On the theory of screening for chronic diseases. *Biometrika* **56,** 601–614.

Chapter–Methods Index

Method–Chapters Index

Subject Index

WILEY SERIES IN PROBABILITY
AND MATHEMATICAL STATISTICS

ESTABLISHED BY WALTER A. SHEWHART AND SAMUEL S. WILKS

Editors
*Vic Barnett, Ralph A. Bradley, Nicholas I. Fisher, J. Stuart Hunter,
J. B. Kadane, David G. Kendall, Adrian F. M. Smith,
Stephen M. Stigler, Jozef L. Teugels, Geoffrey S. Watson*

*Now available in a lower priced paperback edition in the Wiley Classics Library.

*Now available in a lower priced paperback edition in the Wiley Classics Library.

*Now available in a lower priced paperback edition in the Wiley Classics Library.